Pain Management in the Peripartum Period

Editors

RANDALL P. FLICK
JAMES R. HEBL

CLINICS IN PERINATOLOGY

www.perinatology.theclinics.com

Consulting Editor
LUCKY JAIN

September 2013 • Volume 40 • Number 3

ELSEVIER

1600 John F. Kennedy Boulevard • Suite 1800 • Philadelphia, Pennsylvania, 19103-2899

http://www.theclinics.com

CLINICS IN PERINATOLOGY Volume 40, Number 3
September 2013 ISSN 0095-5108, ISBN-13: 978-0-323-18866-1

Editor: Kerry Holland
Developmental Editor: Donald Mumford

Clinics in Perinatology (ISSN 0095-5108) is published quarterly by Elsevier Inc., 360 Park Avenue South, New York, NY 10010-1710. Months of issue are March, June, September, and December. Business and Editorial Offices: 1600 John F. Kennedy Blvd., Ste. 1800, Philadelphia, PA 19103-2899. Customer Service Office: 3251 Riverport Lane, Maryland Heights, MO 63043. Periodicals postage paid at New York, NY and additional mailing offices. Subscription prices are $273.00 per year (US individuals), $401.00 per year (US institutions), $326.00 per year (Canadian individuals), $509.00 per year (Canadian institutions), $400.00 per year (foreign individuals), $509.00 per year (foreign institutions), $129.00 per year (US students), and $186.00 per year (Canadian and foreign students). Foreign air speed delivery is included in all Clinics subscription prices. All prices are subject to change without notice. **POSTMASTER:** Send address changes to *Clinics in Perinatology*, Elsevier Health Sciences Division, Subscription Customer Service, 3251 Riverport Lane, Maryland Heights, MO 63043. **Customer Service: Telephone: 1-800-654-2452** (U.S. and Canada); **1-314-447-8871** (outside U.S. and Canada). **Fax: 1-314-447-8029. E-mail: journalscustomerservice-usa@elsevier.com** (for print support); **journalsonlinesupport-usa@elsevier.com** (for online support).

Reprints. For copies of 100 or more, of articles in this publication, please contact the Commercial Reprints Department, Elsevier Inc., 360 Park Avenue South, New York, NY 10010-1710. Tel. (212) 633-3812; Fax: (212) 482-1935; E-mail: reprints@elsevier.com.

Clinics in Perinatology is also published in Spanish by McGraw-Hill Interamericana Editores S.A., P.O. Box 5-237, 06500 Mexico D.F., Mexico.

Clinics in Perinatology is covered in *MEDLINE/PubMed (Index Medicus) Current Contents, Excepta Medica, BIOSIS* and *ISI/BIOMED.*

Printed and bound by CPI Group (UK) Ltd, Croydon, CR0 4YY

Transferred to digital print 2012

Contributors

CONSULTING EDITOR

LUCKY JAIN, MD, MBA
Richard W. Blumberg Professor and Executive Vice Chairman, Department of Pediatrics;
Medical Director, Emory Children's Center, Emory University School of Medicine, Atlanta,
Georgia

EDITORS

RANDALL P. FLICK, MD, MPH, FAAP
Associate Professor of Anesthesiology and Pediatrics, Mayo Clinic Children's Center,
Mayo Clinic, Rochester, Minnesota

JAMES R. HEBL, MD
Professor of Anesthesiology, Vice-Chair, Clinical Practice, Department of Anesthesiology,
Mayo Clinic, Rochester, Minnesota

AUTHORS

KATHERINE W. ARENDT, MD
Assistant Professor, Department of Anesthesiology, Mayo Clinic College of Medicine,
Rochester, Minnesota

ADRIAN BOSENBERG, MB, ChB, FFA(SA)
Professor, Department Anesthesiology and Pain Management, Faculty Health Sciences,
Seattle Children's Hospital, University Washington, Seattle, Washington

ROLAND BRUSSEAU, MD
Assistant in Anesthesia, Department of Anesthesia, Perioperative and Pain Medicine,
Boston Children's Hospital; Instructor of Anaesthesia, Harvard Medical School, Boston,
Massachusetts

MARSHA CAMPBELL YEO, RN, PhD, NNP-BC
Assistant Professor, School of Nursing, Faculty of Health Professions, Dalhousie
University; Clinician Scientist, Department of Pediatrics, IWK Health Centre, Halifax,
Nova Scotia, Canada

LAURIE A. CHALIFOUX, MD
Assistant Professor, Department of Anesthesiology, Northwestern Feinberg School of
Medicine, Chicago, Illinois

CHRISTOPHER E. COLBY, MD
Assistant Professor, Department of Pediatrics and Adolescent Medicine, The Mayo Clinic,
Rochester, Minnesota

ANDREW DAVIDSON, MBBS, MD, FANNZCA
Associate Professor, Department of Anaesthesia and Pain Management, Royal Children's
Hospital, Parkville, Melbourne, Victoria, Australia

RANDALL P. FLICK, MD, MPH, FAAP
Associate Professor of Anesthesiology and Pediatrics, Mayo Clinic Children's Center, Mayo Clinic, Rochester, Minnesota

MARIA V. FRAGA, MD
Attending Neonatologist, Division of Neonatology, The Children's Hospital of Philadelphia; Assistant Professor of Pediatrics, Department of Pediatrics, Perelman School of Medicine, University of Pennsylvania, Philadelphia, Pennsylvania

LISA A. GILL, MD
Division of Maternal-Fetal Medicine, Department of Obstetrics and Gynecology, Mayo Clinic, Rochester, Minnesota

KENDRA GRIM, MD
Instructor in Anesthesiology, Department of Anesthesiology, College of Medicine, Mayo Clinic, Rochester, Minnesota

TRACY E. HARRISON, MD
Instructor in Anesthesiology, Department of Anesthesiology, College of Medicine, Mayo Clinic, Rochester, Minnesota

ADAM K. JACOB, MD
Assistant Professor of Anesthesiology, Department of Anesthesiology, Mayo Clinic, Rochester, Minnesota

CELESTE JOHNSTON, RN, DEd, FCAHS
Professor Emeritus, Ingram School of Nursing, McGill University, Montreal, Quebec; Scientist, IWK Health Centre, Halifax, Nova Scotia, Canada

BHAVANI SHANKAR KODALI, MD
Associate Professor, Department of Anesthesiology, Brigham and Women's Hospital, Boston, Massachusetts

RUTH LANDAU, MD
Virginia and Prentice Bloedel Professor of Anesthesiology, Director of Obstetric Anesthesia and Clinical Genetics Research, Department of Anesthesiology and Pain Medicine, University of Washington Medical Center, Seattle, Washington

ANNE LAVOIE, MD, FRCPC
Obstetric Anesthesia Fellow, Department of Anesthesiology, Northwestern University, Feinberg School of Medicine, Chicago, Illinois

CARRIE P. MALAVOLTA, MSN, CRNP
Pain Management Nurse Practitioner, Division of Neonatology, The Children's Hospital of Philadelphia, Philadelphia, Pennsylvania

LYNNE G. MAXWELL, MD, FAAP
Associate Professor, Anesthesiology and Critical Care, Perelman School of Medicine, University of Pennsylvania; Senior Anesthesiologist, Department of Anesthesiology and Critical Care Medicine, The Children's Hospital of Philadelphia, Philadelphia, Pennsylvania

CAROL MCNAIR, RN(EC), MN, NP-Pediatrics, NNP-BC
Neonatal Nurse Practitioner, Nursing and Child Health Evaluative Sciences, The Hospital for Sick Children, Toronto, Ontario, Canada

ARIELLE MIZRAHI-ARNAUD, MD
Senior Associate in Anesthesia, Department of Anesthesia, Perioperative and Pain Medicine, Boston Children's Hospital; Assistant Professor of Anaesthesia, Harvard Medical School, Boston, Massachusetts

MICHAEL E. NEMERGUT, MD, PhD
Instructor, Departments of Anesthesiology and Pediatrics and Adolescent Medicine, The Mayo Clinic, Rochester, Minnesota

ADAM D. NIESEN, MD
Assistant Professor of Anesthesiology, Department of Anesthesiology, Mayo Clinic, Rochester, Minnesota

CARL ROSE, MD
Division of Maternal-Fetal Medicine, Department of Obstetrics and Gynecology, Mayo Clinic, Rochester, Minnesota

B. SCOTT SEGAL, MD, MHCM
Chair, Department of Anesthesiology, Tufts Medical Center, Professor of Anesthesiology, Tufts University School of Medicine, Boston, Massachusetts

TODD J. STANHOPE, MD
Division of Maternal-Fetal Medicine, Department of Obstetrics and Gynecology, Mayo Clinic, Rochester, Minnesota

JOHN T. SULLIVAN, MD, MBA
Professor, Department of Anesthesiology, Northwestern Feinberg School of Medicine, Chicago, Illinois

HANS P. SVIGGUM, MD
Assistant Professor, Department of Anesthesiology, Mayo Clinic College of Medicine, Rochester, Minnesota; Obstetric Anesthesia Fellow, Brigham and Women's Hospital, Boston, Massachusetts

ANNA TADDIO, MSc, PhD
Senior Associate Scientist, Child Health Evaluative Sciences, The Hospital for Sick Children; Associate Professor, Clinical, Social and Administrative Pharmacy, Leslie Dan Faculty of Pharmacy, University of Toronto, Toronto, Ontario, Canada

JENNIFER A. TESSMER-TUCK, MD
Instructor, North Memorial Medical Center Laborist Associates, Robbinsdale, Minnesota

PALOMA TOLEDO, MD, MPH
Assistant Professor, Department of Anesthesiology, Northwestern University, Feinberg School of Medicine, Chicago, Illinois

SUELLEN M. WALKER, MBBS, MMed, MSc, PhD, FANZCA, FFPMANZCA
Senior Clinical Lecturer and Consultant in Paediatric Anaesthesia and Pain Medicine, Portex Unit: Pain Research, UCL Institute of Child Health, Great Ormond St Hospital for Children NHS Foundation Trust, London, United Kingdom

ROBERT T. WILDER, MD, PhD
Associate Professor in Anesthesiology, Department of Anesthesiology, College of Medicine, Mayo Clinic, Rochester, Minnesota

MYRON YASTER, MD
Richard J. Traystman Professor, Department of Anesthesiology and Critical Care Medicine and Pediatrics, The Johns Hopkins University, Baltimore, Maryland

Contents

in better patient satisfaction, earlier mobilization, and improved maternal-infant bonding. There are many individual options for treatment of pain; however, multimodal analgesic therapy has become the mainstay of treatment. In this article, the epidemiology of postcesarean delivery pain, pain mechanisms, and the multiple options available to providers for treatment of postoperative pain are discussed.

Accurate pain assessment in preterm and term neonates in the neonatal intensive care unit (NICU) is of vital importance because of the high prevalence of painful experiences in this population, including both daily procedural pain and postoperative pain. Over 40 tools have been developed to assess pain in neonates, and each NICU should choose a limited number of pain assessment tools for different populations and contexts. Only two pain assessment tools have a metric adjustment to account for differences of pain assessment in prematurity. Preterm neonates do not display behavior and physiologic indicators of pain as reliably and specifically as full term infants, and preterm infants are vulnerable to long term sequelae of painful experiences. "Brain-oriented" approaches for more objective measurement of pain in neonates may become available in the future. In the meantime, neonatal pain assessment tools need to be taught, implemented, and their ongoing use optimized to form a consistent, reproducible basis for the safe and effective treatment of neonatal pain.

Nociceptive pathways are functional following birth. In addition to physiological and behavioral responses, neurophysiological measures and neuroimaging evaluate nociceptive pathway function and quantify responses to noxious stimuli in preterm and term neonates. Intensive care and surgery can expose neonates to painful stimuli when the developing nervous system is sensitive to changing input, resulting in persistent impacts into later childhood. Early pain experience has been correlated with increased sensitivity to subsequent painful stimuli, impaired neurodevelopmental outcomes, and structural changes in brain development. Parallel preclinical studies have elucidated underlying mechanisms and evaluate preventive strategies to inform future clinical trials.

All infants undergo painful procedures involving skin puncture as part of routine medical care. Pain from needle puncture procedures is suboptimally managed. Numerous nonpharmacologic interventions are available for these painful procedures, including swaddling, holding, skin-to-skin care, pacifier, sweet-tasting solutions, and breast-feeding. Adoption of nonpharmacologic pain-relieving interventions into routine clinical practice is feasible and should be a standard of care in the delivery of quality health care for infants. This review summarizes current knowledge about the epidemiology of pain from common needle puncture procedures in infants, the effectiveness of nonpharmacologic interventions, implementation considerations, and unanswered questions for future research.

on how brief anesthetic exposure may affect neurodevelopment in the newborn. Good evidence however shows that untreated pain and stress have an adverse effect on neurodevelopment, and therefore, at this stage, providing effective analgesia, sedation, and anesthesia would seem to be more important than concern over neurotoxicity.

Studies on genetic contributions to labor analgesia have essentially evaluated the μ-opioid receptor gene (*OPRM1*), with some evidence that p.118A/G of *OPRM1* influences the response to neuraxial opioids. As for labor progress, the β_2-adrenergic receptor gene (ADRB2) is associated with preterm labor and delivery, and impacts the course of labor. Taken together though, there is no evidence that pharmacogenetic testing is needed or beneficial in the context of obstetric anesthesia; however, realizing the influence of genetic variants on specific phenotypes provides the rationale for a more cautious interpretation of clinical studies that attempt to find a dose-regimen that fits all.

PROGRAM OBJECTIVE

The goal of *Clinics in Perinatology* is to keep practicing perinatologists, neonatologists, obstetricians, practicing physicians and residents up to date with current clinical practice in perinatology by providing timely articles reviewing the state of the art in patient care.

TARGET AUDIENCE

Perinatologists, neonatologists, obstetricians, practicing physicians, residents and healthcare professionals who provide patient care utilizing findings from *Clinics in Perinatology*.

LEARNING OBJECTIVES

Upon completion of this activity, participants will be able to:

1. Review current research evidence and practical considerations of non-pharmacological management of pain during common needle puncture procedures in infants.
2. Discuss nonpharmacologic labor analgesia as well as multimodal post-caesarean delivery analgesia.
3. Recognize and assess pain in the neonate.

ACCREDITATION

The Elsevier Office of Continuing Medical Education (EOCME) is accredited by the Accreditation Council for Continuing Medical Education (ACCME) to provide continuing medical education for physicians.

The EOCME designates this enduring material for a maximum of 15 *AMA PRA Category 1 Credit*(s)™. Physicians should claim only the credit commensurate with the extent of their participation in the activity.

All other health care professionals requesting continuing education credit for this enduring material will be issued a certificate of participation.

DISCLOSURE OF CONFLICTS OF INTEREST

The EOCME assesses conflict of interest with its instructors, faculty, planners, and other individuals who are in a position to control the content of CME activities. All relevant conflicts of interest that are identified are thoroughly vetted by EOCME for fair balance, scientific objectivity, and patient care recommendations. EOCME is committed to providing its learners with CME activities that promote improvements or quality in healthcare and not a specific proprietary business or a commercial interest.

The planning committee, staff, authors and editors listed below have identified no financial relationships or relationships to products or devices they or their spouse/life partner have with commercial interest related to the content of this CME activity:

Katherine W. Arendt, MD; Adrian Bosenberg, MB, ChB, FFA(SA); Roland Brusseau, MD; Laurie Ann Chalifoux, MD; Christopher Colby, MD; Nicole Congleton; Andrew Davidson, MD; Randall P. Flick, MD; Maria V. Fraga, MD; Lisa Gill, MD; Kendra J. Grim, MD; Tracy Harrison, MD; James R. Hebl, MD; Kerry Holland; Brynne Hunter; Adam K. Jacob, MD; Celeste Johnston, RN, DeD, FCAHS; Bhavani Kodali, MD; Sandy Lavery; Anne Lavoie, MD, FRCPC; Carrie P. Malavolta, BSN, MSN; Lynne Maxwell, MD; Carol McNair, CRNP; Jill McNair; Arielle Mizrahi-Arnaud, MD; Palani Murugesan; Michael Nemergut, MD, PhD; Adam D. Niesen, MD; Scott Segal, MD; Todd J. Stanhope, MD; John T. Sullivan, MD; Hans P. Sviggum, MD; Jennifer A. Tessmer-Tuck, MD; Paloma Toledo, MD; Suellen Walker, MBBS, MM (PM), MSc, PhD, FANZCA, FFPMANZCA; Robert Wilder, MD, PhD; and Marsha Campbell Yeo, PhD, NNP-BC, RN.

The planning committee, staff, authors and editors listed below have identified financial relationships or relationships to products or devices they or their spouse/life partner have with commercial interest related to the content of this CME activity:

Ruth Landau, MD has a research grant from Millenium Research Group.

Carl Rose, MD has royalties for Up-To-Date.

Anna Taddio, BScPhm, MSc, PhD has research grants from Pfizer, Natus, and Ferndale.

Myron Yaster, MD is a consultant/advisor for Purdue Pharma, Endo Pharmaceuticals, Cadence Pharmaceuticals and Hospira.

UNAPPROVED/OFF-LABEL USE DISCLOSURE

The EOCME requires CME faculty to disclose to the participants:

1. When products or procedures being discussed are off-label, unlabelled, experimental, and/or investigational (not US Food and Drug Administration (FDA) approved); and
2. Any limitations on the information presented, such as data that are preliminary or that represent ongoing research, interim analyses, and/or unsupported opinions. Faculty may discuss information about pharmaceutical agents that is outside of FDA-approved labelling. This information is intended solely for CME

and is not intended to promote off-label use of these medications. If you have any questions, contact the medical affairs department of the manufacturer for the most recent prescribing information.

TO ENROLL

To enroll in the *Clinics in Perinatology* Continuing Medical Education program, call customer service at 1-800-654-2452 or sign up online at http://www.theclinics.com/home/cme. The CME program is available to subscribers for an additional annual fee of $212 USD.

METHOD OF PARTICIPATION

In order to claim credit, participants must complete the following:

1. Complete enrolment as indicated above.
2. Read the activity.
3. Complete the CME Test and Evaluation. Participants must achieve a score of 70% on the test. All CME Tests and Evaluations must be completed online.

CME INQUIRIES/SPECIAL NEEDS

For all CME inquiries or special needs, please contact elsevierCME@elsevier.com.

CLINICS IN PERINATOLOGY

NOW AVAILABLE FOR YOUR iPhone and iPad

Foreword

Painful Truths About Newborn Pain Management

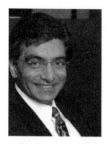

Lucky Jain, MD, MBA
Consulting Editor

Nearly 30 years ago, as I began my training in pediatrics and neonatology, pain management was relatively simple: we had a somewhat rudimentary understanding of neonatal pain and had few agents to treat pain with. The result: pain management varied widely from one neonatologist to the next as did the appreciation of pain in the newborn. Studies in the late 1980s showed that newborns feel pain and do better when given analgesia for painful procedures.[1] This led to a rapid increase appreciation of pain and opioid use worldwide. However, there was little consensus around which medications to use and dosing regimens varied widely; there was also a lack of objective assessment tools for pain, particularly for interventions such as mechanical ventilation.[2]

Basic science and clinical studies since then have greatly enhanced our appreciation of pain and nociception pathways.[3] Our ability to objectively assess pain has similarly improved, as has our understanding of developmental pharmacology. The paucity of therapeutic agents, however, still persists.[2] There are also new and previously unresolved concerns about the safety of existing therapeutic agents such as morphine and fentanyl.[4] Caught in the middle, a busy clinician is once again tasked with balancing the need for adequate pain control with the need to prevent inadvertent harm.

And then there is the chronic problem of underutilization of simple interventions that have proven efficacy but have not gained popularity among clinicians.[5] Studies backing some of these approaches are plagued with design issues and heterogeneity in control interventions. Nevertheless, their safety profile and modest efficacy make them suitable approaches for many neonates: sucrose and breast milk/feeding are perfect examples here.[5]

This issue of the *Clinics in Perinatology* brings together experts from various fields related to pain management and anesthesia in the mother and the newborn. Drs Flick

Clin Perinatol 40 (2013) xv–xvi
http://dx.doi.org/10.1016/j.clp.2013.06.003
0095-5108/13/$ – see front matter © 2013 Published by Elsevier Inc.

perinatology.theclinics.com

and Hebl are to be congratulated for bringing together experts in the field for this state-of-the-art panel of review articles on pain management. I am also grateful to Kerry Holland and Elsevier for their support and to the many authors who have contributed to this important issue of the *Clinics in Perinatology*.

Lucky Jain, MD, MBA
Department of Pediatrics
Emory Children's Center
Emory University School of Medicine
2015 Uppergate Drive
Atlanta, GA 30322, USA

E-mail address:
ljain@emory.edu

REFERENCES

1. Anand KJ, Hickey PR. Pain and its effects in the human neonate and fetus. N Engl J Med 1987;317:1321–9.
2. Van den Anker JN. Treating pain in newborn infants: navigating between Scylla and Charybdis. J Pediatr 2013. [Epub ahead of print]. http://dx.doi.org/10.1016/j.jpeds.2013.04.004.
3. Morton NS. The pain-free ward: myth or reality. Paediatr Anesth 2012;22:527–9.
4. Hall RW, Kronsberg SS, Barton BA, et al, NEOPAIN Trial Investigators Group. Morphine, hypotension, and adverse outcomes among preterm neonates: who's to blame? Secondary results from the NEOPAIN Trial. Pediatrics 2005;115:1351–9.
5. Stevens B, Yamada J, Lee GY, et al. Sucrose for analgesia in newborn infants undergoing painful procedures. Cochrane Database Syst Rev 2013;(1):CD001069.

Preface

Pain Management in the Perinatal Period

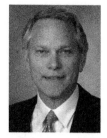 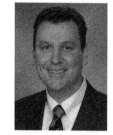

Randall P. Flick, MD, MPH   James R. Hebl, MD
Editors

Pain management in the perinatal period is a topic of immense depth and breadth encompassing the pharmacologic and nonpharmacologic management of pain in the mother, fetus, and neonate, including the use of regional anesthesia techniques. The topic is not limited to pain management but also includes assessment of pain, complications associated with the use of various pain management strategies, chronic pain, sedation, and also the genetic influences that in part predetermine the pain experience.

In this issue of *Clinics in Perinatology,* we have attempted to provide an in-depth overview of an issue that affects all of us who care for mothers and babies in those critical days surrounding birth. Contributors from a wide variety of backgrounds, including anesthesiologists, neonatologists, perinatologists, and pain management specialists in both adults and children, have come together to produce what we think is a wonderful addition to the perinatal literature.

This issue of *Clinics in Perinatology* will carry the reader through the perinatal period and examine pain management throughout that continuum. Beginning with the genetics of obstetric pain and opioid use in pregnancy, the discussion moves to the provision of anesthesia to the mother and fetus during fetal surgery—an area of intense concern and interest in many centers. There is an extensive discussion of both pharmacologic and nonpharmacologic management of pain during delivery. A discussion of regional anesthetic techniques is increasingly relevant in light of increasing evidence of adverse neurodevelopmental consequences of fetal exposure to general anesthetics and sedatives.

Pain, its implications, and its management are extensively covered including discussions of how to assess neonatal pain and how best to provide sedation and nonpharmacologic pain management, and systemic pharmacologic or regional techniques. Of particular interest are the reviews of the potential neurodevelopmental impact of both the treatment and the failure to adequately treat pain in the newborn. This topic

Clin Perinatol 40 (2013) xvii–xviii
http://dx.doi.org/10.1016/j.clp.2013.05.016   **perinatology.theclinics.com**

is receiving an enormous amount of attention from all those who care for children as well as the government and the media.

We are very proud of this issue as it is without a doubt the most up-to-date and comprehensive review of this topic anywhere in the literature. The authors deserve great credit for their work as does the wonderful Elsevier staff. We would especially like to thank Dr Lucky Jain for asking us to undertake this project and Kerry Holland for her infinite patience and skillful editing.

Randall P. Flick, MD, MPH
Departments of Anesthesiology & Pediatrics
Mayo Clinic Children's Center
200 First Street, SW
Rochester, MN 55905, USA

James R. Hebl, MD
Department of Anesthesiology
Mayo Clinic
200 First Street, SW
Rochester, MN 55905, USA

E-mail addresses:
Flick.randall@mayo.edu (R.P. Flick)
Hebl.james@mayo.edu (J.R. Hebl)

Chronic Opioid Use During Pregnancy: Maternal and Fetal Implications

Todd J. Stanhope, MD, Lisa A. Gill, MD, Carl Rose, MD*

KEYWORDS

- Opioid • Narcotic • Pregnancy • Methadone • Buprenorphine

KEY POINTS

- A collaborative, multidisciplinary care approach is essential for pregnancies complicated by chronic narcotic use.
- Management of opioid dependence with either methadone or buprenorphine is appropriate during pregnancy and breastfeeding.
- Detoxification with careful observation is reasonable during pregnancy in appropriately selected patients and is best accomplished during the second or early third trimester.
- Usage of prescription monitoring programs or the evolving Risk Evaluation and Mitigation Strategy (REMS) program may be beneficial in prevention of inappropriate prescribing or diversion.

INTRODUCTION

Concern regarding the use and abuse of both prescription and illicit opioid medications has been a growing medical and societal concern within the United States during the past decade. Since the early 2000s, prescriptions for the opioid, hydrocodone, have exceeded those for either antibiotic or antihypertensive medications.[1] Similar to many chronic medical conditions, this phenomenon is proportionally represented in the pregnant population, with attendant implications for not only the mother but also the unborn child.[2] This article reviews the issues related to prescription and illicit opiate use during pregnancy and proposes strategies for antepartum, intrapartum, and postpartum management.

CLASSIFICATIONS

Opioid medications are defined by the Food and Drug Administration (FDA) as synthetic alkaloid derivatives of the chemical opium and are classified by the Drug

Conflicts of Interest: None.
Division of Maternal-Fetal Medicine, Department of Obstetrics and Gynecology, Mayo Clinic, 200 First Street SW, Rochester, MN 55902, USA
* Corresponding author.
E-mail address: rose.carl@mayo.edu

Clin Perinatol 40 (2013) 337–350
http://dx.doi.org/10.1016/j.clp.2013.05.015   perinatology.theclinics.com

Enforcement Agency (DEA) as schedule II, III, or IV contingent on clinical efficacy and abuse potential (**Table 1**).[3,4] Specialized prescription forms (triplicates) are required in most states for schedule II medications. For obstetric purposes, opioid compounds are classified as either category B or C by the FDA for use during pregnancy, with no confirmed human teratogenic effects reported. The term, *narcotic*, refers to induction of drowsiness or sleep but is also used synonymously in common literature to refer to opioid-category medications from a generic perspective. Specifically, the descriptor, *opiate*, refers to compounds derived directly from natural sources (opium and endogenous opioids), although the words are often used interchangeably.

MECHANISM OF ACTION

All opioids exert their effects primarily through binding to 1 or more of 3 opioid receptors (μ, κ, and Δ), which are widely distributed throughout the body, including the vascular, cardiac, pulmonary, gastrointestinal, and immune systems. The analgesic effect occurs through activation of receptors found in both central and peripheral nervous systems, whereas side effects, such as respiratory depression and decreased

Table 1 Common opioid medications			
Medication	**DEA Schedule**	**FDA Category**	**Duration of Action (h)**
Hydromorphone (Dilaudid)	II	C	3–4
Hydrocodone (Lorcet, Vicodin)	II	C	4–8
Oxycodone (OxyContin, Roxicodone)	II	B	3–6
Meperidine (Demerol)	II	C	2–4
Codeine	II	C	4–6
Morphine (Duramorph, MS Contin)	II	C	4
Tramadol (Ultram)	IV varies by state	C	9
Methadone (Dolophine)	II	C	4–8 Single doses 22–48 Repeat doses
Heroin (not commercially available)	I	Not assigned	3–4
Buprenorphine (Buprenex, Subutex) (combined opioid agonist/antagonist)	III	C	≥6
Naloxone (Narcan) (opioid antagonist)	Not assigned	C	0.5–2

DEA schedules (summarized)[60]: I, no currently accepted medical use and a high potential for abuse; II, high potential for abuse, although less than schedule I—drugs are considered dangerous; III, moderate to low potential for dependence; IV, low potential for abuse and low risk of dependence; and V, lower potential for abuse than schedule IV and contain limited dose of narcotics.

FDA medication pregnancy categories (summarized)[61]: A, adequate studies have failed to demonstrate a risk to the fetus in the first trimester (and there is no evidence of a risk in later trimesters); B, animal reproduction studies have not demonstrated a fetal risk but there are no controlled studies in pregnant women; C, animal studies have demonstrated adverse effects on the fetus and there are no adequate controlled studies in humans—potential benefit may outweigh potential risks for use in pregnant women; D, there is positive evidence of human fetal risk, but the potential benefits from use in pregnant women may be acceptable despite the risk; and X, studies in animals or human have demonstrated fetal abnormalities or there is evidence of fetal risk, and the risk of the use of the drug in pregnant women clearly outweighs any possible benefit.

Data from DEA Drug Scheduling. Retrieved from the United States Drug Enforcement Agency Web site: http://www.justice.gov/dea/druginfo/ds.shtml. Accessed December 17, 2012.

intestinal motility, result from activation of peripheral receptors. The specific formulations differ in agonist or antagonist function as well as duration of action.

Pure opioid agonists activate all receptor types and are commonly used both clinically and illicitly for their analgesic and euphoric effects. Conversely, mixed agonist-antagonist formulations interact differently with each receptor type and were designed to have decreased addictive potential relative to pure agonists. This combination results in a ceiling effect on the maximum analgesia and euphoria experienced by the user, making this class favorable for treating opioid dependence. Opioid antagonists, such as naloxone and its analog naltrexone, function by competitively binding to the μ receptor to inhibit effects at a cellular level and can be used as reversal agents when opioid intoxication is suspected.[5]

Opioid receptor activation may have other effects, such as sedation, pruritus, nausea, and vomiting. Chronic use may lead to hyperalgesia as tachyphylaxis or tolerance develops, requiring escalating doses to provide similar desired analgesic effects.[6] Because individual response to particular medications may vary, the practice of opioid rotation (also known as opioid switching), or the transitioning from one formulation to another, may be of benefit in patients suffering from refractory side effects or inadequate analgesia with one specific drug. Similarly, the use of multiple opioid medications simultaneously (combined therapy) has been suggested to improve synergistic efficacy as well.

PRESCRIPTION MEDICATIONS

Common prescription medications include either pure opioid medications or formulations of an opioid medication combined with a complementary nonopioid analgesic. Such compounded medications usually contain acetaminophen or a nonsteroidal anti-inflammatory drug, such as ibuprofen, for additional analgesia. Most are dispensed in oral or transdermal forms, with intramuscular or intravenous preparations reserved for inpatient settings. Opioid compounds also constitute the primary active ingredient found in several medications prescribed for nonanalgesic indications, including cough suppressants and syrups.

Prescribing Practices

To date, no specific data exist suggesting that alteration of standard prescribing practices is required during pregnancy. Some states do not permit verbal pharmacy orders or facsimile transmission of prescriptions for controlled substances due to concern for diversion, instead mandating that original prescriptions be submitted. Unfortunately, the online pharmaceutical industry is only minimally regulated, particularly for locations outside of the United States. Consequently, so-called nonprescription Web sites illegitimately market opioid and other controlled substances in a semianonymous manner without requiring prescriptions.[7] In 2013, 46 states have operational prescription monitoring programs, with intent to reduce drug diversion practices; however, existing data attesting to their effectiveness remain conflicting.[8] An analysis performed in 2011 showed no difference in opioid mortality when comparing states with tracking programs and those without.[9] From the current data, it is unclear whether these programs alter prescribing practices and, if so, the resulting clinical impact.

In most states, however, where prescription monitoring programs are available, they are used by less than 25% of physicians prescribing narcotic medications.[10] In addition to low usage of the systems where they are available, some states do not permit direct access by the prescribing physicians, instead shifting the responsibility to law enforcement. Additionally, the types of medications that are reported to these databases vary from state to state, with some states tracking only schedule II medications and others tracking schedule II–IV medications.

Methadone

Methadone is a synthetic opioid originally developed in the 1930s and first manufactured in the United States in 1947. Most commonly prescribed for the treatment of heroin addiction, it has also been used in the management of chronic pain syndromes and more recently for prescription opioid abuse.[11] Methadone binds to the μ-opioid receptor as a competitive agonist and also competitively inhibits binding of the neurotransmitter glutamate to the N-methyl D-aspartate receptor within the central nervous system, mitigating some of the physiologic symptoms associated with opioid withdrawal. The elimination half-life of methadone (8–59 hours) is much longer than its analgesic effect (4–8 hours). Classified as a category C medication for use during pregnancy due to concerns for low birthweight and potential teratogenicity, methadone treatment has nevertheless been demonstrated to reduce actions associated with illicit substance use (drug-seeking behavior and prostitution) and provide a more pharmacologically stable fetal environment.[12]

Methadone therapy may be started during any trimester of pregnancy in either an inpatient or outpatient setting. Candidates should undergo standard medical examination, with particular attention to sonographic determination of fetal gestational age, screening for illicit drug use, and serologic studies for infectious diseases (HIV, hepatitis B, and hepatitis C). During the first 24 hours, an initial dose is administered followed by successive lower doses based on maternal symptoms (**Box 1**). During the second day, the cumulative total dose from the first day is administered, with further dosing as required until the patient remains free of withdrawal symptoms for a 24-hour interval (stabilization dose). Typical stabilization doses during pregnancy are 80 mg to 120 mg daily, whereas less than 60 mg daily is likely ineffective. Due to enhanced metabolism during pregnancy, twice-daily or thrice-daily administration may be beneficial in select circumstances.[13,14] Split-dosing regimens also seem to have lessened effects on fetal assessments and may be particularly effective for patients on higher doses who continue to experience symptomatology.[15] Serum trough levels have been described if confirmation of physiologic withdrawal is required.[16] Supplemental opioid analgesics should be avoided if at all possible. Treatment with diacetylmorphine (heroin-assisted treatment) has been described in fewer than 10 patients to date, ostensibly to reduce ongoing illicit substance use, without adverse outcome.[17]

For patients who conceive while enrolled in methadone treatment programs, further titration of dose is usually deferred until after delivery but otherwise follows similar management principles. Surveillance toxicology screening at each prenatal visit is suggested (and may be a legal requirement) to detect concurrent polysubstance abuse. Serial sonography to determine interval fetal growth seems warranted due to a possible increased risk of intrauterine growth restriction.[18] The antepartum dose is usually continued intrapartum and immediately postpartum, although some investigators have suggested decreasing the maintenance dose by 20% to 40% after delivery.[19] Breastfeeding is considered permissible by the American Academy of Pediatrics.[20]

Buprenorphine

Buprenorphine is a partial opioid agonist approved for treatment of opioid dependency by the FDA in 2002. Exclusively buprenorphine (Subutex) formulations are preferred over the buprenorphine/naloxone combination (Suboxone) during

---

Box 1
Methadone and buprenorphine prescribing regimens

Methadone regimens

Initiation (typically as an inpatient)

- Day #1: methadone 20–30 mg loading dose in morning, then 5–10 mg every 3–6 hours PRN for withdrawal symptoms.

- Day #2: cumulative total from day #1 administered as single morning dose with 5–10 mg doses every 3–6 hours as needed for withdrawal symptoms. Typically increase by 10–20 mg per day.

- Continue to escalate dose until no withdrawal symptoms for ≥24 hours (stabilization).

Maintenance

- Continue daily dose previously prescribed.

- Increase dose by 5–10 mg per day every 3–7 days (as required) to prevent withdrawal symptoms. Typical daily dose is 80–120 mg. Doses less than 60 mg are associated with increased relapse.

- Daily dose may be split into 8-h or 12-h intervals (if feasible) for refractory symptoms or during pregnancy.

Buprenorphine regimens

Initiation

- Must be abstinent from opioids for more than 24 hours or risk of withdrawal symptoms.

- Day #1: start 4 mg and observe. If withdrawal symptoms, may repeat dose for total 8 mg.

- Day #2: give prior day dose and observe. May increase by 4 mg increments to maximum 16 mg.

- Titrate by 4–8 mg increments every few days until symptoms resolved (maximum dose 32 mg).

Maintenance

- Continue daily dose as previously prescribed.

- Consider splitting daily dose into 6-h intervals during labor.

Opioid dependence may be managed during pregnancy and lactation with methadone or buprenorphine. Patient response to treatment is variable, so the dosages should be titrated to manage withdrawal symptoms. Due to the long half-life of methadone, incremental changes to maintenance should be made slowly.

---

pregnancy because the latter may precipitate withdrawal symptoms. Although the incidence of neonatal abstinence syndrome (NAS) is reportedly lower in patients treated with buprenorphine, current data do not suggest other specific benefits compared with methadone therapy.[21,22] Typical daily doses range between 8 mg and 16 mg, with a maximum dose of 32 mg (see **Box 1**). Similar to methadone, daily therapy is continued intrapartum, although the total daily dose may be divided to every 6 hours for enhanced analgesic effect. Postpartum, if greater than 48 hours of supplemental opioid therapy is anticipated (as with cesarean delivery or other complex surgical procedure), buprenorphine should be discontinued and therapy reinstituted once acute analgesic requirements have diminished.[23] Breastfeeding seems safe and does not increase risk of neonatal dependence, although data are limited.[24]

DETOXIFICATION DURING PREGNANCY

Although early reports suggested increased risks of spontaneous abortion, preterm delivery, and intrauterine fetal demise associated with opioid detoxification, the most comprehensive series suggests no increased risk of pregnancy complications.[25] Dose reduction and discontinuation of opiates may be attempted in motivated patients to reduce the risk of NAS, optimally during the second or early third trimester. Preexisting fetal growth restriction and oligohydramnios are considered relative contraindications. Choice of agent remains with clinicians because buprenorphine and methadone are both appropriate for use in pregnancy and have equivalent rates of subsequent NAS. In a multicenter randomized controlled trial of 175 pregnant women with opioid dependency, buprenorphine was associated with shorter duration of hospital stay (4.1 vs 9.9 days), decreased antepartum morphine requirements, and shorter neonatal hospital stay (10.0 vs 17.5 days) compared with methadone therapy. Discontinuation of therapy was more common, however, with buprenorphine (33%) than with methadone (18%).[11] Consequently, either medication is appropriate depending on physician comfort and the clinical scenario.

For methadone-naïve patients, a stabilization dose may be achieved followed by dose reductions of 20% every 72 hours. For patients on maintenance methadone therapy, protocols have described reductions of 2 mg to 5 mg every 6 to 16 days, with inpatient admission for taper and discontinuation at daily doses of less than or equal to 20 mg.[26] Unfortunately, the recidivism rate is approximately 40%, tempering the practical applicability of this approach. Only limited protocols for buprenorphine detoxification during pregnancy have been described and do not report adverse maternal or fetal outcomes.[27,28]

ILLICIT SUBSTANCES

Nonmedical use of prescription medications represents the second most common category of illicit drug use after marijuana, with opioid medications representing the majority. Of pregnant women aged 15 to 44, an average of 5% admitted to use of illicit substances in a national survey conducted in 2010–2011. Pregnant women aged 15 to 17 represented the highest risk group, with 20.9% indicating usage.[29] Heroin (diacetylmorphine) is the most commonly abused nonprescription opiate and rates of use, dependence, and death in persons 12 years and older have steadily increased over the past decade. Heroin may be administered nasally, intravenously, or via inhalation and is often compounded or adulterated with other substances, including cocaine, strychnine, quinine, and talc.[30]

The American Congress of Obstetricians and Gynecologists recommends routine screening for substance abuse in pregnancy.[6] Risk factors include adolescent age, single marital status, late or irregular prenatal care, lower level of education completed, history of high-risk sexual behavior, personal or family history of drug dependence, poor weight gain, poor dentition, and history of a mental health disorder. Physical examination may reveal skin lesions, such as track marks along superficial veins, abscesses, or cellulitis. Due to the risk of concomitant infectious disease, serologic testing for HIV, hepatitis B, and hepatitis C should be performed at the initial prenatal visit and repeated during the third trimester. Withdrawal of opioids in dependent patients is generally contraindicated during pregnancy due to risks of withdrawal symptoms and relapse as well as fetal distress or demise.[7,31] Rather, opioid-assisted therapy in the setting of an addiction treatment program is preferable to maintain continuity of care and reduce high-risk behaviors. A medically supervised withdrawal conducted by an experienced provider may be appropriate when a methadone or buprenorphine program is unavailable or if a patient refuses this intervention.

OBSTETRIC COMPLICATIONS

Adverse perinatal outcomes resulting from prescription or illicit substance use comprise a spectrum of maternal and fetal complications through both direct toxicity and engagement in activities and lifestyles related to drug procurement (infectious diseases and trauma).[32] Described specific obstetric complications include preterm delivery, abruptio placenta, fetal growth restriction, and intrauterine fetal demise.[7] Opioid mediations have not traditionally been considered to increase the risk of fetal birth defects, although this has been questioned in a recent review that suggests an increased risk of cardiac malformations.[33,34] Because many patients using illicit substances abuse multiple drugs in varying degrees, isolating the effects of any single drug is often impractical.[35] Although rare, the sharing of contaminated needles for injection can lead to alloimmunization in Rh-negative individuals.

GUIDELINES FOR PREGNANCY MANAGEMENT

Although recognizing that a single strategy may not be applicable to all circumstances and little formal evidence exists to guide various aspects of prenatal care, the authors suggest the following multidisciplinary approach, as practiced in their institution, to management of pregnancy complicated by opioid dependence:

Antepartum

1. At time of initiation of prenatal care, obtain routine prenatal laboratory studies; hepatitis C, gonorrhea, and chlamydia screening; serum/urine toxicology studies; and formal sonography to confirm gestational age.
2. For patients with history or current illicit substance use, consider repeat toxicology screening at each prenatal appointment and repeat HIV, syphilis and gonorrhea, and chlamydial screening at 36 weeks or sooner as clinically indicated.
3. Consultations with Social Work, Psychiatry and Addiction Counseling may be obtained as indicated. Notification of legal authorities is required in some states according to child protection statutes.[36]
4. All prescriptions should be coordinated through a single provider (or practice group) to avoid multiple providers prescribing simultaneously and to limit the potential for medication diversion.
5. If available, online state prescription monitoring programs should be reviewed periodically.
6. Early patient education regarding the potential fetal/neonatal effects of chronic opioid use is critical, with discontinuation or limitation of use as is feasible. Establish clear limits early in gestation in regard to prescriptions provided. As a general rule, the authors' institution has not engaged patients in formal prescribing contracts during pregnancy; however, this may be an option in particularly challenging situations. Rotation of medications may be required in selected circumstances.
7. Consider referral to a pain management or pain rehabilitation provider (if locally available).
8. Perform serial sonography on a monthly basis from 24 weeks' gestation to confirm interval fetal growth.
9. Some authors recommend weekly antenatal surveillance beginning at 32 weeks due to increased risk of fetal demise.

10. Although chronic opioid use has been described to reduce fetal heart rate accelerations and breathing movement on biophysical profile testing, in clinical practice this is not a consistent effect. Methadone has been demonstrated to reduce fetal heart rate with decreased variability and less frequent accelerations.[37,38]
11. Preparation for delivery may be facilitated by Neonatology/Pediatric consultation in the third trimester to discuss implications for nursery care and criteria for infant discharge from the hospital.
12. The provider must recognize that fear of legal revocation of parental custody may preclude some patients from obtaining prenatal care, particularly if they are presently engaged in illicit substance use or active prescription drug diversion.

Intrapartum

1. Notify neonatology/pediatrics and anesthesiology at time of admission.
2. Continuation of the previous antepartum medication regimen is usually feasible during labor. For patients receiving methadone or buprenorphine, confirmation of current dosage with dispensing clinic is suggested.
3. Some patients, particularly those engaged in illicit substance use, may exhibit hyperalgesia to labor discomfort and require substantial doses of intravenous analgesics for relief. Neither methadone nor buprenorphine is typically exclusively sufficient for intrapartum analgesia.
4. Similar to antepartum fetal assessment, although alterations in fetal heart rate patterns have been described, parameters for intrapartum fetal assessment should follow standard obstetric guidelines.[39]

Postpartum

1. Similar to the intrapartum interval, higher doses of analgesic medications may be required postpartum to achieve patient comfort, particularly after cesarean delivery.
2. Anticipated incidence of NAS is approximately 6% to 71% for patients receiving chronic opioid prescriptions.[40] Naloxone is generally avoided in the treatment of neonatal respiratory depression due to concern of precipitating opioid withdrawal seizures.[41]
3. Lactation is permissible in the absence of standard obstetric contraindications (HIV, active tuberculosis, and so forth)
4. Before maternal discharge, a clear plan should be formulated for scheduled subsequent return visits and anticipated postpartum analgesic requirements. If a patient is typically prescribed maintenance opioid therapy from a nonobstetric provider, transitions in prescribing should be discussed in advance with the patient and all involved providers.
5. Postpartum contraceptive options should be discussed.

NEONATAL ABSTINENCE SYNDROME

NAS, also termed neonatal opioid withdrawal, is generally defined as a constellation of physiologic symptoms due to cessation of opioid exposure after interruption of the fetoplacental circulation at time of delivery. Onset may be related to maternal medication elimination half-life but typically occurs within 1 to 10 days of delivery. Symptoms can include dehydration, excessive crying, diarrhea, increased muscle tone, hyperreflexia, fever, congestion, diaphoresis, irritability, difficulty sleeping, or seizures.[42] These effects seem most pronounced in preterm infants or after maternal methadone or heroin use, with some investigators describing rates as high as 71%. Paradoxically, data regarding the risk of NAS do not consistently correlate with methadone dosage.[43,44] Duration of inpatient neonatal observation should be dependent on the specific maternal opioid used during pregnancy.[45]

Minimal data currently exist describing the frequency of NAS occurring in infants born to mothers receiving chronic prescription opioid therapy. A recent review of discharge documentation suggests, however, that a 3-fold increase in NAS has occurred in the United States over the past decade.[46] A recent retrospective investigation from Kellogg and colleagues[40] found that 0.6% of patients were prescribed opioid medications for the duration of pregnancy, with a 6% incidence of NAS. Neonatal outcomes were not stratified by specific maternal dosage. A recent report also suggested 6% of Norwegian pregnant patients are prescribed opioids before conception, during pregnancy, or after delivery, with the majority for short-term indications.[47]

Confirmatory testing of neonatal urine, hair, or meconium samples may be performed but because results are usually not rapidly available, presumptive treatment should be initiated in the interim. Several objective scoring systems have been developed to identify infants requiring treatment and to guide escalation of therapy. Treatment of NAS comprises of avoidance of excess stimulation of the newborn, frequent low-volume/high-calorie feedings, and institution of morphine or methadone therapy contingent on symptoms score (**Table 2**). Phenobarbital may be effective in refractory cases or for infants exposed to multiple illicit substances. Once neonatal condition is stabilized, medication doses are gradually incremental decreased (weaning) over the following days to weeks.

Table 2
Modified Finnegan neonatal abstinence scoring tool

Neonatal Abstinence Scoring System			
Symptom	Score	Symptom	Score
Continuous high pitched (or other) cry	2	Sweating	1
Continuous high pitched (or other) cry	3	Fever 100.4°–101°F (38°–38.3°C)	1
Sleeps <1 h after feeding	3	Fever >101°F (38.3°C)	2
Sleeps <2 h after feeding	2	Frequent yawning (>3–4 times/interval)	1
Sleeps <3 h after feeding	1	Mottling	1
Hyperactive Moro reflex	2	Nasal stuffiness	1
Markedly hyperactive Moro reflex	3	Sneezing (>3–4 times/interval)	1
Mild tremors disturbed	1	Nasal flaring	2
Moderate–severe tremors disturbed	2	Respiratory rate >60/min	1
Mild tremors undisturbed	3	Respiratory rate >60/min with retractions	2
Moderate–severe tremors undisturbed	4	Excessive sucking	1
Increased muscle tone	2	Poor feeding	2
Excoriation (specific area)	1	Regurgitation	2
Myoclonic jerks	3	Projectile vomiting	3
Generalized convulsions	5	Loose stools	2
		Watery stools	3

Modified Finnegan score obtained at 2-hour intervals after delivery. A score ≥8 on 3 or more consecutive occasions generally requires pharmacologic intervention. Blue, central nervous system disturbances; yellow, metabolic/vasomotor/respiratory disturbances; and green, gastrointestinal disturbances.

Developmental outcomes for exposed infants are challenging to definitively categorize, with some epidemiologic studies showing an increased incidence of neurobehavioral issues later in childhood and others demonstrating no differences from age-matched cohorts.[48] A recent report comparing imaging studies in methadone-exposed neonates suggested delayed maturation of cortical neural tracts.[49] Quantification of individual substance effects is difficult to ascertain due to confounding environmental and social factors, which may ultimately play a larger role in determining outcomes.[50]

MANAGEMENT OF ACUTE OPIOID OVERDOSE

Presenting signs of opioid overdose include lethargy, confusion, pupillary constriction, decreased respiratory rate, and, in extreme cases, obtundation or respiratory arrest. Initial efforts should focus on standard cardiopulmonary resuscitation, followed by an initial dose of intravenous naloxone to restore respiratory function.[51] Basic laboratory studies (including serum glucose) should be obtained with ECG, chest radiography, and cranial imaging based on individual clinical scenario (**Fig. 1**).[52,53] Some reports have suggested reversal of buprenorphine overdose may require higher doses of naloxone.[54] Once maternal condition has been stabilized, the patient should be transported to an appropriate obstetric unit for fetal assessment and continued observation.

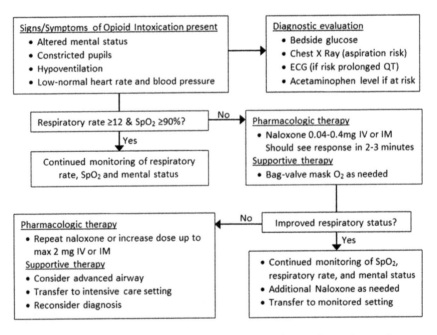

Naloxone use: Goal of treatment is improved respirations, not improved mental status. Excess dose may result in withdrawal symptoms. Duration of action is 45-70 minutes, whereas most ingested opioids last much longer (often 24-72 hours). Repeat doses will likely be required. Continuous intravenous infusion may also be used in such cases.

Fig. 1. Management of acute opioid intoxication. Keys to management of opioid intoxication include supportive therapy and opioid agonists to improve respiratory status.

PREVENTION OF OPIOID ABUSE

Several strategies have been proposed for the prevention of prescription and nonprescription opioid abuse[55–57]:

1. Limitation of prescription refills through specific insurance coverage limitations or restrictions and state prescription monitoring oversight programs to track pharmacy dispensing
2. Creation and enforcement of regulations against doctor shopping or distribution of narcotic medications without adequate medical evaluation
3. Mandatory education of health care providers on evidence-based guidelines regarding appropriate and effective prescribing practices
4. Continuity of care with a single provider

In 2011 the FDA charged all manufacturers of opiate medications to develop and implement a REMS program to educate health care providers regarding the safe prescribing of extended-release/long-acting formulations, with the final protocol released in July 2012.[58,59]

SUMMARY

Prescription and nonprescription chronic opioid abuse represents a growing problem in the United States that will likely increase during the next several years. Strategies for management during pregnancy include discontinuation of narcotic medications with careful observation for withdrawal symptoms, limitation of prescriptions, and medical therapy with methadone or buprenorphine therapy reserved for patients with addiction or dependence—either agent is appropriate for use during pregnancy and breastfeeding, although more data presently exist for methadone treatment. NAS may occur with maternal use of any opioid medication but seems most common with methadone or illicit substance use. Given these multiple challenges, referrals to providers with experience in addiction management, social work, chronic pain, and pediatrics should be made during the antepartum course, with plans for delivery at a facility with availability of adequate resources and staff. Use of prescription monitoring programs or the evolving REMS program may be beneficial in prevention of inappropriate prescribing or diversion, although efforts should be made to create a nonjudgmental environment to reduce risk-taking behaviors and recidivism. Maintaining regular care for opioid-dependent pregnant patients with this multidisciplinary team approach will aid in achieving optimal outcomes for both mothers and their babies in this otherwise challenging scenario.

REFERENCES

1. Herper M. America's most popular drugs. Forbes 2010.
2. Manchikanti L, Helm S, Fellows B, et al. Opioid epidemic in the United States. Pain Physician 2012;15(Suppl 3):ES9–38.
3. Available at: http://www.justice.gov/dea/druginfo/ds.shtml. Accessed January 9, 2013.
4. Code of Federal Regulations title 21. Available at: http://www.accessdata.fda.gov/scripts/cdrh/cfdocs/cfCFR/CFRSearch.cfm?fr=201.57. Accessed January 9, 2013.
5. Yaksh TL, Wallace MS. Opioid analgesics and pain management. In: Brunton L, Chabner B, Knollman B, editors. Goodman and Gilman's the Pharmacological basis of Therapeutics. 12th edition. New York: McGraw-Hill; 2010. p. 481–536.

6. Hoflich AS, Langer M, Jagsch R, et al. Peripartum pain management in opioid dependent women. Eur J Pain 2012;16:574–84.

7. Forman RF, Block LG. The marketing of opioid prescriptions without prescription over the internet. J Publ Pol Market 2006;25(2):133–46.

8. Gugelmann HM, Perrone J. Can prescription drug monitoring programs help limit opioid abuse? JAMA 2011;306(20):2258–9.

9. Paulozzi LJ, Kilbourne EM, Desai HA. Prescription drug monitoring programs and death rates from drug overdose. Pain Med 2011;12(5):747–54.

10. Green TC, Zaller N, Rich J, et al. Revisiting Paulozzi et al.'s "Prescription drug monitoring programs and death rates from drug overdose". Pain Med 2011; 12(6):982–5.

11. American College of Obstetricians and Gynecologists. Opioid abuse, dependence, and addiction in pregnancy. Committee Opinion No. 524. Obstet Gynecol 2012;119(5):1070–6.

12. Mitchell JL. Alcohol and other drug treatment guidelines for pregnant, substance using women. In: Treatment improvement protocol series 2: pregnant, substance-using women. Rockville, Maryland: US Department of Health and Human Services; 1995. p. 14–32.

13. Swift RM, Dudley M, DePetrillo P, et al. Altered methadone pharmacokinetics in pregnancy: implications for dosing. J Subst Abuse 1989;1(4):453–60.

14. DePetrillo PB, Rice JM. Methadone dosing and pregnancy: impact on program compliance. Int J Addict 1995;30(2):207–17.

15. Jansson LM, Dipietro JA, Velez M, et al. Maternal methadone dosing schedule and fetal neurobehaviour. J Matern Fetal Neonatal Med 2009;22(1):29.

16. Drozdick J, Berghella V, Hill M, et al. Methadone trough levels in pregnancy. Am J Obstet Gynecol 2002;187(5):1184–8.

17. Kashiwagi M, Arlettaz R, Lauper U, et al. Methadone maintenance program in a Swiss perinatal center: (I): management and outcome of 89 pregnancies. Acta Obstet Gynecol Scand 2005;84(2):140–4.

18. Liu AJ, Sithamparanathan S, Jones MP, et al. Growth restriction in pregnancies of opioid-dependent mothers. Arch Dis Child Fetal Neonatal Ed 2010;95(4): F258–62.

19. Helmbrecht GD, Thiagarajah S. Management of addiction disorders in pregnancy. J Addict Med 2008;2(1):1–16.

20. Committee on Drugs, American Academy of Pediatrics. The transfer of drugs and other chemicals into human breast milk. Pediatrics 2001;108:776–89.

21. Jones HE, Kaltenbach K, Heil SH, et al. Neonatal abstinence syndrome after methadone or buprenorphine exposure. N Engl J Med 2010;363(24):2320–31.

22. Minozzi S, Amato L, Vecchi S, et al. Maintenance agonist treatments for opiate dependent pregnant women. Cochrane Database Syst Rev 2008;(2):CD006318.

23. Alto WA, O'Connor AB. Management of women treated with buprenorphine during pregnancy. Am J Obstet Gynecol 2011;205(4):302–8.

24. Jones HE, Heil SH, Baewert A, et al. Buprenorphine treatment of opioid-dependent women: a comprehensive review. Addiction 2012;107(Suppl 1): 5–27.

25. Dashe JS, Jackson GL, Olscher DA, et al. Opioid detoxification in pregnancy. Obstet Gynecol 1998;92(5):854.

26. Ward J, Hall W, Mattick RP. Role of maintenance treatment in opioid dependence. Lancet 1999;353(9148):221–6.

27. Comer VG, Annitto WJ. Buprenorphine: a safe method for detoxifying pregnant heroin addicts and their unborn. Am J Addict 2004;13:317–8.

28. Annitto WJ. Detoxification with buprenorphine of a pregnant heroin addict. Am J Addict 2000;9:92–3.
29. Substance Abuse and Mental Health Services Administration. Results from the 2011 National Survey on drug use and health: summary of National Findings. NSDUH Series H-44, HHS Publication No. (SMA) 12–4713. Rockville (MD): Substance Abuse and Mental Health Services Administration; 2012.
30. Doyon S. Chapter 180. Opioids. In: Tintinalli JE, Stapczynski S, Clinc DM, et al, editors. Tintinalli's emergency medicine. 7th edition. New York: The McGraw-Hill Companies, Inc; 2011.
31. Jones HE, O'Grady KE, Malfi D, et al. Methadone maintenance vs. methadone taper during pregnancy: maternal and neonatal outcomes. Am J Addict 2008; 17(5):372–86.
32. Winklbaur B, Jung E, Fischer G. Opioid dependence and pregnancy. Curr Opin Psychiatry 2008;21(3):255–9.
33. Schempf AH. Illicit drug use and neonatal outcomes: a critical review. Obstet Gynecol Surv 2007;62(11):749–57.
34. Broussard CS, Rasmussen SA, Reefhuis J, et al. National birth defects prevention study. Maternal treatment with opioid analgesics and risk for birth defects. Am J Obstet Gynecol 2011;204(4):314.e1–11.
35. Bell J, Harvey-Dodds L. Pregnancy and injecting drug use. BMJ 2008; 336(7656):1303–5.
36. Park EM, Meltzer-Brody S, Suzuki J. Evaluation and management of opioid dependence in pregnancy. Psychosomatics 2012;53:424–32.
37. Jansson LM, Dipietro J, Elko A. Fetal response to maternal methadone administration. Am J Obstet Gynecol 2005;193(3 Pt 1):611–7.
38. Jones HE, Finnegan LP, Kaltenbach K. Methadone and buprenorphine for the management of opioid dependence in pregnancy. Drugs 2012;72(6):747–57.
39. Ramirez-Cacho WA, Flores S, Schrader RM, et al. Effect of chronic maternal methadone therapy on intrapartum fetal heart rate patterns. J Soc Gynecol Investig 2006;13(2):108–11.
40. Kellogg A, Rose CH, Harms RH, et al. Current trends in narcotic use in pregnancy and neonatal outcomes. Am J Obstet Gynecol 2011;204(3):259.e1–4.
41. Rajani AK, Chitkara R, Halamek LP. Delivery room management of the Newborn. Pediatr Clin North Am 2009;56(3):515–35.
42. Jansson LM, Velez M. Neonatal abstinence syndrome. Curr Opin Pediatr 2012; 24(2):252–8.
43. Pizarro D, Habli M, Grier M, et al. Higher maternal doses of methadone does not increase neonatal abstinence syndrome. J Subst Abuse Treat 2011;40(3):295–8.
44. Dashe JS, Sheffield JS, Olscher DA, et al. Relationship between maternal methadone dosage and neonatal withdrawal. Obstet Gynecol 2002;100(6):1244–9.
45. Hudak ML, Tan RC, Committee on Drugs, Committee on Fetus and Newborn. Neonatal drug withdrawal. Pediatrics 2012;129:e540–60.
46. Patrick SW, Schumacher RE, Benneyworth BD, et al. Neonatal abstinence syndrome and associated health care expenditures: United States, 2000-2009. JAMA 2012;307(18):1934–40.
47. Handal M, Engeland A, Rønning M, et al. Use of prescribed opioid analgesics and co-medication with benzodiazepines in women before, during, and after pregnancy: a population-based cohort study. Eur J Clin Pharmacol 2011; 67(9):953–60.
48. Hunt RW, Tzioumi D, Collins E, et al. Adverse neurodevelopmental outcome of infants exposed to opiate in-utero. Early Hum Dev 2008;84(1):29–35.

49. Walhovd KB, Watts R, Amlien I, et al. Neural tract development of infants born to methadone-maintained mothers. Pediatr Neurol 2012;47(1):1–6.

50. Mactier H. The management of heroin misuse in pregnancy: time for a rethink? Arch Dis Child Fetal Neonatal Ed 2011;96(6):F457–60.

51. Deakin CD, Morrison LJ, Morley PT, et al. 2010 International consensus on cardiopulmonary resuscitation and emergency cardiovascular care science with treatment recommendations. Resuscitation 2010;81S:e93–174.

52. Vanden Hoek TL, Morrison LJ, Shuster M, et al. Circulation 2010;122:S829–61.

53. Kosten TR. Chapter 393. Opioid drug abuse and dependence. In: Longo DL, Fauci AS, Kasper DL, et al, editors. Harrison's principles of internal medicine. 18th edition. New York: McGraw-Hill Companies, Inc; 2012.

54. Mégarbane B, Buisine A, Jacobs F, et al. Prospective comparative assessment of buprenorphine overdose with heroin and methadone: clinical characteristics and response to antidotal treatment. J Subst Abuse Treat 2010;38(4):403–7.

55. Paulozzi L, Baldwin G, Franklin G, et al. CDC grand rounds: prescription drug overdoses—a U.S. epidemic. MMWR Morb Mortal Wkly Rep 2012;61(1):10–3.

56. Lembke A. Why doctors prescribe opioids to known opioid abusers. N Engl J Med 2012;367(17):1580–1.

57. Okie S. A flood of opioids, a rising tide of deaths. N Engl J Med 2010;363(21): 1981–5.

58. US Food and Drug Administration Risk Evaluation and Mitigation Strategy (REMS) for Extended-Release and Long-Acting Opioids. Retrieved from the FDA website: http://www.fda.gov/Drugs/DrugSafety/InformationbyDrugClass/ucm309742.htm. Accessed December 17, 2012.

59. Nelson LS, Perrone J. Curbing the opioid epidemic in the United States: the risk evaluation and mitigation strategy (REMS). JAMA 2012;308(5):457–8.

60. DEA Drug Scheduling. Retrieved from the United States Drug Enforcement Agency website: http://www.justice.gov/dea/druginfo/ds.shtml. Accessed December 17, 2012.

61. Howland RH. Categorizing the safety of medications during pregnancy and lactation. J Psychosoc Nurs Ment Health Serv 2009;47(4):17–20.

Nonpharmacologic Labor Analgesia

Katherine W. Arendt, MD[a],*, Jennifer A. Tessmer-Tuck, MD[b]

KEYWORDS

- Nonpharmacologic labor analgesia • Hydrotherapy • Acupuncture • TENS • Yoga
- Hypnosis • Aromatherapy • Sterile water papules

KEY POINTS

- Selection and volunteer bias, differences in cultural and regional acceptance of various nonpharmacologic analgesic options, differences in provider technique, and difficulty in blinding participants provide significant challenges in performing and evaluating the evidence surrounding nonpharmacologic interventions for labor analgesia.
- A woman's satisfaction with her childbirth may or may not be associated with the efficacy of her labor analgesia.
- Overall, there is limited high-quality evidence evaluating nonpharmacologic labor analgesia options; therefore, efficacy remains unclear.
- Although data are limited, acupuncture, acupressure, transcutaneous electrical nerve stimulation (TENS) electrodes applied to acupuncture points, relaxation techniques, yoga, and massage therapy may provide modest analgesic benefit to women in labor.
- Randomized trials do not show benefit for hypnosis, although studies in which women self-select hypnosis indicate benefit from the technique.
- Sterile water papules do not show benefit when compared with saline water papules. When data from studies that compare sterile water papules to other nonpharmacologic treatment modalities (eg, acupuncture or TENS) are included in a meta-analysis, benefit is shown.
- Water immersion may decrease women's requests for regional analgesia during the first stage of labor.
- Continuous personal support for women in labor has robust evidence to support its efficacy of improved obstetric, neonatal, analgesic, and satisfaction outcomes.

Disclosure: Neither Dr Jennifer A. Tessmer-Tuck nor Dr Katherine W. Arendt has interest in any commercial company that has a direct financial interest in the subject matter or materials discussed in the article or with a company making a competing product.

[a] Department of Anesthesiology, Mayo Clinic College of Medicine, 200 First Street SW, Rochester, MN 55905, USA; [b] North Memorial Medical Center Laborist Associates, 3300 Oakdale Avenue North, Robbinsdale, MN 55422, USA
* Corresponding author.
E-mail address: arendt.katherine@mayo.edu

INTRODUCTION

The birth of a child may be one of the most meaningful events of a woman's life. With 9 months to prepare, by the time women reach the labor and delivery unit, most have thought considerably about the impending childbirth. It is important that health care providers accept that an unmedicated childbirth may hold emotional, spiritual, social, cultural, or even religious value to a woman. Each woman has her own ideas and philosophy regarding the significance and value of labor pain. A supportive medical team should be well informed on the various pharmacologic and nonpharmacologic modalities of coping or mitigating labor pain to appropriately support and respectfully care for all patients. Using the rigor of previously published Cochrane systematic reviews, this article summarizes, evaluates, and discusses the efficacy of nonpharmacologic labor analgesic interventions.

CHALLENGES STUDYING NONPHARMACOLOGIC INTERVENTIONS

Scientifically evaluating various nonpharmacologic methods of labor analgesia is difficult. Traditionally, the efficacy of an analgesic intervention is considered by looking at total milligrams of opioid consumed or patient-rated pain scores. The goal of many nonpharmacologic labor interventions, however, is not to lessen pain but to increase a woman's ability to cope with the pain. Therefore, many nonpharmacologic interventions look to evaluate a woman's satisfaction with her birth experience or her willingness to have another birth using the same techniques.

A woman's satisfaction with her childbirth may or may not be associated with the efficacy of pain mitigation. For example, one study evaluated women who had the goal of an unmedicated childbirth.[1] Those who achieved that goal had a greater satisfaction with their childbirth than women who ultimately elected for neuraxial analgesia intrapartum, even though the women who underwent neuraxial analgesia had significantly lower pain scores. Furthermore, although epidural labor analgesia has been shown to improve pain scores and decrease requests for other analgesic agents compared with systemic opioids (**Table 1**), there is no difference in women's ratings of their satisfaction with pain relief.[2]

Further challenges in evaluating the evidence surrounding complementary or alternative interventions include differences in cultural or regional acceptance of various techniques and differences among health care providers as to how interventions are performed.[3,4] Retrospective and observational studies surrounding nonpharmacologic analgesic options are confounded considerably by selection bias. Selection bias is an important consideration, because buy-in from subjects as well as from obstetric providers may be one of the most important factors in the efficacy of a nonpharmacologic technique. For example, a woman who does not believe that acupuncture or massage is helpful is unlikely to find it beneficial. A woman who arrives at the hospital dedicated to an unmedicated birth experience, however, may find even the simplest interventions, from massage to aromatherapy, helpful in assisting her in reaching her goal.

Multiple systematic reviews have been added to the Cochrane Database involving nonpharmacologic interventions for labor analgesia (**Tables 2–11**). Cochrane systematic reviews are particularly scientifically rigorous because the authors and editors work to ensure that evidence fits prespecified eligibility criteria and work to minimize bias by using explicit, systematic methods. Appropriate randomization and blinding of patients, providers, and researchers as much as possible were necessary for an individual study to be included in the Cochrane reviews that are discussed below.

Table 1
Cochrane Database of Systematic Reviews: epidural analgesia versus systemic opioids in labor

Results	Notes and Conclusions[a]
Epidural analgesia was associated with better pain relief than systemic opioids. • 3 Trials; n = 1166 • SMD −3.36, 95% CI, −5.41 to −1.31 Epidural analgesia was associated with a reduction in the need for additional pain relief. • 15 Trials; n = 6019 • RR 0.05; 95% CI, 0.02–0.17 Epidural analgesia was associated with a reduction in the risk of neonatal acidosis. • 7 Trials; n = 3643 • RR 0.80; 95% CI, 0.68–0.94 Epidural analgesia was associated with a reduction in the risk of neonatal naloxone administration. • 10 Trials; n = 2645 • RR 0.15; 95% CI, 0.10–0.23 Epidural analgesia was associated with an increased risk of assisted vaginal birth. • 23 Trials; n = 7935 • RR 1.42; 95% CI, 1.28–1.57 Epidural analgesia was associated with an increased risk of maternal hypotension. • 8 Trials; n = 2789 • RR 18.23; 95% CI, 5.09–63.35 Epidural analgesia was associated with an increased risk of motor blockade. • 3 Trials; n = 322 • RR 31.67; 95% CI, 4.33–231.51 Epidural analgesia was associated with an increased risk of maternal fever. • 6 Trials; n = 2741 • RR 3.34; 95% CI, 2.63–4.23 Epidural analgesia was associated with an increased risk of urinary retention. • 3 Trials; n = 7935 • RR 17.05; 95% CI, 4.82–60.39 Epidural analgesia was associated with an increased length of the second stage of labor. • 13 Trials; n = 4233 • SMD 13.66 min; 95% CI, 6.67–20.66 Epidural analgesia was associated with an increased risk of oxytocin administration. • 13 Trials; n = 5815 • RR 1.19; 95% CI, 1.03–1.39 Epidural analgesia was associated with an increased risk of cesarean section for fetal distress. • 11 Trials; n = 4816 • RR 1.43; 95% CI, 1.03–1.97	Epidural analgesia seems to be effective in reducing pain during labor when compared with systemic opioid analgesia. Epidural analgesia has no significant impact on the risk of cesarean section, maternal satisfaction with pain relief, long-term backache, or neonatal status as determined by APGAR scores.

(continued on next page)

Table 1 (continued)	
Results	**Notes and Conclusions[a]**
Epidural analgesia was NOT associated with an increased risk of cesarean section overall. • 27 Trials; n = 8417 • RR 1.10; 95% CI, 0.97–1.25 Epidural analgesia was NOT associated with an increased risk of long-term backache. • 3 Trials; n = 1806 • RR 0.96; 95% CI, 0.86–1.07 Epidural analgesia was NOT associated with an increased risk of APGAR scores <7 at 5 min. • 18 Trials; n = 6898 • RR 0.80; 95% CI, 0.54–1.20 Epidural analgesia had no impact on maternal satisfaction with pain relief. • 7 Trials; n = 2929 • RR 1.31; 95% CI, 0.84–2.05	

Abbreviation: SMD, standard mean difference.
[a] These are the conclusions of the authors of the Cochrane systematic review.
From Anim-Somuah M, Smyth RM, Jones L. Epidural versus non-epidural or no analgesia in labor. Cochrane Database Syst Rev 2011;12:CD000331; with permission.

OVERVIEW OF EFFICACY OF LABOR ANALGESIA OPTIONS

Multiple randomized trials indicate that epidural and combined spinal epidural analgesia effectively manage the pain of labor with side effects that include hypotension, motor block, urinary retention, pruritus, and fever.[2,5] Results of the Cochrane systematic review regarding epidural analgesia are summarized in **Table 1**. This information may be compared and contrasted to the outcomes associated with nonpharmacologic analgesia (outlined in **Tables 2–11**); Association may not necessarily mean causation, however, and an entire review could be dedicated to each of these associations. Inhaled anesthetics may also decrease pain with side effects that include vomiting, nausea, and dizziness.[5] Nonopioid drugs and local anesthetic peripheral nerve blocks may improve pain management with few side effects.[5]

The efficacy of nonpharmacologic labor analgesia techniques from recently published Cochrane systematic reviews is presented in **Tables 2–11**. An overview of these systematic reviews states, "there is some evidence to suggest that immersion in water, relaxation, acupuncture, (and) massage… may improve management of labor pain with few adverse effects."[5] The investigators go on to state that water immersion, relaxation, and acupuncture improved patient satisfaction with pain relief and water immersion and relaxation may improve a woman's rating of her childbirth experience. They also state that overall there is limited high-quality evidence, and, therefore, the efficacy of nonpharmacologic pain management techniques remains "unclear."[5] This article specifically explores each nonpharmacologic analgesic modality and discusses the results of the specific Cochrane systematic review dedicated solely to that modality.

Many of the nonpharmacologic modalities of pain relief have little risk associated with them, and, therefore, whether they are shown to decrease pain by strict scientific standards may not be important to an individual laboring woman. For example, if she feels that massage, music, or particular smells in the room are helping her cope with

Table 2
Cochrane Database of Systematic Reviews: acupuncture or acupressure for pain management in labor

Results	Notes and Conclusions[a]
Compared with no intervention, acupuncture was associated with less intense pain. • 1 Trial; n = 163 • SMD −1.00, 95% CI, −1.33 to −0.67	Acupuncture and acupressure may have a role in reducing pain, increasing satisfaction with pain management, and reducing the use of pharmacologic treatment modalities.
Compared with placebo, acupressure was associated with less intense pain. • 1 Trial; n = 120 • SMD −0.55, 95% CI, −0.92 to −0.19	No trial was assessed as being low risk of bias for all of the quality domains. There is a need for further research.
Compared with a combined control, acupressure was associated with less intense pain. • 2 Trials; n = 322 • SMD −0.42, 95% CI, −0.65 to −0.18	
Compared with placebo, acupuncture was associated with increased satisfaction with pain relief. • 1 Trial; n = 150 • RR 2.38; 95% CI, 1.78–3.19	
Compared with placebo, acupuncture was associated with reduced use of pharmacologic analgesia. • 1 Trial; n = 136 • RR 0.72; 95% CI, 0.58–0.88	
Compared with standard care, acupuncture was associated with reduced use of pharmacologic analgesia. • 3 Trials; n = 704 • RR 0.68; 95% CI, 0.56–0.83 • Significant heterogeneity	
Compared with standard care, acupuncture was associated with fewer instrumental deliveries. • 3 Trials; n = 704 • RR 0.67; 95% CI, 0.46–0.98 • Significant heterogeneity	

Abbreviation: SMD, standard mean difference.

[a] These are the conclusions of the authors of the Cochrane systematic review.

From Smith CA, Collins CT, Crowther CA, et al. Acupuncture or acupressure for pain management in labor. Cochrane Database Syst Rev 2011;7:CD009232; with permission.

the stress and discomfort of labor, then in most circumstances supporting this woman's desires is the best care—even if scientific evidence may not support the efficacy of the technique via randomized controlled trials (RCTs). Furthermore, pharmacologic techniques, such as regional analgesia and systemic opioids, are very much compatible with most nonpharmacologic techniques. Hydrotherapy is the only notable exception. Labor can be stressful for women even with effective pain control with regional anesthesia, and various deliberate coping techniques chosen by a woman are almost always appropriate.

Table 3
Cochrane Database of Systematic Reviews: hypnosis for pain management in labor and childbirth

Results	Notes and Conclusions[a]
There was no significant difference in use of pharmacologic pain relief between hypnosis and control groups. • 6 Trials, n = 1032 • RR 0.63; 95% CI, 0.39–1.01	All but one trial had a moderate-to-high risk of bias. The control group included women who were taught no hypnotic techniques or had no hypnosis intervention.
There was no significant difference in rate of spontaneous vaginal birth between hypnosis and control groups. • 4 Trials, n = 472 • RR 1.35; 95% CI, 0.93–1.96	There were considerable differences among trials in hypnosis timing and technique. There are still only a few studies assessing the use of hypnosis for labor and childbirth. Although the intervention shows some promise, further research is needed before recommendations can be made regarding its clinical usefulness.
There was no significant difference in satisfaction with pain relief between hypnosis and control groups. • 1 Trial, n = 264. • RR 1.06; 95% CI, 0.94–1.20	
There was no significant difference in satisfaction with the childbirth experience between hypnosis and control groups. • 2 Trials, n = 370 • RR 1.36; 95% CI, 0.52–3.59	
There was no significant difference in admissions to the neonatal ICU between hypnosis and control groups. • 2 Trials, n = 347 • RR 0.58; 95% CI, 0.12–2.89	
There was no significant difference in rates of breastfeeding at discharge from hospital between hypnosis and control groups. • 1 Trial, n = 304 • RR 1.00; 95% CI, 0.97–1.03	

[a] These are the conclusions of the authors of the Cochrane systematic review.

From Madden K, Middleton P, Cyna AM, et al. Hypnosis for pain management during labor and childbirth. Cochrane Database Syst Rev 2012;11:CD009356; with permission.

ACUPUNCTURE AND ACUPRESSURE

Acupuncture is a form of traditional Chinese medicine in which fine needles are inserted along meridians, which are the channels through which energy flow. This energy is called qi, pronounced *chi*, and the needles restore the harmony of its flow. There is no anatomic correlate for meridians or physiologic correlate for qi in traditional Western medicine. It is thought that acupuncture's efficacy may lie in its interaction with the neuroendocrine system.

One difficulty in performing RCTs evaluating acupuncture is the inability to blind an acupuncturist or patient. There are sham acupuncture devices that do not puncture the skin but mimic the procedure and there is also a technique of placing the needles in areas that are not considered acupoints. The former blinds neither the patient nor acupuncturist; the latter blinds only the patient. Also, studies may involve acupuncture, acupressure, or electroacupuncture. The latter involves running a tiny electric current through the needle. A recent electroacupuncture study randomizing to a

Table 4
Cochrane Database of Systematic Reviews: intracutaneous or subcutaneous sterile water injection compared with blinded controls in labor

Results	Notes and Conclusions[a]
There was no significant difference in use of pharmacologic rescue analgesia between sterile water vs saline injections. • 4 Trials, n = 467 • RR 0.86; 95% CI, 0.44–1.69 There was no significant difference in rates of cesarean section between sterile water vs saline injections. • 7 Trials, n = 766 • RR 0.58; 95% CI, 0.33–1.69 There was no significant difference in rates of assisted vaginal (instrumented) delivery between sterile water vs saline injections • 6 Trials, n = 666 • RR 1.31; 95% CI, 0.79–2.18	All studies looked at this intervention to treat low back pain in labor. The control group was isotonic saline injections instead of the more painful sterile water injections. The provider was blinded as to which type of solution was used. The outcomes reported severely limit conclusions for clinical practice. Further large, methodologically rigorous studies are required to determine the efficacy of sterile water to relieve pain in labor.

[a] These are the conclusions of the authors of the Cochrane systematic review.
From Derry S, Straube S, Moore RA, et al. Intracutaneous or subcutaneous sterile water injection compared with blinded controls for pain management in labor. Cochrane Database Syst Rev 2012;1:CD009107; with permission.

control group, a sham group, and an electroacupuncture group found labor pain scores within the electroacupuncture group significantly reduced after 30 minutes of needle retention (control group n = 115, visual analog scale [VAS] 85.43 ± 18.496; sham group n = 117, VAS 81.64 ± 19.159; electroacupuncture group n = 117, VAS 75.97 ± 22.498; $P<.05$) as well as 2 hours after needle withdrawal (control group n = 77, VAS 92.19 ± 12.135; sham group n = 79, VAS 89.46 ± 13.565; electroacupuncture group n = 64; VAS 85.44 ± 15.933; $P<.05$) and 4 hours after needle withdrawal (control group n = 22, VAS 94.5 ± 8.809; sham group n = 37, VAS 91.49 ± 14.36; electroacupuncture group 19 82.42 ± 17.066; $P<.05$).[6]

Table 5
Cochrane Database of Systematic Reviews: transcutaneous electrical nerve stimulation for pain relief in labor

Results	Notes and Conclusions[a]
There was no significant difference in VAS pain scores in women with or without TENS. • 2 Trials, n = 299 • SMD −1.01, 95% CI, −3.00–0.97 Significant heterogeneity There were fewer reports of severe pain in women who received TENS to acupuncture points vs women who did not have any TENS administration. • 2 Trials, n = 190 • RR 0.41; 95% CI, 0.32–0.55	There is limited evidence that TENS reduces pain in labor. TENS does not seem to have any impact (either positive or negative) on other outcomes.

Abbreviation: SMD, standard mean difference.
[a] These are the conclusions of the authors of the Cochrane systematic review.
From Dowswell T, Bedwell C, Lavender T, et al. Transcutaneous electrical nerve stimulation (TENS) for pain relief in labor. Cochrane Database Syst Rev 2009;2:CD007214; with permission.

Table 6
Cochrane Database of Systematic Reviews: water immersion during the first stage of labor

Results	Notes and Conclusions[a]
Water immersion during the first stage of labor reduced the use of epidural/spinal/paracervical analgesia compared with controls • 6 Trials, n = 2499 • RR 0.82; 95% CI, 0.70–0.98 There was no significant difference in assisted vaginal deliveries • 7 Trials, n = 2628 • RR 0.84; 95% CI, 0.66–1.06 There was no significant difference in cesarean section rates • 8 Trials, n = 2709 • RR 1.23; 95% CI, 0.86–1.75 There was no significant difference in maternal infection • 5 Trials, n = 1295 • RR 0.99; 95% CI, 0.50–1.96 There was no significant difference for APGAR score less than 7 at 5 min. • 5 Trials, n = 1834 • RR 1.59; 95% CI, 0.63–4.01 There was no significant difference in neonatal unit admissions. • 3 Trials, n = 1571 • RR 1.06; 95% CI, 0.70–1.62 There was no significant difference in neonatal infection. • 5 Trial, n = 1295 • RR 2.01; 95% CI, 0.50–8.07	Evidence suggests that water immersion during the first stage of labor reduces the use of epidural or spinal analgesia. There is limited information for other outcomes related to water use during the first and second stages of labor due to intervention and outcome variability. There is no evidence of increased adverse effects to the fetus/neonate or to the woman from laboring in water or from water birth.

[a] These are the conclusions of the authors of the Cochrane systematic review.
From Cluett ER, Burns E. Immersion in water in labor and birth. Cochrane Database Syst Rev 2009;2:CD000111; with permission.

As summarized in **Table 2**, acupuncture techniques may be associated with less intense pain, increased satisfaction, decreased use of pharmacologic analgesia, and fewer instrumented deliveries.[7] The differences, however, are modest. A study that randomized 36 women to an electroacupuncture group or a control group found that women in the acupuncture group reported lower pain intensity ($P = .018$) and greater relaxation ($P = .031$) and had greater concentrations of β-endorphin ($P = .037$) and 5-hydroxytryptamine ($P = .030$) in their peripheral blood samples.[8] The availability of such objective physiologic data is rarely seen with other nonpharmacologic techniques of pain management. Furthermore, hormonal differences, such as these, provide a potential mechanistic explanation for acupuncture's efficacy. This makes acupuncture a particularly intriguing subject for future research.

HYPNOSIS

Hypnosis has been described as a state of focused concentration in which a person is relatively unaware of, but not completely blind to, her surroundings. It is generally well accepted by the medical community as a form of pain control. Positron emission

Table 7
Cochrane Database of Systematic Reviews: continuous support for women during childbirth

Results	Notes and Conclusions[a]
Women with continuous labor support were more likely to have a spontaneous vaginal birth. • 19 Trials, n = 14,119 • RR 1.08; 95% CI, 1.04–1.12	Continuous support during labor has clinically meaningful benefits for both women and infants and no known harm. All women should have support throughout labor and birth.
Women with continuous labor support were less likely to use any intrapartum analgesia. • 14 Trials, n = 12,283 • RR 0.90; 95% CI, 0.84–0.96	Subgroup analyses suggest that continuous support was most effective when the support provider was neither part of the hospital staff nor the woman's known social network, and in settings in which epidural analgesia was not routinely available.
Women with continuous labor support were less likely to use regional analgesia. • 9 Trials, n = 11,444 • RR 0.90; 95% CI, 0.88–0.99	
Women with continuous labor support were less likely to report negative feelings about the childbirth experience. • 11 Trials, n = 11,133 • RR 0.69; 95% CI, 0.59–0.79	
Women with continuous labor support were less likely to have a cesarean delivery. • 22 Trials, n = 15,175 • RR 0.78; 95% CI, 0.67–0.91	
Women with continuous labor support were less likely to have an instrumented vaginal delivery. • 19 Trials, n =14,118 • RR 0.90; 95% CI, 0.85–0.96	
Women with continuous labor support were more likely to have a shorter labor. • 12 Trials, n = 5366 • SMD −0.58 hours, 95% CI, −0.85 to −0.31	
Women with continuous labor support were less likely to have a baby with a low 5-min APGAR score. • 13 Trials, n = 12,515 • RR 0.69; 95% CI, 0.50–0.95	

Abbreviation: SMD, standard mean difference.

[a] These are the conclusions of the authors of the Cochrane systematic review.

From Hodnett ED, Gates S, Hofmeyr GJ, et al. Continuous support for women during childbirth. Cochrane Database Syst Rev 2012;10:CD003766; with permission.

tomography has shown that hypnosis modulates pain by suppressing activity within the anterior cingulate gyrus.[9] Studies evaluating the analgesic efficacy of hypnosis during childbirth (also called hypnobirthing) are confounded by differences in the hypnotic techniques used, differences in the intensity of the intervention and lack of randomization, and, therefore, selection bias.

Some hypnosis studies involve the use of audio recordings before and during childbirth. In other studies, women undergo varying types and intensities of hypnosis preparation before childbirth and then proceed with self-hypnosis during labor. Other studies involve working with a practitioner throughout pregnancy and then undergoing

Table 8
Cochrane Database of Systematic Reviews: relaxation techniques for pain management in labor

Results	Notes and Conclusions[a]
Relaxation techniques were associated with a reduction in pain intensity during the latent phase of labor. • 1 Trial, n = 40 • SMD −1.25, 95% CI, −1.97 to −0.53 Relaxation techniques were associated with a reduction in pain intensity during the active phase of labor. • 2 Trials, n = 74 • SMD −2.48, hours, 95% CI, −3.13 to −0.83 Relaxation techniques were associated with increased satisfaction with pain relief. • 1 Trial, n = 40 • RR 8.00; 95% CI, 1.10–58.19 Relaxation techniques were associated with a lower likelihood of assisted vaginal delivery • 2 Trials, n = 86 • RR 0.07; 95% CI, 0.01–0.50 Yoga was associated with reduced pain. • 1 Trial, n = 66 • SMD −6.12, 95% CI, −11.77 to −0.47 Yoga was associated with increased satisfaction with pain relief. • 1 Trial, n = 66 • SMD 7.88, 95% CI, 1.51–14.25 Yoga was associated with increased satisfaction with the childbirth experience. • 1 Trial, n = 66 • SMD 6.34, 95% CI, 0.26–12.42 Yoga was associated with a reduced length of labor when compared with usual care. • 1 Trial, n = 66 • SMD −139.91, 95% CI, −252.50 to −27.32 Yoga was associated with a reduced length of labor when compared with supine position. • 1 Trial, n = 83 • SMD −191.34, 95% CI, −243.72 to −138.93	Relaxation and yoga may have a role in reducing pain, increasing satisfaction with pain relief, and reducing the rate of assisted vaginal delivery. There is need for future research.

Abbreviation: SMD, standard mean difference.
[a] These are the conclusions of the authors of the Cochrane systematic review.
From Smith CA, Levett KM, Collins CT, et al. Relaxation techniques for pain management in labor. Cochrane Database Syst Rev 2011;12:CD009514; with permission.

hypnosis guided by that particular practitioner during labor. Dr Allan Cyna and colleagues[10] who have done much of the research on the efficacy of hypnosis for labor analgesia, measured hypnotizability using the creative imagination scale in the third trimester and between 14 and 28 months postpartum. This group found that women may be more hypnotizable when pregnant compared with when not pregnant (n = 37, pregnant creative imagination scale mean 18.7, SD 6.9; nonpregnant creative imagination scale mean 18.7, SD 6.6; $P<.001$).

Table 9
Cochrane Database of Systematic Reviews: massage for pain management in labor

Results	Notes and Conclusions[a]
Massage was associated with less pain during first stage of labor compared with usual care. • 4 Trials, n = 225 • SMD −0.82, 95% CI, −1.17 to −0.47 Massage was associated with decreased anxiety during first stage of labor compared with usual care. • 1 Trial, n = 60 • SMD −16.27, 95% CI, −27.03 to −5.51 Massage was associated with decreased pain compared with music alone. • 1 Trial, n = 101 • RR 0.40; 95% CI, 0.18–0.89	Massage may have a role in reducing pain and improving women's emotional experience of labor. There is need for further research. No trial was assessed as being low risk for bias.

Abbreviation: SMD; standard mean difference.

[a] These are the conclusions of the authors of the Cochrane systematic review.

From Smith CA, Levett KM, Collins CT, et al. Massage, reflexology and other manual methods for pain management in labor. Cochrane Database Syst Rev 2012;2:CD009290; with permission.

Table 10
Cochrane Database of Systematic Reviews: biofeedback for pain management in labor

Results	Notes and Conclusions[a]
There was no significant difference in assisted vaginal birth between biofeedback and control groups. • 2 Trials, n = 103 • RR 0.75; 95% CI, 0.18–3.10 There was no significant difference in cesarean section between biofeedback and control groups. • 2 Trials, n = 103 • RR 0.41; 95% CI, 0.14–1.15 There was no significant difference in need for augmentation of labor between biofeedback and control groups. • Between biofeedback and control groups 1 trial, n = 55 • RR 1.19; 95% CI, 0.68–2.08 There was no significant difference in the use of pharmacologic pain relief between biofeedback and control groups. • 2 Trials, n = 103 • RR 0.69; 95% CI, 0.23–2.07	Despite some positive results, there is insufficient evidence that biofeedback is effective for the management of pain during labor. All trials were at high risk of bias. Trials in this review greatly differed in diversity of intervention modalities and outcomes measured.

[a] These are the conclusions of the authors of the Cochrane systematic review.

From Barragan Loayza IM, Sola I, Juando Prats C. Biofeedback for pain management during labor. Cochrane Database Syst Rev 2011;6:CD006168; with permission.

Table 11
Cochrane Database of Systematic Reviews: aromatherapy for pain management in labor

Results	Notes and Conclusions[a]
Aromatherapy did not affect the use of pharmacologic pain relief. • 1 Trial, n = 513 • RR 0.35; 95% CI, 0.04–3.32 and • 1 Trial, 22 women • RR 2.50; 95% CI, 0.31–20.45 Aromatherapy did not affect the rate of assisted vaginal birth. • 1 Trial, n = 513 • RR 1.04; 95% CI, 0.48–2.28 and • 1 Trial, 22 women • RR 0.83; 95% CI, 0.06–11.70 Aromatherapy did not affect the rate of cesarean section. • 1 Trial, n = 513 • RR 0.98; 95% CI, 0.49–1.94 and • 1 Trial, 22 women • RR 2.54; 95% CI, 0.11–56.25 Aromatherapy did not affect the rate of spontaneous vaginal delivery. • 1 Trial, n = 513 • RR 1.00; 95% CI, 0.94–1.06 and • 1 Trial, 22 women • RR 0.93; 95% CI, 0.67–1.28 Aromatherapy did not affect the need for labor augmentation. • 1 Trial, n = 513 • RR 1.14; 95% CI, 0.90–1.45	Pain intensity data could not be included in the analysis because only the intervention (and not the control) group was asked to rate their pain after the intervention. Nulliparous (and not multiparous) women rated decreased pain intensity after the aromatherapy intervention. There is a lack of studies evaluating the role of aromatherapy for pain management in labor. Further research is needed. The risk of bias was low in these trials.

[a] These are the conclusions of the authors of the Cochrane systematic review.
From Smith CA, Collins CT, Crowther CA. Aromatherapy for pain management in labor. Cochrane Database Syst Rev 2011;7:CD009215; with permission.

Although initial small studies evaluating hypnosis during childbirth seemed promising,[11–13] the recent Cochrane systematic review, including 6 studies with a nonhypnosis control group, has suggested less favorable effects.[14] As summarized in **Table 3**, there were no significant differences between the hypnosis and control groups in the use of pharmacologic pain relief or a woman's satisfaction with either her pain relief or the childbirth experience overall. All of these studies were deemed, however, at moderate-to-high risk for bias, with a large variation among the trials in the hypnosis timing and technique.

Volunteer bias may be especially pertinent to RCTs evaluating hypnosis because certain types of women may agree to enter a study that involves this intervention. They typically are neither strong advocates nor strong opponents for the technique because such women do not want to risk being randomized in or out of the hypnosis group, respectively. Hypnosis requires a great deal of effort and the willingness of the subject to undergo the intervention is directly related to their ability to achieve a hypnotic state.[15] In comparing studies that use random assignment against those in which women voluntarily select hypnosis, a recent comprehensive review found that the studies that allowed self-selection were more supportive of hypnosis than those that used random assignment (7 of 8 self-selection studies were supportive of hypnosis vs only 3 of 5 random assignment studies).[16]

As a result, an RCT may not be the most appropriate way to study the efficacy of hypnosis in labor. In a recent comprehensive review,[16] 13 randomized and nonrandomized studies were included. The nonrandomized studies used methodology, such as between-subject or mixed-model designs, in which hypnosis was compared with an alternative intervention (eg, supportive counseling, Lamaze method, or childbirth education) or to standard medical care. Here, unlike in the recent Cochrane systematic review, hypnosis techniques were "consistently shown to be more effective than standard medical care, supportive counseling, and childbirth education classes in reducing pain."[16]

In summary, for women who choose a hypnobirthing experience, there is likely benefit. Although it may not be an effective option for all women, respect for the technique and support for the women who choose it remain important.

STERILE WATER PAPULES

Sterile water papules, also called intradermal water blocks, involve the intradermal injection of 4 small papules of water just above the sacrum (**Fig. 1**). Although it is not a widespread practice among obstetricians, midwives have used this technique for women who are experiencing back labor, which is significant low back pain associated with an occiput posterior presenting fetus. The mechanism of analgesia is not known, but the gate control theory is thought to be involved.[17] Individual RCTs have demonstrated decreased back pain (as measured by VAS) at various time points after this technique is used.[17–20] These studies, however, did not show a difference in intravenous opioid[17,18,20] or epidural analgesia use.[17,18] A single study, however, found that women who were randomized to sterile water papules or acupuncture (n = 128) preferred sterile water papules (P<.001) and reported greater pain relief (P<.001) and a greater degree of relaxation (P<.001).[21]

A systematic review and meta-analysis also found favorable outcomes with sterile water papules.[22] In this review, the comparison group was either a saline placebo or another nonpharmacologic treatment modality, such as acupuncture or TENS. Outcomes included a "significant reduction in the pain scores of the sterile water papule group in comparison to the placebo or other intervention group at all time-points following administration of the intervention" as well as a decreased cesarean delivery rate of 4.6% in the sterile water group compared with 9.9% in the comparison group (n = 828; risk ratio[RR] 0.51; 95% CI, 0.30–0.87).[22] The investigators call for a large, double-blinded placebo controlled study to validate their surprising findings of such a significant decrease in cesarean delivery.

A recently published Cochrane systematic review attempted to provide a more tightly controlled meta-analysis on the use of sterile water papules.[23] All studies included in this meta-analysis used intradermal isotonic saline injection as the comparison technique. With this, patients and the providers in individual studies are truly blinded. As summarized in **Table 4**, no significant differences in the use of pharmacologic rescue analgesia or the rates of cesarean or assisted vaginal delivery were found between the 2 groups. Because this systematic review included only studies that compared isotonic saline versus water injections, it does not necessarily disprove the analgesic efficacy of the technique. Specifically, perhaps an intradermal injection of isotonic saline is also effective in decreasing low back pain during labor.

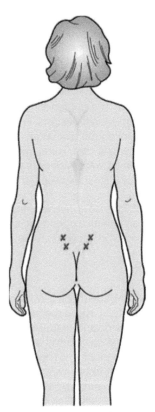

Fig. 1. Location of sterile water papule placement. (*From* Arendt KW, Camann W. Alternative (non-pharmacologic) methods of labor analgesia. In: Suresh MS, Segal BS, Preston RL, et al, editors. Shnider and Levinson's anesthesia for obstetrics. 5th edition. Baltimore (MD): Lippincott Williams & Wilkins; 2013. p. 88; with permission.)

In summary, further investigation is needed to examine the analgesic efficacy of sterile water papules as well as their effect on mode of delivery. Finding answers is difficult, however, because the only way to truly blind the studies involves a similar technique that may also have effect (isotonic saline injection). In the meantime, sterile water papules may provide comfort to some women and have been associated with little harm.

TRANSCUTANEOUS ELECTRICAL NERVE STIMULATION

TENS involves electrodes placed to the low back of laboring women that emit low-voltage electrical impulses. It is thought that this technique may provide analgesia via the gate control theory[24] by increasing endorphin release[25] or providing a parturient with a sense of control or distraction from the pain of labor.[26] Overall, there is little evidence that TENS provides significant labor analgesia.

As summarized in **Table 5**, a Cochrane systematic review reported that there were no significant differences in pain ratings between the TENS and the control group. There were fewer reports of severe pain, however, when TENS electrodes were placed at acupoints. Typically, the TENS electrodes are placed paravertebrally at the levels of T10 to L1 and S2 to S4 bilaterally (**Fig. 2**). In one acupoint study, however, researchers

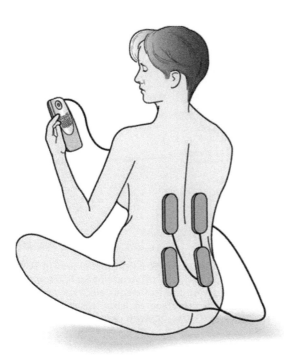

Fig. 2. Location of typical TENS electrode placement for labor analgesia. (*From* Arendt KW, Camann W. Alternative (non-pharmacologic) methods of labor analgesia. In: Suresh MS, Segal BS, Preston RL, et al, editors. Shnider and Levinson's anesthesia for obstetrics. 5th edition. Baltimore (MD): Lippincott Williams & Wilkins; 2013. p. 88; with permission.)

placed much smaller electrodes that used baseline and burst frequency stimulation at acupoints Li 4 (Hegu) and Sp 6 (Sanyinjiao), which are located about the hand and ankle (**Fig. 3**).[27] In this study, the acupoint TENS group experienced a VAS score reduction of greater than or equal to 3 significantly more often than the TENS placebo group (31/50 [62%] vs 7/50 [14%]; $P<.001$). Furthermore, women's willingness to use the same analgesic method for a future childbirth also favored application of TENS to acupoints (TENS 48/50 [96%] vs TENS placebo 33/50 [66%]; $P<.001$). Overall, although the evidence is limited, there may be some analgesic benefit of TENS application to acupoints using specific stimulation techniques.

WATER IMMERSION

Hydrotherapy (or water immersion) for labor pain is theorized to promote relaxation and, therefore, decrease the perception of pain and increase the ability to cope with pain. A typical labor tub is shown in **Fig. 4**. Individual studies have indicated that laboring and birthing in water results in faster labors,[28] fewer requirements for amniotomy or pharmacologic labor augmentation,[29] fewer perineal tears,[28,30] fewer episiotomies,[29] lesser blood loss,[30] decreased incidence of operative delivery,[29] and less requirement for pharmacologic analgesics.[28] Evidence from a Cochrane systematic review supports analgesic benefit of this technique, showing that women randomized to immersion in water during the first stage of labor are significantly less likely to request neuraxial analgesia for pain relief (see **Table 6**). The theory that the technique decreases operative deliveries, however, has not been demonstrated in the literature.

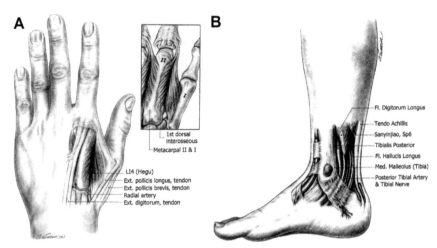

A

1st dorsal interosseous
Metacarpal II & I

LI4 (Hegu)
Ext. pollicis longus, tendon
Ext. pollicis brevis, tendon
Radial artery
Ext. digitorum, tendon

B

Fl. Digitorum Longus
Tendo Achillis
Sanyinjiao, Sp6
Tibialis Posterior
Fl. Hallucis Longus
Med. Malleolus (Tibia)
Posterior Tibial Artery & Tibial Nerve

Fig. 3. Location of acupoints Li 6 (Hegu) and Sp 6 (Sanyinjiao) used in TENS electrode placement for labor analgesia. (*A*) Acupoint Li 6. (*B*) Acupoint Sp 6. (*From* Chaoa A, Chaoa A, Wang T, et al. Pain relief by applying transcutaneous electrical nerve stimulation (TENS) on acupuncture points during the first stage of labor: a randomized double-blind placebo-controlled trial. Pain 2007;127(3):214–20; with permission.)

The Cochrane review demonstrated no significant difference in either the assisted vaginal delivery rate or cesarean section rate for women who underwent hydrotherapy versus those who labored out of the water. Also, it is impossible to blind women and health care providers to this technique.

Pediatricians and obstetricians have expressed concern about water immersion, citing risk for maternal and neonatal infection as well as neonatal water aspiration.[31–35]

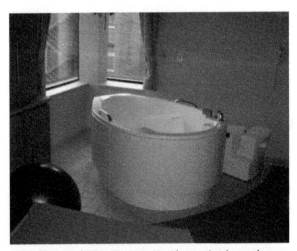

Fig. 4. A labor tub. (*From* Arendt KW, Camann W. Alternative (non-pharmacologic) methods of labor analgesia. In: Suresh MS, Segal BS, Preston RL, et al, editors. Shnider and Levinson's anesthesia for obstetrics. 5th edition. Baltimore (MD): Lippincott Williams & Wilkins; 2013. p. 88; with permission.)

As summarized in **Table 6**, the Cochrane systematic review does not support this increase in risk for women who undergo hydrotherapy during the first stage of labor. Maternal and neonatal infection rates, neonatal APGAR scores, and neonatal unit admission rates are not significantly different between women who labor in water versus those who labor out of water. These data are for women who labored in water, not for women who delivered in water.

The best data on the risk of birthing into water involves a surveillance study of pediatricians in the British Isles and a postal survey of all National Health Service maternity units in England and Wales. The study looked at 4032 deliveries in water (0.6% of all deliveries) between April 1994 and March 1996.[36] Of these 4032 deliveries, no neonatal deaths occurred that could be attributed to delivering in water; however, there were 2 admissions to the neonatal ICU for water aspiration. When they compared the regional data for low-risk normal vaginal deliveries at term, the RR for perinatal mortality associated with delivery in water was 0.9 (99% CI, 0.2–3.6), and the investigators concluded that perinatal mortality is "not substantially higher among babies delivered in water than among those born to low-risk women who delivered conventionally."[36]

CONTINUOUS LABOR SUPPORT

Women who have continuous one-on-one support during labor are more likely to have a shorter labor and spontaneous vaginal birth and are less likely to have intrapartum analgesia, regional analgesia, an instrumented or cesarean delivery, or a baby with low 5-minute APGAR scores.[37] They are also less likely to report negative feelings about the childbirth experience.[37] As summarized in **Table 7**, these data are from RCTs and are relatively robust. One theory explaining these improved outcomes involves the fact that continuous one-on-one support decreases anxiety. Endogenous catecholamine release associated with anxiety may lessen uterine contractions and decrease placental blood flow.[38,39] Supported women, and, therefore, less anxious women and may have improved strength of contractions and enhanced placental blood flow. Furthermore, because anxiety and labor pain are closely related,[40] it is not surprising that supported women have lesser pharmacologic analgesic needs. A single study compared the efficacy of untrained laywomen, trained laywomen (doulas), female relatives, and nurses as labor support providers.[41] One group of support providers was not consistently more effective at supporting parturients than another.

Labor nurses often do not have the luxury of continuously supporting a single woman throughout her entire labor. It is also not uncommon for a partner, friend, or family member to be unable to appropriately support a parturient throughout labor. As a result, some women may hire a doula, who is professionally trained and experienced in labor support. Doulas have been shown to improve outcomes in select circumstances[42] while showing no benefit in others.[43] When more closely evaluating the studies involving one-on-one support, it seems as if cultural and regional differences may influence the efficacy. Two studies[44,45] involving women in a busy Guatemalan hospital and 2 studies[42,46] involving low-income women in American hospitals have indicated improved outcomes. In contrast, a single study of privately insured women in which hospital-based doulas were randomly provided failed to provide benefit.[43] It could be postulated that this may be because the control group already had adequate support, unlike the women of lesser socioeconomic status in Guatemalan or American hospitals. In summary, continuous one-on-one labor support is important for both patient satisfaction and improved labor outcomes, the benefit of which may be greatest in underserved populations.

RELAXATION TECHNIQUES

There are few data on the analgesic benefits of relaxation techniques in labor. Although 11 studies (n = 1374) were included in a Cochrane systematic review, only a few trials met criteria for inclusion.[47] Relaxation techniques included in this review were guided imagery, progressive muscle relaxation, breathing techniques, and meditation. As summarized in **Table 8**, these studies indicated that such techniques may provide a reduction in pain intensity during the latent and active phases of labor, increased satisfaction with pain relief, and decreased likelihood of assisted vaginal delivery.

Yoga is a physical, mental, and spiritual discipline that involves stretching and movement, focused breathing, and mental centering. The Cochrane review found that the use of yoga during labor may reduce pain and increase satisfaction with pain relief and the childbirth experience. It may also reduce the length of labor compared with usual care or the supine position. Improved outcomes with relaxation techniques are speculated to involve a reduction in maternal anxiety that may reduce endogenous catecholamine release (which hinders labor progress and placental blood flow). The prenatal and intrapartum physical movement and stretching involved in yoga may also provide benefit. The literature supporting these techniques, however, is scant and further quality studies need to be performed.

MASSAGE

Currently, there are few data on the analgesic benefit of massage techniques during labor. As summarized in **Table 9**, however, the few data available seem to support the theory that massage may reduce pain and anxiety compared with usual care, including reducing pain, in comparison with music alone.[48] Like continuous labor support, relaxation techniques, and yoga, the outcomes are likely related to decreased anxiety within the parturient.

BIOFEEDBACK AND AROMATHERAPY

Neither biofeedback nor aromatherapy has been shown to improve outcomes in labor when held to the standards of Cochrane systematic reviews (see **Tables 10** and **11**).[49] Through electromagnetic biofeedback, women are informed of their heart rate, body temperature, and muscle tension through an electronic instrument. Through this, anxiety can be recognized and, in response, women can attempt to relax through various techniques, such as focused breathing practices. Aromatherapy uses oils from plants that are massaged into the skin, put into a bath for immersion, or inhaled as a steam or a smoke by using a steam infuser or burning the oil. Such oils may include clary sage, ginger, lemongrass, frankincense, peppermint, lavender, or mandarin. Although little benefit has been found with these interventions, there is likely little harm associated with them, with the exception of a possible allergic reaction.[50]

SUMMARY

Although data are limited, acupuncture, acupressure, TENS electrodes applied to acupuncture points, relaxation techniques, yoga, and massage therapy may provide modest analgesic benefit to women in labor. Water immersion may decrease women's requests for regional anesthesia during the first stage of labor. Randomized trials do not show benefit for hypnosis, although studies in which women self-select suggest some benefit from the technique. Sterile water papules do not show benefit compared with saline water papules but do show benefit when the comparison group includes other nonpharmacologic treatment modalities (such as acupuncture or TENS). Continuous personal support for women in labor has robust evidence to support its efficacy of improved obstetric, neonatal, analgesic, and satisfaction outcomes.

In summary, it is important for health care providers to be cognizant that regardless of proved scientific efficacy, most nonpharmacologic modalities of labor analgesia are associated with little harm. Therefore, for those women who choose to use them, these modalities may assist in coping with the significant stress and pain of labor. Familiarity and respect for such choices allows health care providers to provide respectful and satisfying care for their patients.

REFERENCES

1. Kannan S, Jamison RN, Datta S. Maternal satisfaction and pain control in women electing natural childbirth. Reg Anesth Pain Med 2001;26:468.
2. Anim-Somuah M, Smyth RM, Jones L. Epidural versus non-epidural or no analgesia in labour. Cochrane Database Syst Rev 2011;(12):CD000331.
3. Cardini F, Weixin H. Moxibustion for correction of breech presentation: a randomized controlled trial. JAMA 1998;280:1580.
4. Cardini F, Lombardo P, Regalia AL, et al. A randomised controlled trial of moxibustion for breech presentation. Br J Obstet Gynaecol 2005;112:743-7.
5. Jones L, Othman M, Dowswell T, et al. Pain management for women in labour: an overview of systematic reviews. Cochrane Database Syst Rev 2012;(3): CD009234.
6. Ma W, Bai W, Lin C, et al. Effects of Sanyinjiao (SP6) with electroacupuncture on labour pain in women during labour. Complement Ther Med 2011;19(Suppl 1): S13-8.
7. Smith CA, Collins CT, Crowther CA, et al. Acupuncture or acupressure for pain management in labour. Cochrane Database Syst Rev 2011;(7):CD009232.
8. Qu F, Zhou J. Electro-acupuncture in relieving labor pain. Evid Based Complement Alternat Med 2007;4:125.
9. Rainville P, Duncan GH, Price DD, et al. Pain affect encoded in human anterior cingulate but not somatosensory cortex. Science 1997;277:968.
10. Alexander B, Turnbull D, Cyna A. The effect of pregnancy on hypnotizability. Am J Clin Hypn 2009;52:13-22.
11. Cyna AM, McAuliffe GL, Andrew MI. Hypnosis for pain relief in labour and childbirth: a systematic review. Br J Anaesth 2004;93:505.
12. Cyna AM, Andrew MI, McAuliffe GL. Antenatal hypnosis for labour analgesia. Int J Obstet Anesth 2005;14:365.
13. Cyna AM, Andrew MI, McAuliffe GL. Antenatal self-hypnosis for labour and childbirth: a pilot study. Anaesth Intensive Care 2006;34:464-9.
14. Madden K, Middleton P, Cyna AM, et al. Hypnosis for pain management during labour and childbirth. Cochrane Database Syst Rev 2012;(11):CD009356.
15. Spanos NP, Brett PJ, Menary EP, et al. A measure of attitudes toward hypnosis: relationships with absorption and hypnotic susceptibility. Am J Clin Hypn 1987; 30:139-50.
16. Landolt AS, Milling LS. The efficacy of hypnosis as an intervention for labor and delivery pain: a comprehensive methodological review. Clin Psychol Rev 2011; 31:1022-31.
17. Ader L, Hansson B, Wallin G. Parturition pain treated by intracutaneous injections of sterile water. Pain 1990;41:133-8.

18. Labrecque M, Nouwen A, Bergeron M, et al. A randomized controlled trial of nonpharmacologic approaches for relief of low back pain during labor. J Fam Pract 1999;48:259.

19. Måtensson L, Wallin G. Labour pain treated with cutaneous injections of sterile water: a randomised controlled trial. Br J Obstet Gynaecol 1999;106:633–7.

20. Trolle B, Møller M, Kronborg H, et al. The effect of sterile water blocks on low back labor pain. Am J Obstet Gynecol 1991;164:1277.

21. Mårtensson L, Stener-Victorin E, Wallin G. Acupuncture versus subcutaneous injections of sterile water as treatment for labour pain. Acta Obstet Gynecol Scand 2008;87:171–7.

22. Hutton EK, Kasperink M, Rutten M, et al. Sterile water injection for labour pain: a systematic review and meta-analysis of randomised controlled trials. Br J Obstet Gynaecol 2009;116:1158–66.

23. Derry S, Straube S, Moore RA, et al. Intracutaneous or subcutaneous sterile water injection compared with blinded controls for pain management in labour. Cochrane Database Syst Rev 2012;(1):CD009107.

24. Garrison DW, Foreman RD. Decreased activity of spontaneous and noxiously evoked dorsal horn cells during transcutaneous electrical nerve stimulation (TENS). Pain 1994;58:309–15.

25. Lechner W, Jarosch E, Sölder E, et al. Beta-endorphins during childbirth under transcutaneous electric nerve stimulation. Zentralbl Gynakol 1991;113:439.

26. Simkin P, Bolding A. Update on nonpharmacologic approaches to relieve labor pain and prevent suffering. J Midwifery Womens Health 2004;49:489–504.

27. Chao AS, Chao A, Wang TH, et al. Pain relief by applying transcutaneous electrical nerve stimulation (TENS) on acupuncture points during the first stage of labor: a randomized double-blind placebo-controlled trial. Pain 2007;127:214–20.

28. Odent M. Birth under water. Lancet 1983;322:1476–7.

29. Cluett ER, Pickering RM, Getliffe K, et al. Randomised controlled trial of labouring in water compared with standard of augmentation for management of dystocia in first stage of labour. BMJ 2004;328:314.

30. Geissbühler V, Eberhard J. Waterbirths: a comparative study. A prospective study on more than 2,000 waterbirths. Fetal Diagn Ther 2000;15:291.

31. Rawal J, Shah A, Stirk F, et al. Water birth and infection in babies. BMJ 1994;309:511.

32. Franzin L, Scolfaro C, Cabodi D, et al. Legionella pneumophila pneumonia in a newborn after water birth: a new mode of transmission. Clin Infect Dis 2001;33:e103–4.

33. Nguyen S, Kuschel C, Teele R, et al. Water birth—a near-drowning experience. Pediatrics 2002;110:411.

34. Gilbert R. Water birth—a near-drowning experience. Pediatrics 2002;110:409.

35. Nagai T, Sobajima H, Iwasa M, et al. Neonatal sudden death due to Legionella pneumonia associated with water birth in a domestic spa bath. J Clin Microbiol 2003;41:2227–9.

36. Gilbert RE, Tookey PA. Perinatal mortality and morbidity among babies delivered in water: surveillance study and postal survey. BMJ 1999;319:483.

37. Hodnett ED, Gates S, Hofmeyr GJ, et al. Continuous support for women during childbirth. Cochrane Database Syst Rev 2012;(10):CD003766.

38. Lederman RP, Lederman E, Work BA Jr, et al. The relationship of maternal anxiety, plasma catecholamines, and plasma cortisol to progress in labor. Am J Obstet Gynecol 1978;132:495–500.

39. Lederman RP, Lederman E, Work B Jr, et al. Anxiety and epinephrine in multiparous women in labor: relationship to duration of labor and fetal heart rate pattern. Am J Obstet Gynecol 1985;153:870–7.
40. Curzik D, Jokic-Begic N. Anxiety sensitivity and anxiety as correlates of expected, experienced and recalled labor pain. J Psychosom Obstet Gynaecol 2011;32:198–203.
41. Rosen P. Supporting women in labor: analysis of different types of caregivers. J Midwifery Womens Health 2004;49:24–31.
42. Campbell DA, Lake MF, Falk M, et al. A randomized control trial of continuous support in labor by a lay doula. J Obstet Gynecol Neonatal Nurs 2006;35: 456–64.
43. Gordon NP, Walton D, McAdam E, et al. Effects of providing hospital-based doulas in health maintenance organization hospitals. Obstet Gynecol 1999;93: 422–6.
44. Sosa R, Kennell J, Klaus M, et al. The effect of a supportive companion on perinatal problems, length of labor, and mother-infant interaction. N Engl J Med 1980;303:597–600.
45. Klaus MH, Kennell JH, Robertson SS, et al. Effects of social support during parturition on maternal and infant morbidity. BMJ 1986;293:585.
46. Kennell J, Klaus M, McGrath S, et al. Continuous emotional support during labor in a US hospital. A randomized controlled trial. JAMA 1991;265:2197–201.
47. Smith CA, Levett KM, Collins CT, et al. Relaxation techniques for pain management in labour. Cochrane Database Syst Rev 2011;(12):CD009514.
48. Smith CA, Levett KM, Collins CT, et al. Massage, reflexology and other manual methods for pain management in labour. Cochrane Database Syst Rev 2012;(2):CD009290.
49. Barragan Loayza IM, Sola I, Juando Prats C. Biofeedback for pain management during labour. Cochrane Database Syst Rev 2011;(6):CD006168.
50. Burns EE, Blamey C, Ersser SJ, et al. An investigation into the use of aromatherapy in intrapartum midwifery practice. J Altern Complement Med 2000;6: 141–7.

Combined Spinal-Epidural Versus Epidural Analgesia for Labor and Delivery

Adam D. Niesen, MD, Adam K. Jacob, MD*

KEYWORDS

- Epidural • Combined spinal-epidural • Labor analgesia

KEY POINTS

- Combined spinal-epidural (CSE) analgesia produces more rapid onset of effective analgesia compared with epidural alone, with an average onset difference of approximately 5 minutes.
- There is no difference between epidural and CSE techniques on the progress of labor or risk for instrumented or cesarean delivery.
- Catheters placed with a standard epidural technique have a greater failure rate for labor analgesia, but similar intervention rate for rescue analgesia and similar failure rate for conversion to anesthesia for cesarean delivery.
- CSE results in a greater incidence of dose-related maternal pruritus, maternal hypotension, and fetal bradycardia.
- There is no difference between epidural and CSE techniques in the rates of postdural puncture headache and neuraxial infection.

INTRODUCTION

Labor is considered to be one of the most painful experiences a woman can endure. Furthermore, the anticipation of pain felt during labor and delivery may be a cause of significant anxiety and stress for many women. A variety of factors such as personal expectations, cultural differences, and the relationship with a health care provider may affect a woman's choice of analgesia during labor. Although some women choose to deliver using nonpharmacologic methods, most laboring mothers in the Unites States will request a neuraxial analgesic technique at some point during labor and delivery.[1]

Neuraxial techniques have been shown to provide labor analgesia superior to that achieved with nonpharmacologic methods.[2] However, the rationale for choosing the

Department of Anesthesiology, Mayo Clinic, 200 First Street Southwest, Rochester, MN 55905, USA
* Corresponding author.
E-mail address: jacob.adam@mayo.edu

Clin Perinatol 40 (2013) 373–384
http://dx.doi.org/10.1016/j.clp.2013.05.010
0095-5108/13/$ – see front matter © 2013 Elsevier Inc. All rights reserved.

best neuraxial technique (epidural vs combined spinal-epidural [CSE]) for the initiation of labor analgesia varies widely among anesthesia providers and is usually tailored to the provider, the patient, and the clinical scenario. Dating back to the 1950s, epidural analgesia is considered the gold-standard technique for labor. CSE, also known as a walking epidural, was first described in the early 1990s as an alternative neuraxial technique for labor and cesarean delivery,[3,4] and rapidly became popular for several reasons:

- More rapid onset of analgesia using intrathecal injection techniques
- Potential for decreased motor block
- Presence of an indwelling epidural catheter that could be used once spinal analgesia subsided or for cesarean delivery

The rapid onset of analgesia and improved mobility with CSE techniques has been associated with a higher degree of maternal satisfaction compared with conventional epidural analgesia.[5] However, controversy exists that initiation of labor analgesia with a CSE may be associated with an increased risk for nonreassuring fetal status (ie, fetal bradycardia), and a subsequent need for emergent cesarean delivery.[2] Regardless of the choice of analgesic technique, the perinatal team's primary concern is always the welfare of the mother and fetus.

When evaluating literature comparing traditional epidural techniques with CSE, it is important to be cognizant of the doses and concentrations of medications being used and defined as "traditional" or "conventional" regimens of care. For example, a large body of literature defines traditional epidural analgesia as using bupivacaine 0.25% versus "low-dose" techniques using bupivacaine 0.125% or lower concentrations, with the inclusion of low-dose opioid (eg, fentanyl 2 µg/mL). Because of the significant differences consistently demonstrated in maternal outcomes (eg, mobility, maternal satisfaction, rate of instrumented delivery) with the use of low-dose versus traditional epidural techniques,[6,7] many would argue that a paradigm shift has occurred in modern practice whereby the previous definition of low-dose analgesia has become the new traditional dose used in most labor and delivery units.

INDICATIONS AND CONTRAINDICATIONS

The single greatest indication for neuraxial labor analgesia is maternal request. In the absence of maternal request, establishing early effective neuraxial analgesia may be warranted in some high-risk patients to potentially reduce the need for emergent general anesthesia when such anesthesia might be especially hazardous. Neuraxial analgesia may also be indicated, or strongly recommended, for patients with risk factors that increase the likelihood of either an operative (ie, cesarean) or instrumented vaginal delivery (**Box 1**).

The contraindications to neuraxial labor analgesia are similar to those for any regional anesthetic technique (**Box 2**).

TECHNIQUE AND PROCEDURE

The patient is positioned in the sitting or lateral decubitus position. After sterile skin preparation and draping, a large-bore (17- or 18-gauge) epidural needle is slowly advanced through the skin, subcutaneous tissue, and supraspinous and interspinous ligaments until a loss of resistance is felt in the plunger of a near-frictionless syringe as the needle tip passes through the ligamentum flavum. During conventional epidural placement, a 19- or 20-gauge catheter is advanced through the needle 3 to 5 cm into the epidural space (**Fig. 1**, upper panels). By contrast, during a CSE, a small-bore

---

Box 1
Maternal risk factors for which to consider neuraxial labor analgesia

- Morbid obesity
- Severe preeclampsia
- Fetal macrosomia
- Multiple gestation
- Nonreassuring airway examination
- High risk for operative delivery
- Prior history of anesthesia complications (eg, malignant hyperthermia)

(27-gauge) pencil-point spinal needle is advanced through the epidural needle, puncturing the dura and allowing for the injection of opiate and/or local anesthetic into the intrathecal space before insertion of the epidural catheter (see **Fig. 1**, lower panels).

EFFECT ON COURSE OF LABOR

Epidural analgesia using a local anesthetic concentration of 0.25% bupivacaine or greater has been associated with prolonged second stage of labor, increased use of oxytocin augmentation, and an increased risk for instrumented vaginal delivery.[8] Early evidence suggested that the use of CSE techniques may result in faster rates of cervical dilation and a reduction in the number of instrumented vaginal deliveries.[9,10] A recent Cochrane review was conducted on 27 trials of 3274 women comparing CSE with traditional epidural analgesia as well as low-dose epidural techniques for labor.[11] Traditional was defined for trials in which the epidural local

---

Box 2
Contraindications to neuraxial anesthesia and analgesia

Absolute Contraindications to Neuraxial Anesthesia
- Patient refusal
- Infection at the site of injection
- Coagulopathy (acquired, induced, genetic)
- Uncorrected hypovolemia
- Increased intracranial pressure
- Severe cardiac valvular stenosis
- Allergy to local anesthetic
- Inadequate resuscitative drugs or equipment immediately available

Relative Contraindications to Neuraxial Anesthesia
- Uncooperative patient
- Preexisting neurologic deficits
- Infection distant to the site of injection
- Spinal deformity or previous spinal surgery
- Thrombocytopenia

A Epidural Analgesia

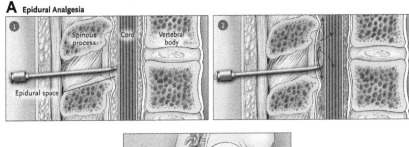

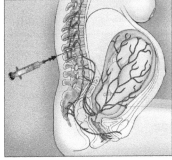

B Combined Spinal–Epidural Analgesia

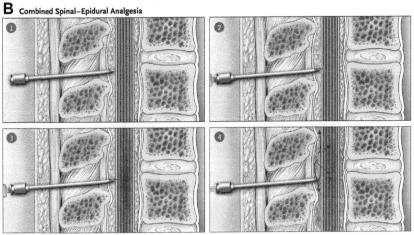

Fig. 1. Technique of epidural analgesia and combined spinal-epidural analgesia. (*From* Eltzschig HK, Lieberman ES, Camann WR. Medical progress: regional anesthesia and analgesic for labor and delivery. N Engl J Med 2003;348:319–32; with permission.)

anesthetic concentration was the equivalent of bupivacaine 0.25% or more; lower concentrations were defined as low-dose. Initiation of analgesia with CSE (opioid only or opioid plus local anesthesia) resulted in a lower incidence of instrumented vaginal delivery compared with traditional epidural analgesia (risk ratio [RR] 0.81, 95% confidence interval [CI] 0.67–0.97). There was no difference detected in the need for labor augmentation or rate of cesarean delivery. However, when CSE was compared with low-dose epidural, there was no significant difference in mode of delivery (instrumented or cesarean) or the need for labor augmentation between the analgesic techniques.

Several studies have investigated the impact of neuraxial analgesia on the rate of cervical change and duration of stage I and stage II labor. Recent evidence would suggest that the type of neuraxial technique does not appear to significantly affect the duration of labor.[6,12–15] In summary, the course of labor does not appear to be significantly affected by the type of neuraxial analgesia, especially if lower-dose (ie, modern-day) epidural infusions are used.

EFFECT ON ANALGESIA AND MATERNAL SATISFACTION

The goal of any analgesic technique is to relieve the discomfort associated with labor. One of the greatest benefits of initiating labor analgesia with a CSE technique in comparison with conventional epidural placement is the onset of analgesia. Numerous studies have reported shorter analgesic onset times with CSE compared with standard epidural techniques.[7,14,16] When CSE was compared with traditional epidural techniques in a pooled meta-analysis of 4 trials, the time from first injection to effective analgesia was less with CSE (mean difference −2.87 minutes, 95% CI −5.07 to −0.67 minutes).[11] When CSE was compared with low-dose epidural in the same meta-analysis (5 trials, 461 women), the average time to onset of effective analgesia with CSE was significantly less than with epidural (mean difference −5.42 minutes, 95% CI −7.26 to −3.59 minutes). When questioned specifically about satisfaction regarding the speed of analgesia onset, women were more satisfied with CSE than with low-dose epidural.[5] Similarly, women felt a greater sense of mobility and were more satisfied with improved mobility with CSE techniques than with low-dose or traditional epidural analgesia.[5] Despite a shorter time to onset of effective analgesia and greater initial mobility, there does not appear to be a significant difference in overall satisfaction between CSE and low-dose epidural techniques.[11] Furthermore, although an average difference of approximately 5 minutes may represent a statistical difference between CSE and low-dose epidural techniques, the clinical significance of this difference in onset time may be irrelevant for most parturients.

EFFECT ON NUMBER OF ANESTHESIA INTERVENTIONS AND RESCUE ANALGESIA

One of the advantages of a continuous regional technique is that additional medications may be given or the infusion rate changed if pain persists despite the initial settings. Depending on the anesthesia staffing model or the workload on the labor and delivery unit, it may be difficult to return to a patient's bedside to make adjustments to the infusion rate or administer rescue analgesia for inadequate labor analgesia. Therefore, a technique that requires a minimal number of interventions by anesthesia personnel may be advantageous for laboring mothers and anesthesia providers alike.

In an efficacy study of 42 patients comparing CSE with conventional epidural placement for labor analgesia, Gomez and colleagues[17] reported that fewer top-up doses were required for rescue analgesia in women randomized to CSE compared with epidural (RR 0.31, 95% CI 0.14–0.70). After initiation of analgesia with epidural loading (8 mL 0.25% bupivacaine) or spinal dose (25 μg fentanyl plus 2.5 mg isobaric bupivacaine with epinephrine), both study groups received the same continuous background infusion of 0.125% bupivacaine plus fentanyl 1 μg/mL without a patient demand option. Studies using a patient-controlled epidural analgesia strategy have reported no significant differences in the number of demand doses or total bupivacaine dose.[14] Furthermore, results of a recent pooled meta-analysis showed no significant difference between CSE and low-dose epidurals with respect to need for rescue analgesia (RR 0.81, 95% CI 0.22–2.98; $P = .75$).[11]

EFFECT ON CATHETER FAILURE RATE

One purported benefit of a technique that intentionally breaches the dura is confirmation of epidural needle position, thus decreasing the likelihood of an improperly positioned epidural catheter; and, secondarily, fewer catheter replacements for ineffective or incomplete analgesia or unsuccessful conversion to anesthesia for cesarean delivery. An analysis of 1495 epidural catheters was conducted to compare the efficacy of catheters placed as a part of an epidural versus a needle-through-needle CSE technique in laboring women.[18] Catheters placed during a CSE technique were more likely to provide bilateral sensory change and effective labor analgesia than those placed after attempting to identify only the epidural space (98.6% vs 98.2%; $P = .02$). Catheters placed as part of a standard epidural technique were also more likely to be produce neither sensory change nor analgesia compared with CSE catheters (1.3% vs 0.2%; $P = .01$). These findings are supported by a 3-year observational study of 19,259 deliveries by Pan and colleagues[19] in which 75% of parturients received either epidural or CSE for labor analgesia. Compared with catheters placed during a CSE technique, catheters placed during conventional epidural placement had:

- Greater overall failure rates (14% vs 10%; $P<.001$)
- Higher incidence of inadequate analgesia (8.4% vs 4.2%; $P<.001$)
- Higher incidence of catheter replacement for inadequate analgesia (7.1% vs 3.2%; $P<.001$)
- Higher incidence of multiple replacements (1.9% vs 0.7%; $P<.001$)

Together, these studies would suggest that the risk for inadequate analgesia, catheter failure, and/or the need for catheter replacement is greater among patients in whom an epidural-only technique is used to initiate labor analgesia.

Although failed labor analgesia is dissatisfying to the mother and disappointing for the anesthesia provider, a greater concern is the need for conversion to general anesthesia because of catheter failure in the event of an urgent or emergent cesarean delivery. A 2002 review of 246 parturients demonstrated that 92% of women developed successful surgical anesthesia using the catheter.[20] Of note, the type of technique (CSE or epidural) did not correlate with catheter failure. An 18-month retrospective review of parturients who received neuraxial labor analgesia and subsequently required intrapartum cesarean delivery was conducted to identify the incidence and predictive factors associated with failed labor epidural augmentation for cesarean delivery. Of the 1025 parturients, 1.7% had failed epidural extension for cesarean delivery, thus requiring conversion to general anesthesia. In addition to prolonged duration of neuraxial labor analgesia ($P = .02$) and 2 or more episodes of breakthrough pain during labor ($P<.001$), the risk for failed epidural anesthesia was greater if labor analgesia was initiated using a standard epidural technique than when CSE was used (odds ratio 5.5, 95% CI 2.1–14.9; $P = .001$).[21] However, a recent systematic review and meta-analysis evaluating risk factors associated with failed conversion of labor epidural analgesia to cesarean-delivery anesthesia pooled the results of the aforementioned studies[20,21] and was unable to conclude that initiating labor analgesia with either technique, epidural or CSE, was more successful in converting epidural analgesia to anesthesia for cesarean delivery.[22]

COMPLICATIONS OF NEURAXIAL LABOR ANALGESIA

Initiation of neuraxial labor analgesia or surgical anesthesia may be associated with several potential side effects or complications:

- Maternal hypotension
- Pruritus

- Postdural puncture headache (PDPH)
- Neuraxial infection
- Neurologic complications
- Fetal bradycardia

Maternal Hypotension

An acute decrease in blood pressure may be seen with both epidural and CSE techniques. This decrease is caused by blockade of sympathetic fibers, causing vasodilation and venous pooling with a subsequent decrease in maternal cardiac output. If this decrease is significant and untreated the patient may experience nausea, lightheadedness, dizziness, or a decreased level of consciousness. In addition, uteroplacental insufficiency with subsequent abnormalities in fetal heart rate may occur. The severity of hypotension may be reduced, but not eliminated, by fluid administration before or during the performance of an epidural or CSE; however, such fluid preloading may reduce the incidence of changes in fetal heart rate observed following block placement.[23] Aortocaval compression by the gravid uterus is a frequent contributor to maternal hypotension, reinforcing the need to avoid a completely supine position.

Close monitoring of maternal blood pressure, assessment for subjective symptoms of hypotension, and prompt administration of vasopressor medications are crucial to optimizing perfusion for both mother and fetus. Although ephedrine was traditionally the vasopressor of choice during labor, it has been associated with decreased pH in the newborn following spinal anesthesia for cesarean section, which was subsequently confirmed in a large meta-analysis of 20 studies including 1069 women.[24] The relative risk of fetal acidosis, defined as a pH of less than 7.20, was 5.29 (95% CI 1.62–17.25) for ephedrine versus phenylephrine ($P = .006$), with a related lower base excess in the ephedrine group. Partial pressure of CO_2 in the umbilical artery was not different between the groups, leading the investigators to conclude that the pH change is not due to a change in CO_2. Although these findings are well studied in patients undergoing cesarean section, it is unclear whether this finding applies to both epidural and CSE analgesia techniques during labor.

The onset of hypotension following spinal anesthesia is typically more rapid and more profound than after epidural anesthesia.[25] An epidural catheter can be slowly injected over a longer period of time to theoretically allow for a more gradual change in blood pressure and more precise control. Earlier studies showed a more rapid and profound degree of hypotension associated with CSE.[26] Intrathecal clonidine improves analgesia, but has been associated with even greater maternal hypotension, an increased need for vasopressor medications, and significantly reduced umbilical artery pH.[27] When the dose of local anesthetic is reduced or eliminated in the spinal component of a CSE for labor, there appears to be no difference in the incidence of hypotension when compared with traditional or low-dose epidural techniques.[11] Slowly dosed epidural analgesia (or anesthesia) has been recommended for parturients with congenital heart defects in whom the rapid hemodynamic changes of spinal anesthesia could be catastrophic. Despite this, there are cases of CSE use in patients with congenital heart defects, although invasive arterial and venous monitors were placed before initiation of blockade to more closely follow and treat alterations in maternal hemodynamic status.[28]

Pruritus

One of the most common side effects of neuraxial opioid administration is pruritus. Although this unpleasant side effect may occur after either epidural or spinal administration, it is much more common after spinal injection than epidural injection.[29] Although modern-day labor analgesic techniques typically include low-dose opiates, the presence of even low-dose opiates such as fentanyl or sufentanil may produce significant maternal itching. Not surprisingly, pruritus is highly dose related.[30] In a recent meta-analysis of trials comparing CSE with epidural, 11 trials measured the incidence of pruritus as a secondary end point with both techniques. Although there was substantial heterogeneity between studies reflecting the marked variability in dosing and outcome definitions, the overall incidence of maternal itching with CSE was greater than with low-dose epidural techniques (49.1% vs 29.7%, respectively; RR 1.80, 95% CI 1.22–2.65).[11]

Postdural Puncture Headache

Unintended dural puncture may occur during any neuraxial procedure. In laboring parturients, the risk of unintended dural puncture during epidural placement ranges from 0.19% to 3.6%.[31–34] If dural puncture does occur with the epidural needle, PDPH rates exceed 50%.[35] Of interest, nearly 40% of PDPHs identified after labor epidural placement are related to an uneventful procedure whereby dural puncture was not readily apparent.[36] In contrast to the high PDPH risk associated with a large, cutting-tip epidural needle, the 27-gauge pencil-point needles typically used for CSE techniques have a PDPH risk of between 0.5% and 1.5%.[37] Although it makes intuitive sense that intentionally puncturing the dura would increase the incidence of PDPH, a large meta-analysis demonstrated no difference between epidural-only and CSE techniques.[11] The reasons for this finding remain unclear.

Neuraxial Infection

Severe infectious complications are uncommon but potentially devastating events following neuraxial blockade. Epidural abscess and meningitis are the most feared infectious complications of neuraxial procedures. Recently, a large national survey of Swedish hospitals identified 13 epidural abscesses and 29 cases of meningitis after 1.7 million neuraxial techniques (ie, 1 infectious complication per 40,000 blocks).[38] This estimated risk (1 per 40,000) was also reported in the third National Audit Project of the Royal College of Anaesthetists, in which 15 epidural abscesses and 3 cases of meningitis were identified after 700,000 neuraxial blocks performed within the United Kingdom.[39] These studies included both obstetric and nonobstetric patients, although a subgroup analysis of these studies and additional investigations have suggested that obstetric patients are less likely than nonobstetric patients to develop neuraxial infection following epidural procedures.[40,41]

Dural puncture has long been considered a risk factor for the development of meningitis, particularly in the presence of immunosuppression, diabetes, or localized or systemic infection.[42] Nevertheless, the incidence of meningitis after dural puncture is exceedingly low, far outpaced by infectious complications following epidural placement.[39] The safety of neuraxial techniques in parturients with chorioamnionitis has been debated, but the limited data available suggest that it is safe.[43] Although intuitively it would seem that CSE techniques would have a higher risk of infectious complications, there is as yet no evidence to support this assertion.

Recent case reports of meningitis following CSE placement in parturients reinforce the need for proper aseptic technique.[44] These measures include cap and mask for all persons in the room (except the patient, who does not need a mask), preprocedural hand hygiene (including removing rings and wristwatch) and sterile gloves for the proceduralist, skin preparation with chlorhexidine in alcohol, and sterile preparation of neuraxial medication infusions according to USP 797 guidelines.[42,44]

Fetal Bradycardia

Concerning tracings of fetal heart rate, including late decelerations and fetal brady-cardia, are well documented following the initiation of neuraxial labor analgesia.[45] The use of intrathecal opioids significantly increases the incidence of abnormalities in fetal heart rate. A large meta-analysis involving 3513 women found a relative risk of 1.81 (95% CI 1.04–3.14) in techniques using spinal opioids versus labor analgesia techniques that did not.[46] The proposed underlying mechanisms of the changes in fetal heart rate include maternal hypotension and uterine hypertonus. The cause of uterine hypertonus is not well understood, and may be related to rapid changes in circulating maternal catecholamine levels or an acute increase in maternal oxytocin levels caused by spinal opioid administration.[47] The occurrence of abnormalities in fetal heart rate appears to be dose related, with 7.5 μg or greater of intrathecal sufen-tanil being associated with a higher likelihood of fetal bradycardia.[26] Although the dose relationship for intrathecal fentanyl is less clear, there is evidence that the incidence of fetal bradycardia with fentanyl is similar to that with sufentanil when equipotent doses are used during CSE.[48] Occasionally the degree of fetal distress is great enough to necessitate cesarean delivery; however, there appears to be no significant difference in the rate of cesarean section between neuraxial and intravenous analgesia, or epidural and CSE techniques.[11,47]

SUMMARY

Epidural and CSE techniques both are safe, effective methods of analgesia in the laboring patient. Epidurals using higher concentrations of local anesthetic were previously associated with a prolonged second stage of labor and higher instrumented delivery rates. However, lower-concentration solutions currently in use do not appear to have these adverse effects, and there appears to be no difference between epidural and CSE techniques for progress of labor or instrumented or cesarean delivery. CSE techniques provide a significantly more rapid onset of analgesia, potentially making this technique advantageous in parturients whose labor is rapidly progressing. Catheters placed with standard epidural techniques appear to have a significantly greater failure rate for labor analgesia, but similar intervention rates for rescue analgesia and similar failure rates for conversion to anesthesia for cesarean delivery.

Despite the shorter onset of effective analgesia, CSE techniques result in a greater incidence of opiate-related maternal pruritus, which is highly dose related. Although intuitively it would seem that CSE would potentially have higher rates of PDPH and neuraxial infection, the evidence has not shown a difference in the rates of these complications.

Box 3
Potential factors to determine epidural versus CSE technique for labor analgesia

CSE

More rapid onset (eg, late-stage labor, rapidly progressing labor)

Confirmation of epidural placement (eg, morbid obesity)

Epidural

Desire for slower onset of analgesia (eg, congenital heart disease)

Lack of equipment for CSE

Lack of experience with CSE

Finally, concerning changes in fetal heart rate may occur following the initiation of neuraxial analgesia. However, these changes are typically transient and do not result in a significantly higher rate of cesarean section. Higher spinal doses of local anesthesia used during CSE are associated with more profound hypotension and the necessity for vasopressor use. Although fluid loading before block performance cannot eliminate hypotension, it may reduce the occurrence of associated changes in fetal heart rate. Intrathecal sufentanil doses of greater than 7.5 µg are associated with the greatest degree of abnormalities in fetal heart rate. Overall, both epidural and CSE techniques possess unique risk/benefit profiles, and the decision to use one technique rather than the other should be determined based on individual patient and clinical circumstances (**Box 3**).

REFERENCES

1. Osterman MJ, Martin JA. Epidural and spinal anesthesia use during labor: 27-state reporting area, 2008. Natl Vital Stat Rep 2011;59:1–16.
2. Jones L, Othman M, Dowswell T, et al. Pain management for women in labour: an overview of systematic reviews. Cochrane Database Syst Rev 2012;(3): CD009234.
3. Eldor J. Combined spinal-extradural anaesthesia in obstetrics. Br J Anaesth 1992;68:634–5.
4. Collis RE, Baxandall ML, Srikantharajah ID, et al. Combined spinal epidural analgesia with ability to walk throughout labour. Lancet 1993;341:767–8.
5. Cooper GM, MacArthur C, Wilson MJ, et al. Satisfaction, control and pain relief: short- and long-term assessments in a randomised controlled trial of low-dose and traditional epidurals and a non-epidural comparison group. Int J Obstet Anesth 2010;19:31–7.
6. Comparative Obstetric Mobile Epidural Trial (COMET) Study Group UK. Effect of low-dose mobile versus traditional epidural techniques on mode of delivery: a randomised controlled trial. Lancet 2001;358:19–23.
7. Wilson MJ, Cooper G, MacArthur C, et al. Randomized controlled trial comparing traditional with two "mobile" epidural techniques: anesthetic and analgesic efficacy. Anesthesiology 2002;97:1567–75.
8. Anim-Somuah M, Smyth RM, Jones L. Epidural versus non-epidural or no analgesia in labour. Cochrane Database Syst Rev 2011;(12):CD000331.
9. Tsen LC, Thue B, Datta S, et al. Is combined spinal-epidural analgesia associated with more rapid cervical dilation in nulliparous patients when compared with conventional epidural analgesia? Anesthesiology 1999;91:920–5.
10. Nageotte MP, Larson D, Rumney PJ, et al. Epidural analgesia compared with combined spinal-epidural analgesia during labor in nulliparous women. N Engl J Med 1997;337:1715–9.
11. Simmons SW, Taghizadeh N, Dennis AT, et al. Combined spinal-epidural versus epidural analgesia in labour. Cochrane Database Syst Rev 2012;(10):CD003401.
12. Norris MC, Fogel ST, Conway-Long C. Combined spinal-epidural versus epidural labor analgesia. Anesthesiology 2001;95:913–20.
13. Pascual-Ramirez J, Haya J, Perez-Lopez FR, et al. Effect of combined spinal-epidural analgesia versus epidural analgesia on labor and delivery duration. Int J Gynaecol Obstet 2011;114:246–50.
14. Sezer OA, Gunaydin B. Efficacy of patient-controlled epidural analgesia after initiation with epidural or combined spinal-epidural analgesia. Int J Obstet Anesth 2007;16:226–30.

15. Skupski DW, Abramovitz S, Samuels J, et al. Adverse effects of combined spinal-epidural versus traditional epidural analgesia during labor. Int J Gynaecol Obstet 2009;106:242–5.
16. Patel NP, Armstrong SL, Fernando R, et al. Combined spinal epidural vs epidural labour analgesia: does initial intrathecal analgesia reduce the subsequent minimum local analgesic concentration of epidural bupivacaine? Anaesthesia 2012; 67:584–93.
17. Gomez P, Echevarria M, Calderon J, et al. The efficacy and safety of continuous epidural analgesia versus intradural-epidural analgesia during labor. Rev Esp Anestesiol Reanim 2001;48:217–22 [in Spanish].
18. Norris MC. Are combined spinal-epidural catheters reliable? Int J Obstet Anesth 2000;9:3–6.
19. Pan PH, Bogard TD, Owen MD. Incidence and characteristics of failures in obstetric neuraxial analgesia and anesthesia: a retrospective analysis of 19,259 deliveries. Int J Obstet Anesth 2004;13:227–33.
20. Riley ET, Papasin J. Epidural catheter function during labor predicts anesthetic efficacy for subsequent cesarean delivery. Int J Obstet Anesth 2002;11:81–4.
21. Lee S, Lew E, Lim Y, et al. Failure of augmentation of labor epidural analgesia for intrapartum cesarean delivery: a retrospective review. Anesth Analg 2009;108: 252–4.
22. Bauer ME, Kountanis JA, Tsen LC, et al. Risk factors for failed conversion of labor epidural analgesia to cesarean delivery anesthesia: a systematic review and meta-analysis of observational trials. Int J Obstet Anesth 2012;21: 294–309.
23. Kinsella SM, Pirlet M, Mills MS, et al. Randomized study of intravenous fluid preload before epidural analgesia during labour. Br J Anaesth 2000;85:311–3.
24. Veeser M, Hofmann T, Roth R, et al. Vasopressors for the management of hypotension after spinal anesthesia for elective caesarean section. Systematic review and cumulative meta-analysis. Acta Anaesthesiol Scand 2012;56:810–6.
25. Ng K, Parsons J, Cyna AM, et al. Spinal versus epidural anaesthesia for caesarean section. Cochrane Database Syst Rev 2004;(2):CD003765.
26. Van De Velde M, Teunkens A, Hanssens M, et al. Intrathecal sufentanil and fetal heart rate abnormalities: a double-blind, double placebo-controlled trial comparing two forms of combined spinal epidural analgesia with epidural analgesia in labor. Anesth Analg 2004;98:1153–9.
27. Missant C, Teunkens A, Vandermeersch E, et al. Intrathecal clonidine prolongs labour analgesia but worsens fetal outcome: a pilot study. Can J Anaesth 2004; 51:696–701.
28. Hamlyn EL, Douglass CA, Plaat F, et al. Low-dose sequential combined spinal-epidural: an anaesthetic technique for caesarean section in patients with significant cardiac disease. Int J Obstet Anesth 2005;14:355–61.
29. Ballantyne JC, Loach AB, Carr DB. Itching after epidural and spinal opiates. Pain 1988;33:149–60.
30. Wong CA, Scavone BM, Slavenas JP, et al. Efficacy and side effect profile of varying doses of intrathecal fentanyl added to bupivacaine for labor analgesia. Int J Obstet Anesth 2004;13:19–24.
31. Berger CW, Crosby ET, Grodecki W. North American survey of the management of dural puncture occurring during labour epidural analgesia. Can J Anaesth 1998;45:110–4.
32. Gleeson CM, Reynolds F. Accidental dural puncture rates in UK obstetric practice. Int J Obstet Anesth 1998;7:242–6.

33. Sprigge JS, Harper SJ. Accidental dural puncture and post dural puncture head-ache in obstetric anaesthesia: presentation and management: a 23-year survey in a district general hospital. Anaesthesia 2008;63:36–43.

34. Stride PC, Cooper GM. Dural taps revisited. A 20-year survey from Birmingham maternity hospital. Anaesthesia 1993;48:247–55.

35. Choi PT, Galinski SE, Takeuchi L, et al. PDPH is a common complication of neu-raxial blockade in parturients: a meta-analysis of obstetrical studies. Can J Anaesth 2003;50:460–9.

36. Van de Velde M, Schepers R, Berends N, et al. Ten years of experience with acci-dental dural puncture and post-dural puncture headache in a tertiary obstetric anaesthesia department. Int J Obstet Anesth 2008;17:329–35.

37. Boyle JA, Stocks GM. Post-dural puncture headache in the parturient—an update. Anaesth Intensive Care Med 2010;11:302–4.

38. Moen V, Dahlgren N, Irestedt L. Severe neurological complications after central neuraxial blockades in Sweden 1990-1999. Anesthesiology 2004;101:950–9.

39. Cook TM, Counsell D, Wildsmith JA. Major complications of central neuraxial block: report on the Third National Audit Project of the Royal College of Anaesthe-tists. Br J Anaesth 2009;102:179–90.

40. Green LK, Paech MJ. Obstetric epidural catheter-related infections at a major teaching hospital: a retrospective case series. Int J Obstet Anesth 2010;19: 38–43.

41. Scott DB, Hibbard BM. Serious non-fatal complications associated with extra-dural block in obstetric practice. Br J Anaesth 1990;64:537–41.

42. Hebl JR. The importance and implications of aseptic techniques during regional anesthesia. Reg Anesth Pain Med 2006;31:311–23.

43. Goodman EJ, Dehorta E, Taguiam JM. Safety of spinal and epidural anesthesia in parturients with chorioamnionitis. Reg Anesth 1996;21:436–41.

44. Centers for Disease Control and Prevention. Bacterial meningitis after intrapartum spinal anesthesia - New York and Ohio, 2008-2009. MMWR Morb Mortal Wkly Rep 2010;59:65–9.

45. Stavrou C, Hofmeyr GJ, Boezaart AP. Prolonged fetal bradycardia during epidural analgesia. Incidence, timing and significance. S Afr Med J 1990;77: 66–8.

46. Mardirosoff C, Dumont L, Boulvain M, et al. Fetal bradycardia due to intrathecal opioids for labour analgesia: a systematic review. BJOG 2002;109:274–81.

47. Van De Velde M. Neuraxial analgesia and fetal bradycardia. Curr Opin Anaesthe-siol 2005;18:253–6.

48. Nelson KE, Rauch T, Terebuh V, et al. A comparison of intrathecal fentanyl and sufentanil for labor analgesia. Anesthesiology 2002;96:1070–3.

The Association Between Epidural Labor Analgesia and Maternal Fever

Katherine W. Arendt, MD[a],*, B. Scott Segal, MD, MHCM[b]

KEYWORDS

- Labor • Hyperthermia • Intrapartum fever • Maternal temperature
- Epidural analgesia

KEY POINTS

- Observational, retrospective, before-and-after, and randomized controlled trials that randomize to intravenous opioid or epidural analgesia indicate that epidural analgesia is associated with maternal fever.
- Criticisms of the studies demonstrating an association between epidural and fever include selection bias, bias in obstetric practice, crossover and protocol violation, and the potential that systemic mu-opioid agonists mitigate an inflammatory febrile response.
- Randomized controlled trials that randomize to epidural analgesia initiated in early versus late labor indicate that the patients who get an early epidural are not more likely to develop a fever. The absence of a "dose-effect" for the association between epidurals and fever is puzzling, but leads some to believe that there may be "trigger effect."
- Previously, it was thought that all women who had epidural analgesia had a gradual elevation of core body temperature. The current thinking is that only about 20% of those that receive epidural labor analgesia develop a fever and the remaining women have no increase in core body temperature with labor.
- A recent observational study evaluated the temperature slope of parturients throughout labor before and after the initiation of labor analgesia. They excluded any woman who developed a fever and therefore did not study the population affected by the phenomenon.
- Neonatal consequences of maternal fever in labor may involve low fetal tone, lower Apgar scores, assisted ventilation, tracheal intubation, cardiopulmonary resuscitation, supplemental oxygen requirements in the nursery, early onset neonatal seizures, and a greater likelihood of receiving a neonatal septic evaluation and antibiotic treatment.

Continued

Disclosure: Neither Dr B. Scott Segal nor Dr Katherine W. Arendt have interest in any commercial company that has a direct financial interest in the subject matter or materials discussed in the article or with a company making a competing product.
[a] Department of Anesthesiology, Mayo Clinic, 200 First Street SW, Rochester, MN 55905, USA;
[b] Department of Anesthesiology, Tufts Medical Center, Tufts University School of Medicine, 800 Washington Street, Mailbox 298, Boston, MA 02111, USA
* Corresponding author.
E-mail address: arendt.katherine@mayo.edu

Clin Perinatol 40 (2013) 385–398
http://dx.doi.org/10.1016/j.clp.2013.06.002   **perinatology.theclinics.com**

Continued

- Maternal consequences of fever in labor may involve an increased likelihood of receiving intrapartum antibiotics and undergoing a cesarean or assisted vaginal delivery.
- Multiple proposed mechanisms exist to explain the association between labor epidurals and fever but the involvement of noninfectious inflammation mediated by proinflammatory cytokines is supported most consistently by current evidence.
- The next steps in studying this association and its clinical consequences involve delineating the mechanism of the noninfectious inflammatory state and exactly how epidurals cause it; examining whether noninfectious inflammation is as harmful to the neonate as infectious inflammation is known to be; and determining how to block this febrile response safely.

INTRODUCTION

In 1989, Gleeson and colleagues[1] described a greater elevation of body temperature in women laboring with epidural analgesia than those without. Subsequently, a large body of research has been produced examining the relationship between epidural labor analgesia and maternal hyperthermia. This article focuses on the current literature associating epidural labor analgesia with fever organized by research methodology (**Table 1**) and discusses the criticisms of these studies (**Box 1**). Described are the proposed mechanisms, the consequences, and previous attempts to block or treat epidural-associated fever. Finally, the next steps for obstetricians and anesthesiologists in preventing the potential harmful effects of epidural-associated fever are discussed.

PROSPECTIVE OBSERVATIONAL AND RETROSPECTIVE STUDIES

Prospective observational trials in which women self-select their analgesia illustrate that women with epidural analgesia experience a higher incidence of fever or a modest elevation in temperature compared with women who select systemic opioids. Fusi and colleagues[2] compared 18 women who selected epidural analgesia with 15 women who selected intramuscular meperidine and metoclopramide. Although the vaginal temperatures of the nonepidural group remained unchanged throughout labor, the average vaginal temperature of the epidural group increased by 1°C over 7 hours. Camann and colleagues[3] also showed that women who selected epidural labor analgesia (randomized to infusions with or without epidural fentanyl) instead of intravenous nalbuphine had an increase in tympanic temperature of 0.07°C per hour on average. This study confirmed that the increased incidence of fever as observed by Fusi and colleagues was not an artifact of measuring temperature vaginally. Interestingly, the temperature increase began after 5 hours of epidural analgesia and there was no difference between the groups that did or did not receive epidural fentanyl.

Retrospective analyses also indicate that women who labor with epidural analgesia compared with those that do not are more likely to experience clinical fever, defined as a temperature greater than 37.8°C,[4] or 38°C.[5-8] The data in many of these studies are quite dramatic. For example, Kaul and colleagues[6] prospectively collected data for a quality improvement database and found that 61 out of 922 primiparous women who received epidural labor analgesia developed a fever of greater than 38°C, compared

Table 1
Incidence of fever with epidural labor analgesia

Study Author, Year	Design	Fever Definition (°C)	Epidural Group (% [n/N])	Nonepidural Group (% [n/N])	P Value
Vinson et al,[64] 1993	Observational	≥37.5	26.8 (11/41)	8.3 (3/36)	.05
		>38	14.6 (6/41)	0 (0/36)	.03
Herbst et al,[7] 1995	Observational	≥38	6.4 (44/683)	1.1 (28/2426)	<.001
Ploeckinger et al,[5] 1995	Observational	>38	1.6 (17/1056)	0.2 (11/6261)	<.005
Ramin et al,[13] 1995	RCT[a]	≥38	22.7 (98/432)	4.8 (21/437)	<.001
Lieberman et al,[8] 1997	Observational	>38	14.5 (152/1047)	1 (6/610)	<.001
Mayer et al,[4] 1997	Observational	≥37.8	20.4 (39/191)	2.1 (2/96)	<.001
Sharma et al,[14] 1997	RCT	>38	23.9 (58/243)	6.2 (16/259)	<.0001
Dashe et al,[31] 1999	Observational[b]	≥38	46.3 (37/80)	26.1 (18/69)	.01
Kaul et al,[6] 2001	Observational	>38	6.6 (61/922)	0 (0/255)	<.001
Lucas et al,[16] 2001	RCT[c]	≥38	20.4 (76/372)	7.1 (26/366)	<.001
Yancey et al,[12] 2001	Before-after study[d]	≥37.5	26.2 (150/572)	8.2 (41/498)	<.01
		≥38	11.0 (63/572)	0.6 (3/498)	<.01
Sharma et al,[15] 2002	RCT[a]	≥38	33.2 (75/226)	6.9 (16/233)	<.001
Agakidis et al,[65] 2011	Observational	≥38	11 (54/480)	0.8 (4/480)	<.0001
de Orange et al,[66] 2011	RCT[e]	≥38	14.3 (5/35)	0 (0/35)	.027
Riley et al,[37] 2011	Observational	>38	22.7 (34/150)	6.0 (3/50)	.009
Greenwell et al,[47] 2012	Observational	>37.5	44.8 (1246/2784)	14.6 (62/425)	<.0001
		>38	19.2 (535/2784)	2.4 (10/425)	<.0001

Abbreviation: RCT, randomized controlled trial.
[a] Fever reported for protocol-compliant women only.
[b] All patients had ruptured membranes more than 6 hours and included fever up to 6 hours postpartum.
[c] Patients with pregnancy-induced hypertension; percentages recalculated from n/N reported in the original publication.
[d] Epidural group reported as "after" period, in which 83% of women received epidural analgesia; nonepidural group reported as "before" period, in which 1% received epidural analgesia.
[e] Patients with combined-spinal or nonpharmacologic analgesia.
Modified from Segal S. Labor epidural analgesia and maternal fever. Anesth Analg 2010;111:1467–75; with permission.

Box 1
Criticisms of epidural fever studies

- Artifact of averaging
  - The epidural group in observational studies and randomized controlled trials (RCTs) may contain a small group of women who develop higher fever than those without epidurals and a larger group of women who do not develop fever at all.
- Selection bias
  - Women who have longer labors are more likely to get chorioamnionitis (and therefore a fever) and are more likely to request an epidural.
  - Women with subclinical chorioamnionitis or placental infection may be more likely to select epidural analgesia for labor.
- Crossover and dropout
  - Some RCTs have high rates of women leaving a nonepidural group and receiving epidural analgesia. These women more commonly have complicated labors.
  - Some RCTs have high rates of women dropping out of the epidural group because of rapid, uncomplicated vaginal deliveries. This reduces uncomplicated labors in the epidural group.
- Unknown temperature effects of intravenous opioids
  - Most studies randomize to epidural or intravenous opioid labor analgesia. There are no studies randomizing women to unmedicated childbirth. It seems that intravenous opioids may have antipyretic effects.
- Obstetric management bias
  - It is impossible to mask the obstetrician or other providers to the presence or absence of an epidural.
  - Women randomized to epidural groups may have increased frequency of cervical examinations, use of oxytocin, or artificial rupture of membranes, which may increase their temperature.
- Temperature measurement flaws
  - Women without epidurals are more likely to hyperventilate during labor, artificially cooling an oral temperature measurement.
  - Vaginal temperature measurements involve measuring below the level of the sympathectomy, which could falsely increase temperature measurements in women with epidural analgesia.

---

with none of the 255 nonepidural nulliparous women ($P = .000$). Also, Herbst and colleagues[7] performed a retrospective case-control study in which 44 (61.1%) of the 72 women who developed a fever had epidural analgesia, whereas only 639 (21%) of the 3037 women who were afebrile had an epidural ($P<.001$).

Frolich and colleagues[9] recently performed an observational study in which they reported the time-temperature slope of 81 parturients selecting epidural analgesia in labor. The change in temperature over time was calculated before and after initiation of epidural analgesia. Although a longer duration of rupture of membranes and elevated body mass index was associated with a more positive temperature trend, epidural analgesia was not. The authors suggest this observation exonerates epidural labor analgesia as a cause of intrapartum fever. However, it seems that women with "chorioamnionitis" (defined as temperature >38°C[9]) were excluded from analysis.

Excluding the population of women who develop clinical fever is a serious limitation. Previous studies have shown that the overall increase in temperature demonstrated in groups of women who labor with epidurals may be an "averaging artifact."[10,11] There seems to be a small group (about 20%) of women with an elevated inflammatory state[10] who have a significant increase in temperature when laboring with an epidural. When the temperatures of these women are averaged with the remaining cohort, most of whom have no change in temperature, a gradual increase in temperature is demonstrated for all women laboring with epidural analgesia. However, because Frolich and colleagues[9] excluded the small subset of women who eventually develop clinical fever, they may have excluded the group who explain the entire effect of epidural analgesia on temperature. Thus, the authors may have simply confirmed the lack of an effect of epidural analgesia on temperature among the large proportion of women who remain clinically afebrile throughout labor, as previously shown.[10,11] Any further work in evaluation of the association between fever and epidural labor analgesia needs to focus on this approximately 20% of women who eventually do become febrile.

The data from observational and retrospective studies are clear: women who choose epidural analgesia are more likely to develop intrapartum fever. There is no need to perform further retrospective or observational studies comparing maternal temperature in labor of women who do or do not choose epidural labor analgesia. It is possible that the reason why these women choose epidural analgesia may be the reason that they are experiencing fever. Women who have clinical or subclinical chorioamnionitis or, perhaps more generally, an elevated inflammatory state may experience greater labor pain (and greater labor pain earlier in labor) and are therefore more likely to request epidural analgesia. Therefore, because of selection bias one should not presume that epidural labor analgesia causes maternal fever from these retrospective and observational data, no matter how dramatic the differences observed between the epidural and nonepidural groups.

BEFORE-AND-AFTER STUDY

A single before-and-after study evaluated maternal temperature within a cohort of term nulliparous patients before and then after the implementation of a continuous epidural analgesia service.[12] In this retrospective cohort analysis, the frequency of epidural analgesia increased from 1% to 83% in approximately 1 year, and the incidence of a temperature of greater than 38°C was 3 (0.6%) out of 498 before and 63 (11%) out of 572 after the implementation (relative risk, 18.2; 95% confidence interval, 7–86; $P<.001$). The overall maximum intrapartum temperature was 98.6°F $\pm$ 0.7°F versus 99°F $\pm$ 1.1°F ($P<.01$). Because other factors may have also changed during the period of introduction of epidural analgesia, the authors attempted to account for any bias by reporting no significant differences in the frequency of artificial rupture of membranes (55.5% vs 57.2%); the number of vaginal examinations in labor; and the length of first stage of labor (14.3 vs 13.6 hours). Of note, there was a significant difference in the length of second stage of labor (0.7 vs 1.1 hours; $P<.01$). This study design is beneficial in that it is not complicated by crossover between groups as the RCTs demonstrate. Furthermore, although women in the "after" group self-select their analgesia, their temperatures are compared with the women in the "before" group who did not self-select. As a result, selection bias is more limited than in retrospective or observational studies.

RANDOMIZED CONTROLLED TRIALS: EPIDURAL ANALGESIA VERSUS INTRAVENOUS OPIOIDS

Multiple randomized controlled trials (RCTs) have been performed that consistently illustrate the presence of epidural-associated fever. Here, women are randomized to receive epidural or nonepidural analgesia. Ramin and colleagues[13] randomized 1330 women of mixed parity to epidural analgesia or intravenous meperidine. Unfortunately, the trial was analyzed on a protocol-compliant basis only, excluding one-third of subjects who did not receive the randomized analgesia. Nonetheless, 98 (23%) of 432 subjects who received epidural analgesia developed fever greater than 38°C, compared with 21 (5%) of 437 in the meperidine group ($P<.001$).

Sharma and colleagues,[14,15] from the same institution, were able to avoid such a high rate of crossover in two consecutive studies, which were analyzed on an intention-to-treat basis. In the first,[14] they randomized 715 women of mixed parity to either epidural analgesia or intravenous meperidine. Of the 358 women randomized to epidural analgesia, 243 received epidural analgesia, and 115 did not, with 78 women progressing too rapidly to receive the block. Of the 357 women randomized to intravenous meperidine, 259 followed protocol and 98 did not with 73 receiving no analgesia because of rapid delivery, 20 refusing analgesia, and 5 women requesting epidural analgesia because of inadequate analgesia from the meperidine. Of the 243 women in the epidural group, 58 (24%) developed a fever of 38°C or greater. Of the 259 women in the meperidine group, 16 (6%) developed fever ($P<.0001$). In a subsequent study,[15] they randomized 459 nulliparous women in spontaneous labor to epidural or intravenous meperidine. Of the 226 randomized to epidural analgesia, 214 followed protocol. Of the 233 randomized to meperidine, 207 followed protocol, with 14 women crossing over to epidural analgesia because of inadequate pain relief. Of the 226 women randomized to epidural analgesia, 75 (33%) developed a fever of 38°C or greater, whereas only 16 (7%) of the intravenous meperidine group became febrile ($P<.001$).

Lucas and colleagues[16] published an RCT that showed no significant differences in length of the first stage of labor, no significant differences in oxytocin augmentation, and little crossover. Here, 372 women with pregnancy-induced hypertension were randomized to epidural analgesia and 366 to intravenous meperidine and promethazine. Only three women in the meperidine group crossed over. However, there were overall 51 protocol violations in the epidural group and 26 in the meperidine group. An intent-to-treat analysis found that 76 (22%) of those randomized to the epidural group developed an intrapartum fever, compared with only 26 (8%) of those in the meperidine group ($P<.001$).

All of these RCTs are criticized because obstetric providers cannot be truly masked to whether a parturient is laboring with or without epidural analgesia. Therefore, bias is likely present. Both of the studies performed by Sharma and colleagues[14,15] report a higher rate of oxytocin augmentation in the epidural groups (33% vs 15%, $P<.0001\%$; 45% vs 34%, $P = .01$). Both report a longer interval from the initiation of epidural analgesia to the discovery of complete cervical dilation (260.3 ± 188 vs 199 ± 171 minutes, $P<.001$; 302 ± 189 vs 261 ± 188 minutes, $P = .03$). Further obstetric management questions remain, such as the potential differences in the frequency of cervical examinations in patients laboring with an epidural compared with those without epidural analgesia, or the allowance of women comfortable enough with an epidural to delay pushing after complete cervical dilation. This could lead to increased likelihood of fever from causes other than epidural analgesia and make the RCT study design in which women are randomized to epidural or nonepidural analgesia suboptimal in studying the presence of epidural-associated fever.

Finally, as discussed later, a few studies have indicated that systemic mu-opioid agonists may suppress fever.[17,18] Therefore, RCTs may suffer from some bias when comparing an epidural analgesia group with a systemic opioid analgesia group. There are no studies that compare epidural analgesia with no analgesia whatsoever, and it would be difficult and perhaps unethical to carry out such a study.

RANDOMIZED CONTROLLED TRIALS: EARLY VERSUS LATE EPIDURAL ANALGESIA

When women are randomized to receive epidural analgesia early or later in labor, no difference in temperatures is observed. Wong and colleagues[19] randomized 750 women to either early combined spinal epidural with intrathecal opioid (N = 366), or systemic hydromorphone analgesia and delayed combined spinal epidural placement (N = 362). The maximal oral temperature of both groups was 37.3 ± 0.5 (P = .06). A similar result was observed by the same group in induced labor in nulliparous women (incidence of fever >38°C, 12.7% in the early group vs 10.3% in the late group; P = .32).[20] Likewise, Wang and colleagues[21] randomized 12,793 nulliparous women to early epidural analgesia (N = 6394) or systemic meperidine and delayed epidural analgesia until cervical dilation was at least 4 cm (N = 6399). The median duration of epidural analgesia was 12.6 hours in the early epidural group and 4.8 hours in the delayed-epidural group and the overall length of labor was not significantly different between the groups. The average oral temperature during labor was not different at 37.4°C ± 0.4°C versus 37.2°C ± 0.3°C (P = .52).

In a different type of design, Wang and colleagues[22] randomized women to receive combined spinal epidural labor analgesia with 2 mg bupivacaine and 20 μg fentanyl and either immediate epidural analgesia (N = 26) or delayed epidural analgesia after the return of pain (N = 28). Three patients (11.5%) in the immediate epidural group developed a temperature greater than 38°C, whereas only two patients (7.1%) in the delayed epidural group developed a temperature greater than 38°C. This difference was not significant (P = .66). Because a previous study reported that intermittent epidural boluses resulted in a lesser incidence of maternal fever compared with continuous infusion epidural analgesia,[23] it seemed that a similar result would follow in the study by Wang and coworkers, although it was admittedly underpowered.

Taken together, the RCTs that randomize women to epidural analgesia initiated in early versus late labor indicate that patients who have a longer duration of epidural analgesia are not more likely to develop a fever. The absence of a "dose-effect" for the association between epidurals and fever leads some to suggest that there may be a "trigger effect." In this view, epidural analgesia interacts with an inflammatory state in susceptible women to initiate a febrile response shortly after the block is begun.

PROPOSED MECHANISMS

It is important to address the proposed mechanisms of this phenomenon if it is to be possible to avoid or appropriately treat hyperthermia with epidural labor analgesia. Unlike nonlaboring patients who receive epidural anesthesia and experience heat loss because of well-understood redistribution of heat from the core to the periphery,[24,25] the observational, before-and-after, and randomized controlled studies discussed previously illustrate that some women in labor who receive epidural analgesia experience an elevation of core body temperature. The proposed theories behind this observation are as follows:

- High ambient temperatures in delivery rooms.[2]

- A decrease in heat-dissipating hyperventilation with effective pain relief.[26]
- Altered thermoregulation,[27] which may involve an elevated sweating threshold below the level of the block[28] or an increased likelihood of heat-producing shivering.[1]
- A difference in the patient population requesting epidurals such that they are more likely to have subclinical chorioamnionitis at presentation, or more likely to have longer labors requiring multiple interventions, increasing the risk of chorioamnionitis throughout labor.[7,29]
- A difference in obstetric management in women with effective analgesia, such as increased use of oxytocin, or more frequent cervical examinations.[30]
- Antipyretic effects of systemic opioid analgesia, the group to which patients who do not receive epidural analgesia are randomized in RCTs.[17]
- An exaggerated noninfectious inflammatory response by proinflammatory cytokines in women laboring with an epidural.[31–37]

One theory is that epidural analgesia does not increase temperature, but systemic mu-opioid agonists may decrease the incidence of fever. Negishi and colleagues[17] induced fever by intravenous interleukin (IL)-2 in eight nonpregnant subjects on 4 separate days each randomized to one of the following four groups on different days: (1) a control day with no opioid or epidural, (2) epidural analgesia with ropivacaine, (3) epidural analgesia with ropivacaine and 2 μg/mL fentanyl, or (4) intravenous fentanyl at a target plasma concentration of 2.5 ng/mL. Intravenous fentanyl halved the pyrogenic response to the IL-2 injection compared with the control day, whereas epidural ropivacaine with and without fentanyl did not inhibit fever. Although this phenomenon was not present in a large retrospective review using the opioid agonist-antagonist nalbuphine,[38] the clinical effects of systemic mu-agonists is a question that remains unanswered, and potentially undermines the value of RCTs that involve groups that receive systemic opioid agonists, such as meperidine.

The most intriguing mechanism of epidural-induced fever involves the theory that the fever is not infectious in origin but is associated with an inflammatory state.[32–37] Riley and colleagues[37] compared the rate of placental infection and the degree of maternal inflammatory response in women with and without epidural labor analgesia. Similar, but very low, rates of placental infection as measured by placental cultures and polymerase chain reaction analysis were present in the epidural and nonepidural groups (4.7% vs 4%; $P > .99$). However, fever was more common in the epidural group (22.7% vs 5%; $P = .009$), and the risk of fever in those women laboring with epidurals was greater in women who presented with elevated IL-6 levels at admission (relative risk, 2.3; 95% confidence interval, 1.2–4.4). Experts believe that "these data support a non-infectious inflammatory theory for explaining epidural-associated maternal fever among women with an 'activated' immune system."[39] Other studies have shown that women who develop an epidural-associated fever do so immediately,[10] almost as if they are primed or activated to do so. This theory is also supported by studies that have shown the overall gradual increase in temperature demonstrated in groups of women who labor with epidurals[3,12] may be an "averaging artifact."[10,11] There seems to be a small group of women with elevated inflammatory states who have a significant increase in temperature when laboring with an epidural.[10,11] The "averaging artifact" occurs when the temperatures of these women are averaged with the remaining cohort (most of whom have no change in temperature). A resultant gradual increase in temperature is demonstrated for all women laboring with epidural analgesia.

Kozlov[40] recently proposed a role for the TRPV1 receptor (also known as the capsaicin receptor). The author hypothesized that local anesthetics act as agonists/antagonists at this receptor and that antagonist actions may cause hyperthermia through changes in thermoregulation and that agonist action may cause release of IL-6 and other inflammatory cytokines, which are known to cause fever. Much work needs to be done to investigate the possibility and the exact role of a potential receptor in the spine that could link the association between labor epidural and fever.

Some evidence does suggest thermoregulatory and other mechanisms of epidural-associated fever. Most evidence, however, supports the potential involvement of noninfectious inflammation. It is possible that women with elevated inflammatory states are more likely to get epidurals because of greater pain in labor. Whether epidural labor analgesia actually causes or induces an elevation of a maternal inflammatory state has not yet been entirely determined. There are no simple animal models of epidural labor analgesia, and thus evidence is indirect. It is most likely that an epidural interacts with a pre-existing inflammatory state and as a result unveils fever that may not have otherwise been observed.[37]

CONSEQUENCES

The observation that epidural labor analgesia may be associated with an elevation of maternal core body temperature was once dismissed as a physiologic curiosity. The consequences, however, are potentially dire. The development of maternal fever is debatably associated with indirect clinical effects, such as increasing a woman's likelihood of receiving intrapartum antibiotics and undergoing a cesarean or assisted vaginal delivery,[41] and the neonate's likelihood of receiving a neonatal septic evaluation and antibiotic treatment.[8] The latter association, however, is not consistent and seems to be related to neonatal practice style.[6]

Most ominously, however, maternal fever results in fetal hyperthermia. Although some studies show no differences in neonatal well-being (Apgar scores, umbilical cord gas, and acid-base measurements) with fetuses born greater than 38°C,[42] most indicate that intrapartum maternal fever is associated with a poor neonatal condition, including low fetal tone, lower Apgar scores, bag mask ventilation, tracheal intubation, cardiopulmonary resuscitation, supplemental oxygen requirements in the nursery, and neonatal seizure.[43–46] Most recently, Greenwell and colleagues[47] found that the rate of neonatal adverse outcomes increased directly with maximum maternal temperature in low-risk women receiving epidural labor analgesia. Compared with women with a maximum temperature of 37.5°C or less, babies born to mothers with temperatures greater than 38°C were more likely to have early onset neonatal seizures (adjusted odds ratio, 6.5); 5-minute Apgar score less than 7 (adjusted odds ratio, 4.8); prolonged neonatal hypotonia greater than 15 minutes (adjusted odds ratio, 3.1); and require assisted ventilation (adjusted odds ratio, 2.1).

The current theory that epidural fever is associated with an elevated maternal inflammatory state is worrisome. Recent animal studies indicate that intrauterine inflammation results in fetal brain inflammation and neurotoxicity.[48] Even more worrisome, one animal model that induced only subclinical placental inflammation still caused fetal brain injury.[49] Historically, the association between intrapartum infection and cerebral palsy has been well established.[50–54] The destructive contribution of the inflammatory state alone is debatably significant,[52] as is the destructive contribution of the hyperthermic state alone.[55–58]

TREATMENT

Goetzl[59] has stated that "obstetricians and anesthesiologists should partner in eluci-dating the mechanism of epidural fever and in developing effective mechanism-based interventions rather than seeking to discourage epidural analgesia." Unfortunately, all attempts to date have been unsuccessful or impractical. Goetzl's group attempted such an approach, randomizing 42 afebrile women requesting epidural analgesia to receive 650 mg of rectal acetaminophen or placebo. They found no differences in the incidence of fever, the mean maximal temperature, or the change in temperature over time.[60] This result is not surprising given the weak anti-inflammatory effect of acetaminophen. Evron and colleagues[18] randomized laboring women to receive intra-venous remifentanil only (N = 44); epidural ropivacaine only (N = 50); intravenous remifentanil and epidural ropivacaine (N = 49); or epidural ropivacaine with intrave-nous acetaminophen (N = 49). Although there was a significantly lesser maximal in-crease from baseline temperature in the remifentanil-only group (P = .013), no other significant differences in temperature change were found. The acetaminophen group had an insignificantly reduced incidence of hyperthermia than the epidural ropivacaine-only group (4 [8%] of 49 vs 7 [14%] of 15), and the epidural ropivacaine and remifentanil group had an insignificantly reduced incidence compared with the epidural ropivacaine-only group (4 [8%] of 49 vs 7 [14%] of 15). It is likely that this study was underpowered to detect these differences and that intravenous opioid and intravenous acetaminophen could have a therapeutic benefit alone, or in combi-nation, in preventing epidural-associated fever.

Goetzl and colleagues[61] did successfully prevent fever associated with epidural analgesia with systemic maternal steroids. At the time of epidural placement, women were randomized to placebo (N = 100), intravenous 25-mg methylprednisolone every 8 hours (N = 50), or 100 mg every 4 hours (N = 49). Fever occurred in 22 (21.8%), 17 (34%), and 1 (2%) of the placebo, low-dose steroid, and high-dose steroid groups, respectively. High-dose steroids decreased the incidence of epidural-associated fe-ver by 90% (P<.001). However, neonatal bacteremia was present in none of the pla-cebo group, one (2.1%) of the low-dose group, but four (9.3%) of the high-dose group (P = .005). This complication renders this therapy impractical clinically but sup-ports the inflammatory nature of epidural-associated fever.

Preliminary work on the potential differing effects on the incidence of fever of various types of epidural local anesthesia (0.08% ropivacaine vs 0.06% levobupivacaine) re-veals the potential for a series of studies to find the least pyrogenic labor epidural cocktail.[62] Goetzl[59] believes that proactive labor management that shortens labor may also play a role in reduction of intrapartum fever. Epidural dexamethasone also shows some promise of potential benefit. Wang and colleagues[63] randomized women to epidural solutions with or without 0.2 mg/mL dexamethasone. They found that the group receiving the epidural solution without dexamethasone had an increase in maternal temperature and IL-6 levels, whereas the epidural dexamethasone group did not. There was, however, no difference in the incidence of fever between the groups. The appropriate epidural dexamethasone dose and the therapy's potential ef-fects on neonatal bacteremia require further study.

SUMMARY

Epidural analgesia is strongly associated with maternal intrapartum fever, and the effect does not seem to be merely attributable to selection bias. The most likely mechanism involves noninfectious inflammation, although the pathophysiology is incompletely understood. The direct effects of maternal fever are significant but, as yet, not definitely linked to epidural-caused fever. The next steps in studying this association and the clinical consequences of it involve delineating the mechanism of the noninfectious inflammatory state and exactly how epidurals cause it; examining whether epidural-triggered noninfectious inflammation is as harmful to the neonate as other causes of maternal fever; and finally determining how safely to block, or at least minimize, this febrile response.

REFERENCES

1. Gleeson NC, Nolan KM, Ford MR. Temperature, labour, and epidural analgesia. Lancet 1989;2:861–2.
2. Fusi L, Steer PJ, Maresh MJ, et al. Maternal pyrexia associated with the use of epidural analgesia in labour. Lancet 1989;1:1250–2.
3. Camann WR, Hortvet LA, Hughes N, et al. Maternal temperature regulation during extradural analgesia for labour. Br J Anaesth 1991;67:565–8.
4. Mayer DC, Chescheir NC, Spielman FJ. Increased intrapartum antibiotic administration associated with epidural analgesia in labor. Am J Perinatol 1997;14: 83–6.
5. Ploeckinger B, Ulm MR, Chalubinski K, et al. Epidural anaesthesia in labour: influence on surgical delivery rates, intrapartum fever and blood loss. Gynecol Obstet Invest 1995;39:24–7.
6. Kaul B, Vallejo M, Ramanathan S, et al. Epidural labor analgesia and neonatal sepsis evaluation rate: a quality improvement study. Anesth Analg 2001;93: 986–90.
7. Herbst A, Wolner-Hanssen P, Ingemarsson I. Risk factors for fever in labor. Obstet Gynecol 1995;86:790–4.
8. Lieberman E, Lang JM, Frigoletto F Jr, et al. Epidural analgesia, intrapartum fever, and neonatal sepsis evaluation. Pediatrics 1997;99:415–9.
9. Frolich MA, Esame A, Zhang K, et al. What factors affect intrapartum maternal temperature? A prospective cohort study: maternal intrapartum temperature. Anesthesiology 2012;117:302–8.
10. Goetzl L, Rivers J, Zighelboim I, et al. Intrapartum epidural analgesia and maternal temperature regulation. Obstet Gynecol 2007;109:687–90.
11. Gelfand TP, Tsen LC, Segal S. Warming in parturients with epidurals is an averaging artifact. Anesthesiology 2007;106:A5.
12. Yancey MK, Zhang J, Schwarz J, et al. Labor epidural analgesia and intrapartum maternal hyperthermia. Obstet Gynecol 2001;98:763–70.
13. Ramin SM, Gambling DR, Lucas MJ, et al. Randomized trial of epidural versus intravenous analgesia during labor. Obstet Gynecol 1995;86:783–9.
14. Sharma SK, Sidawi JE, Ramin SM, et al. Cesarean delivery: a randomized trial of epidural versus patient-controlled meperidine analgesia during labor. Anesthesiology 1997;87:487–94.
15. Sharma SK, Alexander JM, Messick G, et al. Cesarean delivery: a randomized trial of epidural analgesia versus intravenous meperidine analgesia during labor in nulliparous women. Anesthesiology 2002;96:546–51.
16. Lucas MJ, Sharma SK, McIntire DD, et al. A randomized trial of labor analgesia in women with pregnancy-induced hypertension. Am J Obstet Gynecol 2001; 185:970–5.
17. Negishi C, Lenhardt R, Ozaki M, et al. Opioids inhibit febrile responses in humans, whereas epidural analgesia does not: an explanation for hyperthermia during epidural analgesia. Anesthesiology 2001;94:218–22.

18. Evron S, Ezri T, Protianov M, et al. The effects of remifentanil or acetaminophen with epidural ropivacaine on body temperature during labor. J Anesth 2008;22: 105–11.

19. Wong CA, Scavone BM, Peaceman AM, et al. The risk of cesarean delivery with neuraxial analgesia given early versus late in labor. N Engl J Med 2005;352: 655–65.

20. Wong CA, McCarthy RJ, Sullivan JT, et al. Early compared with late neuraxial analgesia in nulliparous labor induction: a randomized controlled trial. Obstet Gynecol 2009;113:1066–74.

21. Wang F, Shen X, Guo X, et al. Epidural analgesia in the latent phase of labor and the risk of cesarean delivery: a five-year randomized controlled trial. Anesthesiology 2009;111:871–80.

22. Wang LZ, Chang XY, Hu XX, et al. The effect on maternal temperature of delaying initiation of the epidural component of combined spinal-epidural analgesia for labor: a pilot study. Int J Obstet Anesth 2011;20:312–7.

23. Mantha VR, Vallejo MC, Ramesh V, et al. The incidence of maternal fever during labor is less with intermittent than with continuous epidural analgesia: a randomized controlled trial. Int J Obstet Anesth 2008;17:123–9.

24. Holdcroft A, Hall GM, Cooper GM. Redistribution of body heat during anaesthesia. A comparison of halothane, fentanyl and epidural anaesthesia. Anaesthesia 1979;34:758–64.

25. Matsukawa T, Sessler DI, Christensen R, et al. Heat flow and distribution during epidural anesthesia. Anesthesiology 1995;83:961–7.

26. Hagerdal M, Morgan CW, Sumner AE, et al. Minute ventilation and oxygen consumption during labor with epidural analgesia. Anesthesiology 1983;59:425–7.

27. Goodlin RC, Chapin JW. Determinants of maternal temperature during labor. Am J Obstet Gynecol 1982;143:97–103.

28. Glosten B, Savage M, Rooke GA, et al. Epidural anesthesia and the thermoregulatory responses to hyperthermia: preliminary observations in volunteer subjects. Acta Anaesthesiol Scand 1998;42:442–6.

29. Vallejo MC, Kaul B, Adler LJ, et al. Chorioamnionitis, not epidural analgesia, is associated with maternal fever during labour. Can J Anaesth 2001;48:1122–6.

30. Dolak JA, Brown RE. Epidural analgesia and neonatal fever. Pediatrics 1998; 101:492 [author reply: 493–4].

31. Dashe JS, Rogers BB, McIntire DD, et al. Epidural analgesia and intrapartum fever: placental findings. Obstet Gynecol 1999;93:341–4.

32. Goetzl L, Evans T, Rivers J, et al. Elevated maternal and fetal serum interleukin-6 levels are associated with epidural fever. Am J Obstet Gynecol 2002;187:834–8.

33. Gonen R, Korobochka R, Degani S, et al. Association between epidural analgesia and intrapartum fever. Am J Perinatol 2000;17:127–30.

34. De Jongh RF, Bosmans EP, Puylaert MJ, et al. The influence of anaesthetic techniques and type of delivery on peripartum serum interleukin-6 concentrations. Acta Anaesthesiol Scand 1997;41:853–60.

35. Smulian JC, Bhandari V, Vintzileos AM, et al. Intrapartum fever at term: serum and histologic markers of inflammation. Am J Obstet Gynecol 2003;188:269–74.

36. Evron S, Parameswaran R, Zipori D, et al. Activin betaA in term placenta and its correlation with placental inflammation in parturients having epidural or systemic meperidine analgesia: a randomized study. J Clin Anesth 2007;19:168–74.

37. Riley LE, Celi AC, Onderdonk AB, et al. Association of epidural-related fever and noninfectious inflammation in term labor. Obstet Gynecol 2011;117:588–95.

38. Gross JB, Cohen AP, Lang JM, et al. Differences in systemic opioid use do not explain increased fever incidence in parturients receiving epidural analgesia. Anesthesiology 2002;97:157–61.

39. Butwick AJ. 2012 Gerard W. Ostheimer Lecture–What's new in obstetric anesthesia? Int J Obstet Anesth 2012;21:348–56.

40. Kozlov I. Why labor epidural causes fever and why lidocaine burns on injection? Role of TRPV1 receptor in hyperthermia: possible explanation of mechanism of hyperthermia during labor epidural and burning sensation on injection of local anesthetics. Open J Anesthesiol 2012;2:134–7.

41. Lieberman E, Cohen A, Lang J, et al. Maternal intrapartum temperature elevation as a risk factor for cesarean delivery and assisted vaginal delivery. Am J Public Health 1999;89:506–10.

42. Macaulay JH, Bond K, Steer PJ. Epidural analgesia in labor and fetal hyperthermia. Obstet Gynecol 1992;80:665–9.

43. Lieberman E, Lang J, Richardson DK, et al. Intrapartum maternal fever and neonatal outcome. Pediatrics 2000;105:8–13.

44. Perlman JM. Maternal fever and neonatal depression: preliminary observations. Clin Pediatr (Phila) 1999;38:287–91.

45. Shalak LF, Perlman JM, Jackson GL, et al. Depression at birth in term infants exposed to maternal chorioamnionitis: does neonatal fever play a role? J Perinatol 2005;25:447–52.

46. Lieberman E, Eichenwald E, Mathur G, et al. Intrapartum fever and unexplained seizures in term infants. Pediatrics 2000;106:983–8.

47. Greenwell EA, Wyshak G, Ringer SA, et al. Intrapartum temperature elevation, epidural use, and adverse outcome in term infants. Pediatrics 2012;129: e447–54.

48. Burd I, Brown A, Gonzalez JM, et al. A mouse model of term chorioamnionitis: unraveling causes of adverse neurological outcomes. Reprod Sci 2011;18: 900–7.

49. Elovitz MA, Brown AG, Breen K, et al. Intrauterine inflammation, insufficient to induce parturition, still evokes fetal and neonatal brain injury. Int J Dev Neurosci 2011;29:663–71.

50. Eastman NJ, Deleon M. The etiology of cerebral palsy. Am J Obstet Gynecol 1955;69:950–61.

51. Grether JK, Nelson KB. Maternal infection and cerebral palsy in infants of normal birth weight. JAMA 1997;278:207–11.

52. Yoon BH, Romero R, Park JS, et al. Fetal exposure to an intra-amniotic inflammation and the development of cerebral palsy at the age of three years. Am J Obstet Gynecol 2000;182:675–81.

53. Wu YW, Colford JM Jr. Chorioamnionitis as a risk factor for cerebral palsy: a meta-analysis. JAMA 2000;284:1417–24.

54. Wu YW, Escobar GJ, Grether JK, et al. Chorioamnionitis and cerebral palsy in term and near-term infants. JAMA 2003;290:2677–84.

55. Milunsky A, Ulcickas M, Rothman KJ, et al. Maternal heat exposure and neural tube defects. JAMA 1992;268:882–5.

56. Li DK, Janevic T, Odouli R, et al. Hot tub use during pregnancy and the risk of miscarriage. Am J Epidemiol 2003;158:931–7.

57. Mishima K, Ikeda T, Yoshikawa T, et al. Effects of hypothermia and hyperthermia on attentional and spatial learning deficits following neonatal hypoxia-ischemic insult in rats. Behav Brain Res 2004;151:209–17.

58. Wang W, Dow KE, Flavin MP. Hyperthermia amplifies brain cytokine and reactive oxygen species response in a model of perinatal inflammation. Neurosci Lett 2008;445:233–5.

59. Goetzl L. Epidural analgesia and maternal fever: a clinical and research update. Curr Opin Anaesthesiol 2012;25:292–9.

60. Goetzl L, Rivers J, Evans T, et al. Prophylactic acetaminophen does not prevent epidural fever in nulliparous women: a double-blind placebo-controlled trial. J Perinatol 2004;24:471–5.

61. Goetzl L, Zighelboim I, Badell M, et al. Maternal corticosteroids to prevent intra-uterine exposure to hyperthermia and inflammation: a randomized, double-blind, placebo-controlled trial. Am J Obstet Gynecol 2006;195:1031–7.

62. Lee HL, Lo LM, Chou CC, et al. Comparison between 0.08% ropivacaine and 0.06% levobupivacaine for epidural analgesia during nulliparous labor: a retrospective study in a single center. Chang Gung Med J 2011;34:286–92.

63. Wang LZ, Hu XX, Liu X, et al. Influence of epidural dexamethasone on maternal temperature and serum cytokine concentration after labor epidural analgesia. Int J Gynaecol Obstet 2011;113:40–3.

64. Vinson DC, Thomas R, Kiser T. Association between epidural analgesia during labor and fever. J Fam Pract 1993;36:617–22.

65. Agakidis C, Agakidou E, Philip Thomas S, et al. Labor epidural analgesia is independent risk factor for neonatal pyrexia. J Matern Fetal Neonatal Med 2011; 24:1128–32.

66. de Orange FA, Passini R Jr, Amorim MM, et al. Combined spinal and epidural anaesthesia and maternal intrapartum temperature during vaginal delivery: a randomized clinical trial. Br J Anaesth 2011;107:762–8.

Anesthetic Management of External Cephalic Version

Laurie A. Chalifoux, MD[a],*, John T. Sullivan, MD, MBA[b]

KEYWORDS

- External cephalic version • Breech presentation • Cesarean delivery
- Neuraxial anesthesia

KEY POINTS

- ECV offers an opportunity to avoid planned cesarean delivery in parturients with singleton breech presentation at term.
- Tocolysis increases the likelihood of ECV procedural success.
- Because ECV is associated with a significant degree of maternal pain, neuraxial anesthesia during the procedure provides a superior maternal experience when compared with systemic intravenous analgesia or no analgesia.
- Neuraxial anesthesia has been reported to increase the success of ECV procedures when surgical anesthetic dosing is used.
- Although ECV and neuraxial blockade have associated side effects and increased costs, it is likely justified given the potential effect of reducing cesarean delivery rates.

INTRODUCTION

External cephalic version (ECV) is the process of applying external pressure maneuvers to the maternal abdomen with the purpose to convert a breech or transverse fetal presentation to a vertex presentation (**Fig. 1**). This procedure is performed to increase the likelihood of a vertex vaginal birth while avoiding the adverse fetal outcomes associated with vaginal breech delivery and the increased maternal complications that may result from cesarean delivery.

BREECH PRESENTATION

Breech presentation is the most common abnormal fetal presentation. In this longitudinal position relative to the maternal axial skeleton, the fetal buttocks or lower

[a] Department of Anesthesiology, Northwestern Feinberg School of Medicine, 251 East Huron Street F5-704, Chicago, IL 60611, USA; [b] Section of Obstetric Anesthesiology, Department of Anesthesiology, Northwestern Feinberg School of Medicine, 251 East Huron Street F5-704, Chicago, IL 60611, USA
* Corresponding author.
E-mail address: l-chalifoux@md.northwestern.edu

Clin Perinatol 40 (2013) 399–412
http://dx.doi.org/10.1016/j.clp.2013.06.001   **perinatology.theclinics.com**
0095-5108/13/$ – see front matter © 2013 Elsevier Inc. All rights reserved.

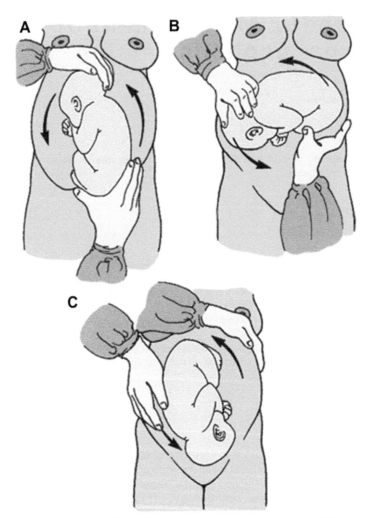

Fig. 1. Anesthesia for external cephalic version. (*A–C*) Fetus is converted from breech to vertex presentation. (*From* Beckmann CR, Frank W. Obstetrics and gynecology, 5th edition. Philadelphia: Lippincott Williams & Wilkins; 2006. Copyright © 2006 Lippincott Williams & Wilkins; with permission.)

extremities lie at the pelvic brim, while the fetal head occupies the upper pole of the uterus. There are several types of breech presentation defined by the position of the fetal lower extremities (**Fig. 2**). The diagnosis of breech presentation is made by either physical or ultrasound examination. Physical evidence of breech presentation may be observed by palpation of the maternal abdomen (Leopold maneuvers) or cervical examination to determine the presenting fetal part. Ultrasound examination may confirm this diagnosis while allowing the obstetrician to estimate fetal weight and screen for major fetal or placental abnormalities.

Epidemiology

The overall incidence of breech fetal presentation is inversely related to gestational age. Breech type also varies with gestational age. For example, during early

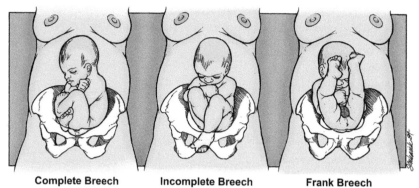

Complete Breech   **Incomplete Breech**   **Frank Breech**

Fig. 2. Frank breech: both hips flexed, both knees extended. Complete breech: both hips and knees are flexed. Incomplete breech: intermediate deflexion of one or both hips and knees. Other variations: footling breech (one or both feet are the presenting part) or kneeling breech (one or both knees are the presenting part). (*From* Lanni SM, Seeds JW. Malpresentations and shoulder dystocia. In: Gabbe SG, Niebyl JR, et al, eds. Obstetrics: normal and problem pregnancies, 6th edition. Philadelphia: Elsevier; 2012; with permission.)

pregnancy the fetus remains mobile and may change positions frequently in its relatively large volume of amniotic fluid. By 32 to 34 weeks' gestation, most fetuses have turned to a vertex presentation. By term, only 3% to 4% of fetuses present in the breech position.[1]

There are several other maternal and fetal factors that have been associated with breech presentation. Several conditions may interfere with the normal fit of the fetal head as it descends into a vertex position within the maternal pelvis (**Box 1**).

Obstetric Complications

Breech presentation is associated with an increased risk of intrapartum complications (**Table 1**). Obstetricians may elect cesarean delivery to mitigate some of the fetal risk; however, cesarean breech delivery incurs maternal risk associated with the surgery and subsequent risk in future pregnancies and deliveries. Vaginal breech delivery is an option in some cases, but the increased neonatal risk must be weighed against any maternal benefit.

Management Options

Obstetricians faced with breech presentation may choose to deliver the breech fetus vaginally, plan a cesarean delivery, or attempt to convert the presentation to vertex. The American Congress of Obstetricians and Gynecologists recommends that obstetricians offer ECV whenever possible to all women near term with a breech fetal presentation.[2] Additionally, other international organizations including the Royal College of Obstetricians and Gynecologists promote ECV as a safe procedure that should be offered to eligible patients in the absence of contraindication.[3–7]

Alternative management options include moxibustion, acupuncture, and postural maneuvers. However, these alternative and relatively low-risk methods of managing breech presentation have little definitive evidence of efficacy.[8]

Moxibustion is a traditional Chinese therapy whereby herbs are burned in proximity to the skin either alone or in combination with acupuncture. A meta-analysis of eight trials involving 1346 women found limited evidence to support the use of moxibustion alone to convert a breech presentation to vertex.[9] Compared with no treatment,

---

Box 1
Maternal and fetal conditions associated with breech presentation

Uterine factors
- Distention
  - Multiparity
  - Polyhydraminios
- Abnormal uterine shape
  - Space-occupying lesions (leiomyomata, pelvic tumors)
  - Pelvic or uterine contracture
  - Bicornuate or septate uterus[33]

Fetal factors
- Fetal anomaly
  - Anencephaly, hydrocephaly, fetal masses
- Decreased fetal mobility
  - Fetal asphyxia
  - Short umbilical cord[34]
  - Multiple gestations

Obstetric factors
- Previous breech delivery[35]
- Placenta previa or cornual-fundal placenta[36]
- Fetal growth restriction
- Oligohydramnios
- Heredity[37]

---

moxibustion was not found to reduce the number of breech presentations at birth. However, when combined with acupuncture or postural techniques, moxibustion did result in fewer noncephalic presentations at birth and fewer cesarean deliveries compared with no treatment. An additional large randomized controlled trial published after the systematic review reported evidence for the efficacy of moxibustion alone.[10]

Postural management of breech presentation involves repeated, short duration, maternal positioning (eg, knee to chest, elevated pelvis) to augment the effect of gravity on fetal presentation. A meta-analysis of six randomized and quasi-randomized studies involving 417 patients demonstrated no difference in the rates of noncephalic births or cesarean deliveries.[11]

In the case of a fetus remaining breech at term, the debate between vaginal breech delivery versus cesarean is complex and represents a comparison of fetal and maternal risks. The largest randomized, multicenter study conducted by the Term Breech Trial Collaborative Group demonstrated an increase in the composite outcome of perinatal and neonatal mortality and serious neonatal morbidity in the group assigned to planned vaginal as compared with planned cesarean delivery (1.6% vs 5%; relative risk, 0.33; 95% confidence interval, 0.19–0.56; $P<.0001$).[12] Maternal mortality and serious maternal morbidity were not statistically different between groups (3.9% vs 3.2%; 1.24 [0.79–1.95]; $P = .35$) but the study was likely underpowered to address this composite of secondary outcomes.

Table 1
Risk associated with breech presentation at term

Incidence of Complications Seen with Breech Presentation	
Complication	Incidence
Intrapartum fetal death	Increased 16-fold[23]
Perinatal mortality	1.3%[20]
Intrapartum asphyxia	Increased 3.8-fold[31]
Cord prolapse	Increased 5- to 20-fold[14,15] 1.3%[20]
Birth trauma	Increased 13-fold[14] 1.4%[20]
Dystocia, difficulty delivering head	4.6%[20] to 8.8%[14]
Spinal cord injuries with extended head	21%
Major anomalies	6%–18%[31]
Prematurity	16%–33%[22,25]
Hyperextension of head	5%
Fetal heart rate abnormalities	15.2%[20]

From Lanni SM, Seeds JW. Malpresentations and shoulder dystocia. In: Gabbe SG, Niebyl JR, et al, eds. Obstetrics: normal and problem pregnancies, 6th edition. Philadelphia: Elsevier; 2012; with permission.

Although some obstetricians continue to offer vaginal breech delivery, it has become an increasingly uncommon practice in the United States, especially among younger practitioners. In 2006 and 2010 committee opinions, the American Congress of Obstetricians and Gynecologists stated that breech vaginal delivery remains a reasonable option in appropriate cases, but added that the decision to proceed with a trial of labor and vaginal breech delivery should be based on the experience of the practitioner.[13]

There are several considerations when proceeding directly to a planned cesarean delivery for breech presentation. The rising cesarean delivery rate in the United States and internationally is a problem that continues to challenge health care providers. Cesarean section is the most commonly performed surgery in the United States. In 2009, the cesarean delivery rate in the United States reached 32.3%, for a total of more than 1.3 million cesarean sections preformed. The cesarean delivery rate continues to rise, with a 50% increase since 1996, of which the contribution of reduced planned vaginal breech delivery has been significant (**Fig. 3**).[14]

The associated maternal risks of cesarean delivery include hemorrhage; infection; damage to adjacent organs; and postsurgical complications, such as thromboembolism, acute and chronic pain, and death. In the past, it has been widely accepted that cesarean delivery leads to an increased maternal mortality rate compared with vaginal delivery. However, several factors must be considered when assessing mortality related to cesarean delivery. For example, mortality rate seems to differ based on the urgency of the surgery; intrapartum versus antepartum timing of the delivery; coexisting maternal disease; and the availability of resources at the institution (eg, blood products, specialists). Importantly, there is little strong evidence on maternal mortality rates comparing cesarean with vaginal delivery. Because of the rare nature of maternal death, especially in the developed world, the existing studies are heterogeneous in design, likely underpowered, and differ widely in their conclusions.[15] Additional risk is also incurred for future pregnancies because of the increased rate of

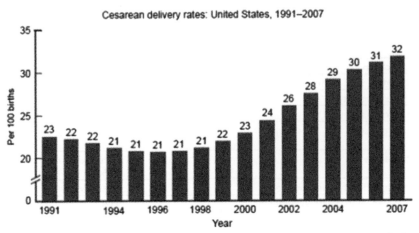

Fig. 3. Cesarean delivery rate in the United States. (*From* Natl Vital Stat Rep 2009;57(12); and *Courtesy of* Centers for Disease Control/NCHS, National Vital Statistics System.)

abnormal placentation, including placental abruption, placenta previa, and placenta accreta, increta or percreta, and catastrophic uterine complications.

EXTERNAL CEPHALIC VERSION
Definition

ECV involves using external manual force on the maternal abdomen to rotate the fetus from breech to cephalic presentation (see **Fig. 1**). The goal of ECV is to decrease the number of term breech presentations and more importantly decrease the number of vaginal breech extractions and cesarean deliveries and their associated fetal and maternal morbidity and mortality. ECV has been identified as the only clinical intervention with conclusive evidence to support the overall reduction in cesarean delivery rates.[16]

Success of ECV

The success rates of ECV have been reported from 35% to 86%, reflecting not only a range in practitioner capability but also heterogeneity in study methodology.[3,5–7] Several factors have been reported to be associated with increased ECV success (**Box 2**).[17–19] Optimal timing for successful ECV remains unclear. It has been

---

Box 2
Factors associated with increased ECV success

- Multiparity
- Non-obesity
- Relaxed uterus
- Suprapelvic presenting fetal part
- Lateral fetal spine position
- Complete breech presentation
- Palpable fetal head
- Normal amniotic fluid volume

suggested that conducting ECV at 34 to 35 weeks' gestation may result in the higher incidence of vertex breech presentation at birth; however, the fetus may revert back to breech position before the onset of labor. For this reason, and because of concerns of fetal lung immaturity, many practitioners prefer to wait until 37 to 39 weeks' gestation to proceed with ECV attempts.[20]

ECV success can be facilitated with uterine relaxation. β_2 Agonists, including terbutaline (subcutaneous or intravenous), are commonly administered to achieve this goal. A meta-analysis of published studies demonstrates an increased ECV success rate with β agonists but not with nitroglycerine or calcium channel blockers.[8,21] Intravenous nitroglycerine, despite being recognized as a potent uterine relaxant in other clinical settings (eg, uterine tachysystole and prolapse), has not been associated with an increase in ECV success in limited published studies. However, it is possible that study methodology may not have accounted for the very short duration of action of nitroglycerine relative to terbutaline, which may have accounted for these negative results.

Contraindications

There are several contraindications to ECV (**Box 3**). The decision to pursue ECV typically follows careful consideration of the risks and benefits to the mother and fetus. Conditions that are considered contraindications to ECV reflect not only circumstances associated with increased risks (eg, placenta previa and hemorrhage) but also conditions associated with decreased procedural success (eg, oligohydramnios and obesity).

Complications of ECV

Numerous complications have been reported in association with attempts at ECV (**Box 4**).[18,22] The incidence of each of these complications has not been well established; however, the most severe ones, including fetal death, are rare. Transient fetal bradycardia is very common and occasionally persists to the point of requiring emergent delivery. One of the advantages of neuraxial anesthesia is that it may facilitate rapid cesarean delivery without the use of general anesthesia.

Box 3
Contraindications to ECV

- Nonreassuring fetal status
- Placenta previa
- Placental abruption
- Intrauterine growth restriction
- Isoimmunization
- Severe preeclampsia
- Significant fetal or uterine anomalies

Relative contraindications (caused by decreased likelihood of ECV success)

- Oligohydramnios
- Maternal obesity
- Small for gestational age fetus (<10%)
- Ruptured membranes

Box 4
Complications associated with ECV procedures

- Fetal bradycardia
- Fetomaternal transfusion
- Vaginal bleeding
- Umbilical cord prolapse
- Fetal spinal cord injury
- Fetal intracranial hemorrhage
- Fetal death

ECV AND NEURAXIAL ANALGESIA
Maternal Pain and ECV

ECV is associated with significant maternal discomfort and anxiety. The maternal pain experience during this noninvasive, transient procedure is often significant; median maternal pain scores during unanesthetized ECV has been reported to be 5.6 on a 10-cm visual analog scale (interquartile range, 2.7–6.8).[23] This is perceived to be a barrier to achieving success during the procedure because increased maternal pain is inversely associated with procedural success. This is perhaps caused by either anatomic conditions resulting in a more difficult version procedure, splinting of abdominal muscles, or simply the obstetrician's premature termination of ECV because of maternal discomfort.

Neuraxial analgesia (encompassing spinal, epidural, or combined spinal epidural techniques) has been used by anesthesiologists to make ECV procedures more comfortable for women. Maternal pain and satisfaction are significantly improved even with "analgesic" (ie, subanesthetic) density blockade (**Fig. 4**). The administration of neuraxial analgesia may also help facilitate fetal movement by maximizing maternal abdominal muscle relaxation. Another possible benefit of neuraxial placement for ECV is the ability to dose an epidural catheter for surgical anesthesia, and thus avoid the

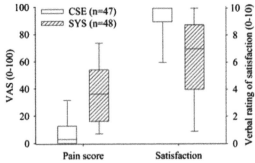

Fig. 4. Maternal satisfaction rating. Visual analog scale (VAS) pain scores (0–100 mm) and verbal rating scale scores of satisfaction (0–10) during external cephalic version. CSE, combined spinal-epidural; SYS, systemic analgesia. $P<.05$ between groups. (*From* Sullivan JT. A randomized controlled trial of the effect of combined spinal-epidural analgesia on the success of external cephalic version for breech presentation. Int J Obstet Anesth 2009;18(4):328–34; with permission.)

risks of airway management and general anesthesia should an emergent cesarean delivery become necessary during attempts to reposition the fetus.

In the past, critics of the use of neuraxial anesthesia for ECV have raised the concern that it may allow the obstetrician to use excessive force during the procedure, thus increasing the risk fetal morbidity. However, a meta-analysis of randomized controlled trials of neuraxial anesthesia versus intravenous or no analgesia does not suggest any difference in serious complications, such as placental abruption, between these groups. This lack of difference may be considered supportive, but not conclusive, of the safety of the use of neuraxial anesthesia for ECV (**Table 2**).

Procedural Success

Several randomized controlled trials have been conducted to address the relationship between neuraxial analgesia and the success of ECV. The anesthetic techniques and other investigative methodology differ subtly among these studies (**Table 3**); but allow for conclusions to be made. For example, differences among the studies have revealed important insights about medication dosing of the neuraxial technique. In all of the studies, tocolysis was used to facilitate ECV success.

When systematically reviewed, the six published, randomized controlled trials demonstrate an increase in the success rate of ECV with neuraxial anesthesia compared with intravenous analgesia or no analgesia (59.7% vs 37.6%; relative risk, 1.58; 95% confidence interval, 1.29–1.93).[24] The number needed to treat with neuraxial analgesia for one additional successful ECV was found to be five. The use of neuraxial anesthesia was also associated with an 11% reduction in cesarean delivery (from 59.3%–48.4%), although this did not reach statistical significance. However, the pooled studies were likely underpowered with regard to this more important clinical outcome. As the results of the last of these trials were published, an important dose-response effect emerged; specifically, that increased success was associated with denser neuraxial blockade (**Fig. 5**).[25] The local anesthetic dosing used in trials with a positive ECV outcome was equivalent to that used for surgical anesthesia during cesarean delivery.[26–28] Less dense (ie, "analgesic") blockade used within negative ECV outcome trials was equivalent to doses of local anesthetic used during labor analgesia.[25,29] When considering only those trials that used denser blockade, the effect on

Table 2		
Significant adverse events reported in randomized controlled trials with neuraxial anesthesia for ECV		
Principal Investigator, Year	Adverse Events- Treatment Group	Adverse Events-Control Group
Schorr et al,[26] 1997	0	0
Dugoff et al,[29] 1999	0	1 urgent cesarean delivery 3 h post-ECV for prolonged fetal heart rate deceleration ultimately diagnosed as placental abruption
Mancuso et al,[27] 2000	0	0
Weiniger et al,[28] 2007	0	0
Sullivan et al,[25] 2009	1 emergent cesarean delivery, fetal status	1 emergent cesarean delivery, fetal status
Weiniger,[38] 2010	0	0

Table 3
Methodology and results of randomized controlled trials of neuraxial anesthesia for ECV

Principal Investigator, Year	Sample Size	Anesthetic Technique	Success Treatment Group	Success Control Group	P Value	Notes
Schorr et al,[26] 1997	69	Epidural, lidocaine 2% with epinephrine (volume to obtain T6 level)	24/35 69%	11/34 32%	.01	—
Dugoff et al,[29] 1999	102	Spinal, bupivacaine 2.5 mg, sufentanil 10 μg	44%	42%	.863	—
Mancuso et al,[27] 2000	108	Epidural, lidocaine 2% with epinephrine 13 mL	59%	33%	<.05	—
Weiniger et al,[28] 2007	74	Spinal, bupivacaine 7.5 mg	67%	32%	.004	Nulliparous
Sullivan et al,[25] 2009	95	CSE spinal, bupivacaine 2.5 mg, fentanyl 25 μg	47%	31%	.14	Control: intravenous fentanyl 50 μg
Weiniger,[38] 2010	64	Spinal, bupivacaine 7.5 mg	87%	58%	.009	Parous

procedural success and vaginal delivery rates becomes more compelling. This dose-response phenomenon is further supported when two additional unpublished and non–peer-reviewed manuscripts are included in the analysis.[30]

One proposed methodology to approach ECV has been to escalate the intensity (and risk) of interventions with each successive failed attempt to turn the fetus. For example, an initial attempt at ECV (or series of attempts) could be made with tocolysis alone and without analgesia. If those attempts fail, subsequent attempts could be made with systemic analgesia, neuraxial anesthesia, and even escalating tocolysis. A high success rate has been reported with this methodology[31]; however, the manpower resource intensity of such a prolonged procedure may be a considerable disadvantage.

Neuraxial Anesthesia Complications and Resource Considerations

Denser anesthetic blockade is also associated with a greater degree of sympathectomy, hypotension, and need for more prolonged vigilance from the anesthetic team. This, in turn, requires greater resource use compared with less dense neuraxial techniques, systemic intravenous analgesia, or no anesthesia. Many ECVs are conducted in labor and delivery rooms, as opposed to operating suites, and it is unclear whether denser blockade necessitates escalating the procedure location to an operating room.

There has been a wide range of hypotension reported in conjunction with ECV using neuraxial anesthesia (8%[29] to 63%[25]). Factors that may be associated with this incidence include nonlaboring status, superimposed sympathectomy, and compression of the uterus against the inferior vena cava even amid adequate left uterine displacement. Vigilance of maternal hemodynamics and therapeutic or prophylactic

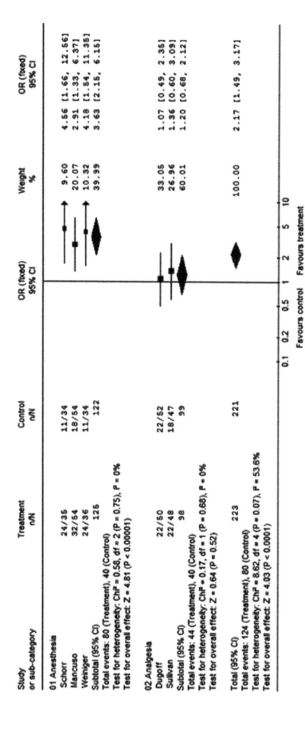

Study or sub-category	Treatment n/N	Control n/N	OR (fixed) 95% CI	Weight %	OR (fixed) 95% CI
01 Anesthesia					
Schorr	24/35	11/34		9.60	4.56 [1.66, 12.56]
Mancuso	32/54	18/54		20.07	2.91 [1.33, 6.37]
Weiniger	24/36	11/34		10.32	4.18 [1.54, 11.35]
Subtotal (95% CI)	125	122		39.99	3.63 [2.15, 6.15]
Total events: 80 (Treatment), 40 (Control)					
Test for heterogeneity: Chi² = 0.58, df = 2 (P = 0.75), I² = 0%					
Test for overall effect: Z = 4.81 (P < 0.00001)					
02 Analgesia					
Dugoff	22/50	22/52		33.05	1.07 [0.49, 2.35]
Sullivan	22/48	18/47		26.96	1.36 [0.60, 3.09]
Subtotal (95% CI)	98	99		60.01	1.20 [0.68, 2.12]
Total events: 44 (Treatment), 40 (Control)					
Test for heterogeneity: Chi² = 0.17, df = 1 (P = 0.68), I² = 0%					
Test for overall effect: Z = 0.64 (P = 0.52)					
Total (95% CI)	223	221		100.00	2.17 [1.49, 3.17]
Total events: 124 (Treatment), 80 (Control)					
Test for heterogeneity: Chi² = 8.62, df = 4 (P = 0.07), I² = 53.6%					
Test for overall effect: Z = 4.03 (P < 0.0001)					

0.1   0.2   0.5   1   2   5   10

Favours control   Favours treatment

Fig. 5. Meta-analysis of randomized controlled trials comparing neuraxial anesthesia versus analgesia for success of external cephalic version. Neuraxial treatment interventions were as follows: Schorr[26]: epidural lidocaine 2% to achieve T6 anesthesia; Mancuso[27]: epidural 2% lidocaine with epinephrine 1:200000, 13 mL; Weiniger[28]: intrathecal bupivacaine 7.5 mg; Dugoff[29]: intrathecal sufentanil 10 lg plus bupivacaine 2.5 mg; Present study: intrathecal fentanyl 15 lg plus bupivacaine 2.5 mg. The meta-analysis was performed using Review Manager (RevMan) [Computer program]. Version 4.2 for Windows. Copenhagen: The Nordic Cochrane Centre, The Cochrane Collaboration, 2003.

vasopressor strategies during ECV should be used. Naturally, all other reported complications from neuraxial anesthesia can occur during these antepartum procedures and their management generally does not significantly influence subsequent obstetric or anesthetic care.[28]

Economic Considerations

ECV and neuraxial anesthesia used to facilitate the success of ECV are likely cost-effective interventions.[32] Given the disparate system costs (including complications and subsequent pregnancy outcomes) between vaginal and cesarean delivery, the economic justification for ECV and anesthetic intervention become more favorable.

SUMMARY

ECV offers an opportunity to avoid planned cesarean delivery in parturients with singleton breech presentation at term. Tocolysis increases the likelihood of ECV procedural success. Because ECV is associated with a significant degree of maternal pain, neuraxial anesthesia during the procedure provides a superior maternal experience compared with systemic intravenous analgesia or no analgesia. Neuraxial anesthesia has been reported to increase the success of ECV procedures when surgical anesthetic dosing is used. Although ECV and neuraxial blockade have associated side effects and increased costs, it is likely justified given the potential effect of reducing cesarean delivery rates.

REFERENCES

1. Hickok DE. The frequency of breech presentation by gestational age at birth: a large population-based study. Am J Obstet Gynecol 1992;166(3):851–2.
2. Committee on Obstetric Practice. ACOG committee opinion. Mode of term singleton breech delivery. Number 265, December 2001. American College of Obstetricians and Gynecologists. Int J Gynaecol Obstet 2002;77(1):65–6.
3. Hofmeyr GJ. Interventions to help external cephalic version for breech presentation at term. Cochrane Database Syst Rev 2002;(2):CD000184.
4. Hofmeyr GJ. External cephalic version facilitation for breech presentation at term. Cochrane Database Syst Rev 2000;(2):CD000184.
5. Bewley S. The introduction of external cephalic version at term into routine clinical practice. Eur J Obstet Gynecol Reprod Biol 1993;52(2):89–93.
6. Yogev Y. Changing attitudes toward mode of delivery and external cephalic version in breech presentations. Int J Gynaecol Obstet 2002;79(3):221–4.
7. Caukwell S. Women's attitudes towards management of breech presentation at term. J Obstet Gynaecol 2002;22(5):486–8.
8. Cluver C. Interventions for helping to turn term breech babies to head first presentation when using external cephalic version. Cochrane Database Syst Rev 2012;(1):CD000184.
9. Coyle ME, Smith CA, Peat B. Cephalic version by moxibustion for breech presentation. Cochrane Database Syst Rev 2012;(5):CD003928.
10. Vas J. Using moxibustion in primary healthcare to correct non-vertex presentation: a multicentre randomised controlled trial. Acupunct Med 2012;31:31–8.
11. Hofmeyr GJ, Kulier R. Cephalic version by postural management for breech presentation. Cochrane Database Syst Rev 2012;(10):CD000051.
12. Hannah ME. Planned caesarean section versus planned vaginal birth for breech presentation at term: a randomised multicentre trial. Term Breech Trial Collaborative Group. Lancet 2000;356(9239):1375–83.

13. ACOG Committee on Obstetric Practice. ACOG Committee Opinion No. 340. Mode of term singleton breech delivery. Obstet Gynecol 2006;108(1):235–7.
14. Martin JA. Births: final data for 2009. Natl Vital Stat Rep 2011;60(1):1–70.
15. Vadnais M, Sachs B. Maternal mortality with cesarean delivery: a literature review. Semin Perinatol 2006;30(5):242–6.
16. Walker R, Turnbull D, Wilkinson C. Strategies to address global cesarean section rates: a review of the evidence. Birth 2002;29(1):28–39.
17. Kok M. Clinical factors to predict the outcome of external cephalic version: a metaanalysis. Am J Obstet Gynecol 2008;199(6):630.e1–7 [discussion: e1–5].
18. Zhang J, Bowes WA Jr, Fortney JA. Efficacy of external cephalic version: a review. Obstet Gynecol 1993;82(2):306–12.
19. Fortunato SJ, Mercer LJ, Guzick DS. External cephalic version with tocolysis: factors associated with success. Obstet Gynecol 1988;72(1):59–62.
20. Hutton EK, Hofmeyr GJ. External cephalic version for breech presentation before term. Cochrane Database Syst Rev 2006;(1):CD000084.
21. Wilcox CB, Nassar N, Roberts CL. Effectiveness of nifedipine tocolysis to facilitate external cephalic version: a systematic review. BJOG 2011;118(4): 423–8.
22. Collaris RJ, Oei SG. External cephalic version: a safe procedure? A systematic review of version-related risks. Acta Obstet Gynecol Scand 2004;83(6):511–8.
23. Fok WY. Maternal experience of pain during external cephalic version at term. Acta Obstet Gynecol Scand 2005;84(8):748–51.
24. Goetzinger KR. Effect of regional anesthesia on the success rate of external cephalic version: a systematic review and meta-analysis. Obstet Gynecol 2011; 118(5):1137–44.
25. Sullivan JT. A randomized controlled trial of the effect of combined spinal-epidural analgesia on the success of external cephalic version for breech presentation. Int J Obstet Anesth 2009;18(4):328–34.
26. Schorr SJ, Speights SE, Ross EL, et al. A randomized trial of epidural anesthesia to improve external cephalic version success. Am J Obstet Gynecol 1997;177(5): 1133–7.
27. Mancuso KM, Yancey MK, Murphy JA, et al. Epidural analgesia for cephalic version: a randomized trial. Obstet Gynecol 2000;95(5):648–51.
28. Weiniger CF, Ginosar Y, Elchalal U, et al. External cephalic version for breech presentation with or without spinal analgesia in nulliparous women at term: a randomized controlled trial. Obstet Gynecol 2007;110(6):1343–50.
29. Dugoff L, Stamm CA, Jones OW 3rd, et al. The effect of spinal anesthesia on the success rate of external cephalic version: a randomized trial. Obstet Gynecol 1999;93(3):345–9.
30. Lavoie A, Guay J. Anesthetic dose neuraxial blockade increases the success rate of external fetal version: a meta-analysis. Can J Anaesth 2010;57(5):408–14.
31. Cherayil G. Central neuraxial blockade promotes external cephalic version success after a failed attempt. Anesth Analg 2002;94(6):1589–92 [table of contents].
32. Tan JM. Cost-effectiveness of external cephalic version for term breech presentation. BMC Pregnancy Childbirth 2010;10:3.
33. Ben-Rafael Z. Uterine anomalies. A retrospective, matched-control study. J Reprod Med 1991;36(10):723–7.
34. Soernes T, Bakke T. The length of the human umbilical cord in vertex and breech presentations. Am J Obstet Gynecol 1986;154(5):1086–7.
35. Ford JB. Recurrence of breech presentation in consecutive pregnancies. BJOG 2010;117(7):830–6.

36. Fianu S, Vaclavinkova V. The site of placental attachment as a factor in the aetiology of breech presentation. Acta Obstet Gynecol Scand 1978;57(4): 371–2.

37. Nordtveit TI. Maternal and paternal contribution to intergenerational recurrence of breech delivery: population based cohort study. BMJ 2008;336(7649):872–6.

38. Weiniger CF, Ginosar Y, Elchalal U, et al. Randomized controlled trial of external cephalic version in term multiparae with or without spinal analgesia. Br J Anaesth 2010;104(5):613–8.

Maternal Anesthesia for Fetal Surgery

Hans P. Sviggum, MD[a,b,]*, Bhavani Shankar Kodali, MD[b]

KEYWORDS

- Fetal surgery • Obstetric anesthesia • Fetal anesthesia • EXIT procedure

KEY POINTS

- Fetal surgery is increasingly becoming a beneficial intervention for many fetal anomalies diagnosed in utero.
- Physiologic and anatomic changes related to pregnancy may require adaptations of surgical and anesthetic techniques.
- Open fetal procedures and ex utero intrapartum therapy (EXIT) procedures typically are performed under general anesthesia, whereas minimally invasive procedures are routinely performed under neuraxial or local anesthesia.
- Maternal complications associated with fetal surgery include difficulties in airway management, hemorrhage, infection, preterm labor, premature membrane separation, thromboembolism, and pulmonary edema.
- Anesthesiologists must consider the anesthetic requirements of the fetus, including immobility and analgesia.
- A multidisciplinary approach with input and communication between nursing, obstetrics, pediatrics, surgery, maternal-fetal medicine, and anesthesiology optimizes coordinated care of both mother and fetus.

INTRODUCTION

Fetal surgery (**Box 1**) has evolved into a mainstream mode of therapy, giving many fetuses with significant anomalies an increased chance of survival.[1] Improvements in diagnostic and therapeutic technology, along with advances in understanding fetal pathophysiology and the natural history of many of these conditions, have opened the

Funding Sources: None.
Conflict of Interest: None.
[a] Department of Anesthesiology, Mayo Clinic College of Medicine, 200 First Street Southwest, Rochester, MN 55905, USA; [b] Department of Anesthesiology, Brigham and Women's Hospital, 75 Francis Street, CWN-L1, Boston, MA 02115, USA
* Corresponding author. Department of Anesthesiology, Mayo Clinic College of Medicine, 200 First Street SW, Rochester, MN 55905.
E-mail address: sviggum.hans@mayo.edu

Box 1
Fetal surgery overview

Techniques

1. Open fetal surgery

2. Minimally invasive fetal surgery

3. EXIT procedure: distinct fetal surgical technique, which includes a fetal procedure at the time of cesarean delivery

Goals

1. Correct or improve a fetal anomaly

2. Minimize the risks posed to the mother

---

door for prenatal surgical interventions to prevent irreversible organ damage or fetal demise.

It is estimated that approximately 1000 fetal surgeries were performed in 2012 in the United Sates, and this number likely will rise substantially in the near future.[2] Currently, only certain fetal anomalies are amenable to in utero intervention during pregnancy whereas other conditions are better managed at or after delivery. Fetal surgery is a reasonable option if several specific conditions are met (**Box 2**).

Providing anesthesia for fetal surgery presents a unique challenge, because more than one patient needs to be considered. The parturient has been referred to as an "innocent bystander," who is exposed to surgical and postpartum risk but receives no health benefits.[3] The mother should always be protected from undue risks.[4,5]

MATERNAL ANESTHETIC ASPECTS OF FETAL SURGERY

An understanding of maternal physiologic and anatomic changes during pregnancy helps anesthesiologists safely care for the mother. Although these changes are usually well tolerated, even subtle disturbances can have an impact on management. There are several changes that occur during pregnancy that can influence anesthetic management (**Table 1**).

Inhalational anesthetics have a long history of successful outcomes in pregnancy. Local and regional anesthetic techniques are often used, however, in pregnant patients for the following reasons[6]:

Box 2
Conditions that must be met for fetal surgery to be a reasonable option

- Informed consent obtained from parent(s)

- Correct diagnosis of a significant isolated fetal anomaly

- Accurate assessment of fetal anomaly, both in severity and prognosis

- Maternal risks of surgery and anesthesia acceptably low

- Reason to believe that neonatal outcome would be improved more by in utero intervention than by postnatal surgery

- Multidisciplinary team in agreement regarding the treatment plan

- Patients with access to high-level medical, bioethical, and psychosocial care

---

Table 1
Important systemic changes of pregnancy

System	Changes	Notes
Cardiovascular	Cardiac output increases 30%–50% Systemic vascular resistance decreases 30%	Due to increases in both heart rate and stroke volume
Respiratory	Minute ventilation increases 40%–50% Oxygen consumption increases 20%–40% Function residual capacity is reduced 20% Normal $Paco_2$ is 28–32 mm Hg	Mostly due to increased tidal volume Leads to rapid progression to hypoxia on apnea Alveolar-arterial gradient is lower
Gastrointestinal	Upward rotation of stomach Progesterone effect Increased incidence of reflux	Relaxation of lower esophageal sphincter tone Increased risk of aspiration
Hematologic	Plasma volume increases more than red blood cell volume increases Most clotting factors increase Protein and albumin levels decrease	Physiologic anemia (hematocrit 33%–36%) Consider thromboprophylaxis Increased risk for edema
Renal	Renal blood flow and glomerular filtration rate increase	Normal serum creatinine values are lower (0.5–0.8)
Nervous	Minimal alveolar concentration decreases 30%–40% More extensive block after neuraxial anesthesia	Reduce doses for spinal and epidural anesthesia
Anatomic	Weight gain, soft tissue edema, increased vascularity of mucous membranes Enlarging gravid uterus, polyhydraminos	Each contributes to difficult airway management Leads to aortocaval compression

- Improved pain control
- Reduced need for airway management
- Reduced fetal drug exposure
- Increased maternal safety
- Patient preference

Fetal surgery is most often performed in the latter part of the second trimester or early in the third trimester of pregnancy, with the exception of EXIT procedures that are performed at the time of cesarean delivery. Patients undergoing fetal surgery safely undergo general, neuraxial, or local anesthesia, depending on the type of procedure. Although care should be adapted to individual patients, there are a few generalities that apply to nearly all patients undergoing fetal surgery (**Box 3**).

Prevention of preterm labor is an essential part of fetal surgery.[7] Tocolytic agents are used before, during, and after surgery, depending on the risk for preterm labor. Although well tolerated by most patients, they can contribute to maternal complications, including the development of pulmonary edema.[8] Other essential components of fetal surgery include blood pressure management (**Box 4**) and airway management (**Box 5**).

Women with pregnancy-induced disease states (eg, preeclampsia) or other significant comorbidities are usually not considered candidates for fetal interventions.

Box 3
Considerations for all patients undergoing fetal surgery

- Aspiration prophylaxis with multiple agents
- Left lateral decubitus positioning to prevent aortocaval compression
- Restrictive use of intravenous (IV) fluids to limit pulmonary edema
- Maintenance of end-tidal CO_2 in normal range for pregnancy (30–34 mm Hg)
- Aggressive blood pressure treatment to maintain uteroplacental perfusion
- Developing a plan for adequate postoperative pain control
- Necessary equipment and personnel available should delivery become imminent

---

Although there are no clear guidelines for the exclusion of candidates for fetal surgery, any coexisting disease that places the mother at a greater surgical or anesthetic risk may be reason to withdraw her from consideration for the procedure. Anesthesiologists must participate in multidisciplinary presurgical assessment efforts to determine whether maternal risk is acceptably low for the potential fetal benefit.

FETAL ANESTHETIC ASPECTS OF FETAL SURGERY

Maternal anesthesia can have both direct (**Box 6**) and indirect effects on the fetus. Intrauterine asphyxia is the most important fetal risk, and anything that disrupts maternal oxygenation, ventilation, perfusion, or acid-base status is a potential threat to the fetus. Although transient mild decreases in maternal oxygenation or blood pressure are usually well tolerated by the fetus, maintenance of normal maternal hemodynamic parameters is critical to maintaining adequate uteroplacental blood flow. In addition, maternal hypercapnia can lead to fetal acidosis whereas hyperventilation can decrease maternal cardiac output, create uteroplacental vasoconstriction, and cause

---

Box 4
Blood pressure management

Rationale: maintaining normal or baselinematernal blood pressure during fetal surgery is vital for ensuring adequate uteroplacental perfusion.

Agents: historically, ephedrine has been the vasopressor of choice during pregnancy. Recent experience has shown, however, both phenylephrine and ephedrine are safe and effective at maintaining maternal blood pressure.[9,10]

Clinical pearls: the decision to use phenylephrine, ephedrine, or both in combination should be individualized and guided by the maternal heart rate, suspected cause of hypotension, and fetal heart rate tracing. Regardless of the agent used, therapy should be administered as soon as the blood pressure begins to decrease rather than after the occurrence of clinically significant hypotension.

Adjuncts: noninvasive cardiac output monitoring may be useful in guiding blood pressure management and optimizing treatment.

Data from Cooper DW, Carpenter M, Mowbray P, et al. Fetal and maternal effects of phenylephrine and ephedrine during spinal anesthesia for cesarean delivery. Anesthesiology 2002;97:1582–90; and Lee A, Ngan Kee WD, Gin T. A quantitative systematic review of randomized controlled trials of ephedrine versus phenylephrine for the management of hypotension during spinal anesthesia for cesarean delivery. Anesth Analg 2002;94:920–6.

Box 5
Airway management

Pregnant patients have a higher incidence of difficult airway management than nonpregnant patients, with the rates of difficult and failed intubation approaching 3.3% and 0.4% of cases, respectively.[11]

A recent study confirmed that the expected incidence of failed tracheal intubation is approximately 8 times higher in pregnant patients (1:224) than in the general population.[12]

Pregnant patients are also at higher risk for gastric aspiration.[13] In addition, they have a reduced functional residual capacity and an increased metabolic rate that can result in a rapid progression to hypoxia on induction of general anesthesia.[14]

Recent advances in video laryngoscopy have increased intubation success,[15] and this likely holds true in the pregnant population as well.[16]

---

a leftward shift of the oxyhemoglobin dissociation curve—all of which can compromise fetal oxygenation.

The question of whether a fetus experiences pain continues to be a challenge.[20] Fetuses undergoing procedures at mid to late gestation may have the requisite neural development and the hormonal and hemodynamic stress responses to noxious stimuli to indicate they are capable of experiencing pain.[29–31] Despite ongoing debate regarding fetal experiences of pain, fetal anesthesia and analgesia are warranted for fetal surgical procedures because they serve additional purposes unrelated to pain reduction,[29] including

---

Box 6
Anesthetic effects on the fetus

Volatile anesthetics

These have direct depressant effects on fetal cardiovascular system. Low concentrations (1–1.5 minimal alveolar concentration) have minimal fetal effects in animal models.[17] Higher concentrations may result in fetal acidosis,[18] although prolonged or deep maternal inhalation anesthesia has not been shown to cause fetal hypoxia or acidosis clinically.[19]

Intravenous agents

Induction agents and opioids can decrease fetal heart rate variability but do not lead to fetal morbidity as long as maternal hemodynamic parameters remain stable.[20]

Teratogenicity

There is no evidence of teratogenicity of anesthetic agents used at clinical concentrations and doses in pregnant women undergoing surgery.[21] Several early retrospective studies linked first-trimester diazepam use with an increased incidence of cleft palate; however, the current consensus is that benzodiazepines are safe for clinical use.[22,23]

Neurodevelopmental consequences

Some animal studies show that an exposure of an immature brain to anesthetic agents can cause neurodegeneration, decreased spatial recognition, impaired memory, and subsequent learning problems.[24,25] This evidence is weak, however, and mixed within human studies.[26] These adverse neurodevelopmental consequences may be attenuated or blocked by providing adequate fetal analgesia and anesthesia.[27]

A recent review suggests changes in clinical practice should not be based on animal studies and that a change in current practice is currently unwarranted.[28]

- Inhibiting fetal movement
- Achieving uterine relaxation
- Preventing hormonal stress responses associated with poor fetal outcomes
- Possibly preventing adverse effects on long-term neurodevelopment and behavior responses to pain

The current consensus is to provide fetal analgesia and anesthesia during all potentially painful fetal interventions.[32]

Fetal anesthesia and analgesia can be achieved by placental transfer of agents given to the mother or by direct fetal administration intramuscularly or through umbilical vessels. Intra-amniotic administration of agents can potentially be effective,[33] although this is not routinely used in practice. Fetal anesthesia helps prevent fetal movements and has also been shown to blunt fetal stress responses to noxious stimuli.[34] Medications that may be used for fetal anesthesia, immobility, or resuscitation include

- Fentanyl (10–50 μg/kg)
- Vecuronium (0.1–0.3 mg/kg) or pancuronium (0.1–0.3 mg/kg)
- Atropine (0.02 mg/kg)
- Epinephrine (1 μg/kg)

These medications should be ready for the surgeon to administer in single-dose syringes to avoid accidental overdosing.[19] If the clinical situation dictates, O-negative, cytomegalovirus-negative, leukocyte-depleted blood should be available in 5 mL/kg to 10 mL/kg aliquots in case fetal transfusion becomes necessary.

Open Fetal Surgery

Open surgery involves a hysterotomy. An epidural is placed for postoperative pain control but is not dosed before surgery to avoid any contribution to intraoperative hypotension. Preoperative intrathecal opioids can be used as an alternative to epidural analgesia. After a rapid sequence induction and intubation, volatile anesthetics are used for anesthetic maintenance because they produce dose-dependent uterine relaxation desired for optimal surgical exposure and placental gas exchange.[20,35] Isoflurane is less potent than desflurane or sevoflurane in producing uterine relaxation,[36] although all 3 agents have been used successfully. Early institution of high concentrations of volatile agents for long periods of time before hysterotomy may cause hypotension and has also resulted in the development of intraoperative fetal bradycardia, especially with the use of desflurane.[37] It may be prudent to use supplemental IV anesthesia initially and only increase the volatile anesthetic concentrations to 2 to 3 minimal alveolar concentration to achieve the desired uterine tone just before hysterotomy. An arterial line is usually placed after induction for close monitoring of blood pressure. Central venous access is rarely needed.

The surgeon assesses uterine tone for adequate relaxation before hysterotomy. IV nitroglycerin boluses (50–100 μg IV) or infusion (0.5–1 μg/kg/min IV) can be used for uterine relaxation when placental transfer of volatile agent is not sufficient to obtain optimal uterine tone. In cases when neuraxial anesthesia is used, IV nitroglycerin can be used as the sole agent for intraoperative uterine relaxation.[38,39] This technique may be associated with greater maternal morbidity, including hypotension, reflex tachycardia, methemoglobinemia, tachyphylaxis, headache, and pulmonary edema.[40,41] After ensuring placental positioning, the uterine incision is made with a stapling device to prevent excessive bleeding and seal the membranes to the endometrium. Amnioinfusion with warm lactated Ringer solution is used to keep the fetus warm, maintain uterine volume, and prevent umbilical cord compression.[40] Vasopressors are commonly needed to maintain adequate maternal blood pressure (maintaining utero-placental perfusion), particularly with the use of high concentrations of volatile anesthetics. IV fluids should be limited to reduce risk of postoperative pulmonary edema.[5]

Fetal well-being can be assessed intraoperatively with fetal pulse oximetry, intermittent or continuous fetal echocardiography, fetal scalp electrodes, and umbilical blood sampling.[35] Although placental transfer of inhalational agents may provide adequate fetal anesthesia and immobility, fentanyl and a muscle relaxant are commonly administered directly to the fetus (intramuscularly) (discussed previously). After uterine closure, the volatile agent can be greatly reduced or discontinued to limit its effect on uterine tone. Anesthesia can be maintained with IV agents (eg, propofol) and/or nitrous oxide. The epidural catheter is activated after ensuring hemostasis and hemodynamic stability, facilitating a timely, comfortable emergence. Coughing or straining during emergence should be avoided to prevent disruption of the uterine closure.

Adequate postoperative pain control is associated with lower maternal concentrations of oxytocin,[42] reducing the risks of uterine contractions and preterm labor. If needed, systemic opioids can supplement a functioning epidural catheter. Preoperative rectal indomethacin (50 mg) and postprocedure magnesium sulfate (4–6 g IV loading dose, followed by 1–2 g/h IV infusion) are administered for tocolysis.[43] If uterine contractions persist, additional tocolysis with indomethacin, nifedipine, or terbutaline may be used.[7] Magnesium potentiates the effects of nondepolarizing muscle relaxants, and diligent monitoring of neuromuscular function is required (**Box 7**).

Emergence from anesthesia is a critical time period. A review of maternal deaths at cesarean delivery under general anesthesia revealed that no maternal deaths occurred during induction or maintenance of anesthesia; all the deaths occurred during extubation and emergence from anesthesia.[45] Extubation should only occur when a patient is fully awake and responsive and when muscle relaxation has been reversed to minimize the chance of gastric aspiration or loss of airway tone.

Mothers undergoing open fetal surgery are typically not allowed to labor in current or future pregnancies due to increased risk of uterine rupture after vertical uterine incisions, rates of which are comparable to those after classic cesarean section.[46] Other potential maternal risks of open fetal surgery include[5]

- Pulmonary edema
- Hemorrhage
- Premature rupture of membranes

Box 7
Neuromuscular blockade

Neuromuscular blocking drugs do not readily cross the placental barrier. They do not produce uterine relaxation.

Despite increased hepatic clearance, pregnant patients are more sensitive to nondepolarizing neuromuscular blocking drugs.

The duration of succinylcholine-induced block may be reduced due to an increased volume of distribution (despite reduced plasma cholinesterase), although clinical dosing for intubation is the same as in nonpregnant patients.

Despite both being quaternary compounds, neostigmine may cross the placenta more readily than glycopyrrolate due to its low molecular weight. If there is concern about neostigmine-induced fetal bradycardia during reversal of neuromuscular blockade, atropine can be used instead of glycopyrrolate because it freely crosses the placenta.[44]

- Chorion-amnion membrane separation
- Preterm labor
- Preterm delivery (and subsequent complications of prematurity)
- Fetal demise
- Chorioamnionitis
- Placental abruption
- Increased need for maternal transfusion at the time of delivery

Most mothers tolerate surgery well, however, and ICU admissions are generally not necessary.

Minimally Invasive Fetal Surgery

To reduce maternal and fetal morbidity, surgical approaches without large incisions or a hysterotomy have been developed, which reduce the stresses inflicted on mother and fetus compared with open surgery.[1] These minimally invasive endoscopic, percutaneous, and image-guided procedures on the fetus, placenta, or membranes have evolved from largely diagnostic procedures into therapeutic modalities that have proved successful for treating many fetal conditions, including

- Twin-twin transfusion syndrome: laser ablation of vessels[47]
- Obstructive uropathy: shunt insertion and valve ablation[48]
- Aortic or pulmonary stenosis: valvuloplasty (**Fig. 1**)[49]
- Cyanotic heart disease: atrial septostomy[50]
- Congenital diaphragmatic hernia: tracheal balloon occlusion[51]
- Spina bifida: fetoscopic closure of the malformation[52]
- Twin reversed arterial perfusion: radiofrequency ablation[53]

Maternal anesthetic management for minimally invasive surgery has both similarities and differences compared with open fetal surgery and EXIT procedures (**Box 8, Table 2**).

When using local or regional anesthesia, the fetus does not receive any anesthesia, analgesia, or immobility.[55] Many minimally invasive procedures (eg, selective laser

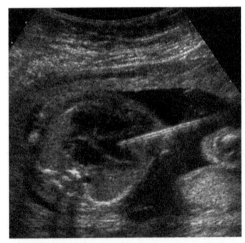

Fig. 1. Ultrasound-guided needle placement into fetal left ventricle. A balloon catheter was subsequently placed through the needle across the aortic valve for performance of aortic valvuloplasty.

Box 8
Anesthesia for minimally invasive surgery

General, neuraxial, and local anesthetic techniques have been used successfully for minimally invasive surgeries.[54]

If general anesthesia is used, less volatile anesthetic is needed compared with open surgery because uterine relaxation is not necessary.

Profound uterine relaxation can make maintaining correct fetal position difficult.

Maternal hemodynamic stability may be achieved more easily with neuraxial anesthesia for fetoscopic fetal surgery.

Neuraxial anesthesia is chosen over local anesthesia based on the following factors[20]:

1. Anatomic location of surgery

2. Length and complexity of procedure

3. Desire for postoperative analgesia

4. Probability of progressing to cesarean delivery

---

photocoagulation of communicating vessels) do not require fetal immobilization or anesthesia, whereas others do to prevent fetal movement, responses to noxious stimuli, and pain (eg, aortic valvuloplasty). Supplemental maternal sedation and analgesia with IV opioids, benzodiazepines, and/or low-dose propofol can provide varying

---

Table 2
Comparing management of different types of fetal surgery

	Open Surgery	Minimally Invasive	EXIT
Gestational age	Late 2nd/early 3rd trimester	Late 2nd/early 3rd trimester	Time of delivery
Maternal anesthesia	General, epidural for postoperative analgesia	Local or neuraxial anesthesia[a] ± IV sedation	General, ± epidural for postoperative analgesia
Desired uterine tone	Complete relaxation	Minimal relaxation	Complete relaxation
Fetal anesthesia	Transplacental inhalation agents, direct (IM or umbilical cord) opioids and muscle relaxants	Direct (IM or umbilical cord) opioids and muscle relaxants or transplacental opioids[b]	Transplacental inhalation agents, direct (IM or umbilical cord) opioids and muscle relaxants
Preterm labor risk	Increased	Minimal	Not applicable
Invasive blood pressure monitoring	Yes	No	Yes
Amnioinfusion	Yes	No	Yes
Future labor allowed	No	Yes	Yes

Abbreviation: IM, intramuscular.
  [a] Local anesthesia is used mostly for surgery on the placenta or membranes. Neuraxial anesthesia is used for more complex fetoscopic procedures.
  [b] Remifentanil is most reliable.

degrees of fetal immobility and anesthesia via placental transfer. Specifically, remifentanil has been shown to provide adequate maternal sedation and fetal immobilization.[56] Direct intramuscular or umbilical vein administration of a nondepolarizing muscle relaxant results in onset of fetal paralysis in approximately 2 minutes, lasting for 1 to 2 hours.[57] Similarly, direct opioid administration to the fetus supplements any medications given to the mother. Atropine is often coadministered to prevent fetal bradycardia. At the authors' institution, ultrasound-guided intramuscular fentanyl and vecuronium are given for fetal immobility and anesthesia for all fetoscopic procedures performed under maternal regional anesthesia.

Unlike with open fetal surgery, patients undergoing minimally invasive surgery are usually allowed to labor in their current and future pregnancies. Compared with open fetal surgery, there is a reduced risk of preterm labor and delivery due to less uterine manipulation and trauma. Risks of chorion-amnion membrane separation, preterm rupture of membranes, infection, and bleeding remain as well as morbidity associated with improper endoscope or needle placements.[7]

Ex utero Intrapartum Treatment Procedures

The EXIT procedure is a modification of cesarean delivery. Although placental support is maintained, the baby is partially (head and upper torso) or, less often, completely delivered. Procedures needed for the infant's survival are performed before clamping the umbilical cord and completing the delivery (**Figs. 2** and **3**). The EXIT procedure is primarily performed in cases of potential airway compromise to allow for continuing placental perfusion and oxygenation until a definitive airway has been established. Most procedures last a matter of minutes (eg, tracheal intubation), but procedures lasting more than 2 hours have been successfully performed.[58] Although pregnancy should be extended close to term to decrease the complications of prematurity, the EXIT procedure is ideally performed before onset of labor or development of fetal compromise.

Most EXIT procedures are performed with the mother under general anesthesia, using high concentrations of volatile anesthetics at the time of hysterotomy for uterine relaxation.[40] Uterine relaxation is important not only to facilitate delivery of fetal head but also to prevent placental separation and to preserve uteroplacental flow during the procedure. An arterial line for close blood pressure monitoring and judicious use of vasoactive medications to maintain normotension and adequate uteroplacental blood flow are imperative, similar to open fetal surgery.

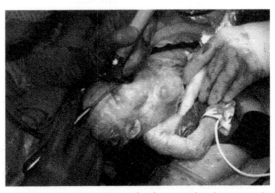

Fig. 2. EXIT procedure showing intubation of a fetus with a large cervical teratoma.

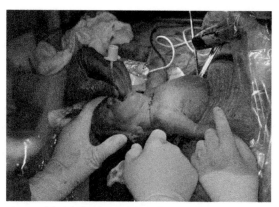

Fig. 3. EXIT procedure with intubation and neck incision for extracorporeal membrane oxygenation initiation in a fetus with severe congenital heart disease.

An epidural catheter may be placed preoperatively for postoperative analgesia. Rapid sequence induction and intubation are used to secure the airway, as described previously for open fetal surgery. Amnioinfusion with warm lactated Ringer solution is provided to keep the fetus warm, maintain uterine volume, and prevent umbilical cord compression.[40] Fetal analgesia and anesthesia can be directly administered as previously described, either before (under ultrasound guidance) or after (under direct vision) hysterotomy. When neuraxial anesthesia is performed, IV nitroglycerin is used for profound and transient uterine relaxation (described previously).[38,39]

Ideally, a second anesthesiologist dedicated to the baby ensures that there is necessary equipment (eg, pulse oximeter) and medications for the fetus. A second adjacent operating room should be available if additional surgery should be needed on the baby after delivery. Increased uterine blood flow during pregnancy, reduced uterine tone from volatile anesthetics and tocolytics, and possible need for vertical uterine incision all increase the risk of hemorrhage, particular during lengthy procedures.[59,60] Blood products for both mother and baby should be available for administration.

After complete delivery of the baby, uterine tone should be prioritized to prevent excessive bleeding from uterine atony and the placental bed. Reducing or eliminating volatile anesthesia in favor of IV agents with or without nitrous oxide and administering oxytocin can accomplish this. Additional uterotonic agents should be available in case uterine atony persists.[40] After ensuring hemodynamic stability, the epidural catheter may be loaded with a bolus of local anesthetic and opioid to ensure patient comfort at the time of emergence. With adequate preparation and vigilance, maternal outcomes after EXIT procedures are comparable to those after cesarean delivery.[58,61]

Postoperative Management

Postoperative maternal management of patients undergoing fetal surgery includes

- Close monitoring of fetal heart rate and uterine activity during the immediate postoperative period after minimally invasive surgery and for the first 24 to 48 hours after open fetal surgery
- Adequate analgesia using a multimodal regimen with acetaminophen, opioids (oral, parenteral, or neuraxial), neuraxial and local anesthetics, nonpharmacologic modalities, or a combination of these

- Consideration of venous thromboprophylaxis, especially in those patients with limited mobility
- Postoperative tocolytic administration as part of a regimen designed to prevent preterm labor

SUMMARY

Maternal fetal surgery is a multidisciplinary effort that requires vigilant communication between teams of physicians and nurses. Maternal anesthetic care can be demanding because of the physiologic and anatomic changes associated with pregnancy. Maintenance of adequate blood pressure, prevention of hypoxia and acidosis, and providing adequate analgesia are the cornerstones of creating a safe environment for the fetus. In addition to providing maternal anesthesia, it is recommended to provide adequate fetal anesthesia and analgesia during potentially painful procedures during in utero life.

Not all infants benefit from early intervention and fetal surgery. More work is needed to determine whether baseline characteristics can predict which fetuses are more or less likely to benefit from prenatal surgery and in developing less traumatic approaches to fetal interventions.[62] Further studies are also needed to determine the optimal anesthetic technique that ensures maternal and fetal cardiovascular stability, optimal uteroplacental perfusion, necessary uterine relaxation, adequate fetal anesthesia and immobility, minimal fetal myocardial depression, and adequate blockade of the fetal stress response.

REFERENCES

1. Deprest JA, Flake AW, Gratacos E, et al. The making of fetal surgery. Prenat Diagn 2010;30:653–67.
2. Zoler M. Myelomeningocele repair drives changes in fetal surgery. Pediatr News 2012;1–5.
3. Farmer D. Fetal surgery. BMJ 2003;326:461–2.
4. Longaker MT, Golbus MS, Filly RA, et al. Maternal outcome after open fetal surgery: a review of the first 17 human cases. JAMA 1991;265:737–41.
5. Golombeck K, Ball RH, Lee H, et al. Maternal morbidity after maternal-fetal surgery. Am J Obstet Gynecol 2006;194:834–9.
6. Rollins M, Lucero J. Overview of anesthetic considerations for cesarean delivery. Br Med Bull 2012;101:105–25.
7. Gupta R, Kilby M, Cooper G. Fetal surgery and anaesthetic implications. Contin Educ Anaesth Crit Care Pain 2008;8:71–5.
8. Ogunyemi D. Risk factors for acute pulmonary edema in preterm delivery. Eur J Obstet Gynecol Reprod Biol 2007;133:143–7.
9. Cooper DW, Carpenter M, Mowbray P, et al. Fetal and maternal effects of phenylephrine and ephedrine during spinal anesthesia for cesarean delivery. Anesthesiology 2002;97:1582–90.
10. Lee A, Ngan Kee WD, Gin T. A quantitative systematic review of randomized controlled trials of ephedrine versus phenylephrine for the management of hypotension during spinal anesthesia for cesarean delivery. Anesth Analg 2002; 94:920–6.
11. McDonnell NJ, Paech MJ, Clavisi OM, et al. Difficult and failed intubation in obstetric anaesthesia: an observational study of airway management and complications associated with general anaesthesia for cesarean section. Int J Obstet Anesth 2008;17:292–7.

12. Quinn AC, Milne D, Columb M, et al. Failed tracheal intubation in obstetric anaesthesia: 2 yr national case-control study in the UK. Br J Anaesth 2013; 110:74–80.

13. Engelhardt T, Webster NR. Pulmonary aspiration of gastric contents in anaesthesia. Br J Anaesth 1999;83:453–60.

14. McClelland SH, Bogod DG, Hardman JG. Apnoea in pregnancy: an investigation using physiological modeling. Anaesthesia 2008;63:264–9.

15. Aziz MF, Dillman D, Fu R, et al. Comparative effectiveness of the C-MAC video laryngoscope versus direct laryngoscopy in the setting of the predicted difficult airway. Anesthesiology 2012;116:629–36.

16. Aziz MF, Kim D, Mako J, et al. A retrospective study of the performance of video laryngoscopy in an obstetric unit. Anesth Analg 2012;115:904–6.

17. Okutomi T, Whittington RA, Stein DJ, et al. Comparison of the effects of sevoflurane and isoflurane anesthesia on the maternal-fetal unit in sheep. J Anesth 2009;23:392–8.

18. Palahniuk RJ, Shnider SM. Maternal and fetal cardiovascular and acid-base changes during halothane and isoflurane anesthesia in the pregnant ewe. Anesthesiology 1974;41:462–72.

19. Rosen MA. Anesthesia for fetal surgery and other intrauterine procedures. In: Chestnut DH, editor. Obstetric anesthesia. 4th edition. Philadelphia: Mosby Elsevier; 2009. p. 123–40.

20. Van de Velde M, De Buck F. Fetal and maternal analgesia/anesthesia for fetal procedures. Fetal Diagn Ther 2012;31:201–9.

21. Mazze RI, Kallen B. Reproductive outcome after anesthesia and operation during pregnancy: a registry study of 5405 cases. Am J Obstet Gynecol 1989;161: 1178–85.

22. Dolovich LR, Addis A, Vaillancourt JM, et al. Benzodiazepine use in pregnancy and major malformations or oral cleft: meta-analysis of cohort and case-control studies. BMJ 1998;317:839–43.

23. Wikner BN, Stiller CO, Bergman U, et al. Use of benzodiazepines and benzodiazepine receptor agonists during pregnancy: neonatal outcome and congenital malformations. Pharmacoepidemiol Drug Saf 2007;16:1203–10.

24. Creeley C. The young: neuroapoptosis induced by anesthetics and what to do about it. Anesth Analg 2010;110:442–8.

25. Jevtovic-Todorovic V, Hartman RE, Izumi Y, et al. Early exposure to common anesthetic agents causes widespread neurodegeneration in the developing rat brain and persistent learning deficits. J Neurosci 2003;23:876–82.

26. Wilder RT. Is there any relationship between long-term behavior disturbance and early exposure to anesthesia? Curr Opin Anaesthesiol 2010;23:332–6.

27. Lowery CL, Hardman MP, Manning N, et al. Neurodevelopmental changes of fetal pain. Semin Perinatol 2007;31:275–82.

28. Stratmann G. Neurotoxicity of anesthetic drugs in the developing brain. Anesth Analg 2011;113:1170–9.

29. Lee SJ, Peter Ralston HJ, Drey EA, et al. Fetal pain: a systematic multidisciplinary review of the evidence. JAMA 2005;294:947–54.

30. Giannakoulopoulos X, Sepúlveda W, Kourtis P, et al. Fetal plasma cortisol and betaendorphin response to intrauterine needling. Lancet 1994;344:77–81.

31. Teixeira JM, Glover V, Fisk NM. Acute cerebral redistribution in response to invasive procedures in the human fetus. Am J Obstet Gynecol 1999;181:1018–25.

32. Ramírez MV. Anestesiaparacirugía fetal. Rev Colomb Anestesiol 2012;40: 268–72.

33. Strumper D, Durieux ME, Gogarten W, et al. Fetal plasma concentrations after intraamniotic sufentanil in chronically instrumented pregnant sheep. Anesthesiology 2003;98:1400–6.

34. Fisk NM, Gitau R, Teixeira JM, et al. Effect of direct fetal opioid analgesia on fetal hormonal and hemodynamic stress response to intrauterine needling. Anesthesiology 2001;95:828–35.

35. De Buck F, Deprest J, Van de Velde M. Anesthesia for fetal surgery. Curr Opin Anaesthesiol 2008;21:293–7.

36. Yoo KY, Lee JC, Yoon MH, et al. The effects of volatile anesthetics on spontaneous contractility of isolated human pregnant uterine muscle: a comparison among sevvoflurane, desflurane, isoflurane, and halothane. Anesth Analg 2006;103:443–7.

37. Boat A, Mahmoud M, Michelfelder EC, et al. Supplementing desflurane with intravenous anesthesia reduces fetal cardiac dysfunction during open fetal surgery. Paediatr Anaesth 2010;20:748–56.

38. Clark KD, Viscomi CM, Lowell J, et al. Nitroglycerin for relaxation to establish a fetal airway (EXIT procedure). Obstet Gynecol 2004;103:113–5.

39. George RB, Melnick AH, Rose EC, et al. Case series: combined spinal epidural anesthesia for cesarean delivery and ex utero intrapartum treatment procedure. Can J Anaesth 2007;54:218–22.

40. Olutoye OO, Olutoye OA. EXIT procedure for fetal neck masses. Curr Opin Pediatr 2012;24:386–93.

41. Garcia PJ, Olutoye OO, Ivey RT, et al. Case scenario: anesthesia for maternal-fetal surgery. Anesthesiology 2011;114:1446–52.

42. Santolaya-Forgas J, Romero R, Mehendale R. The effect of continuous morphine administration on maternal plasma oxytocin concentration and uterine contractions after open fetal surgery. J Matern Fetal Neonatal Med 2006;19:231–8.

43. Adzick NS. Open fetal surgery for life-threatening fetal anomalies. Semin Fetal Neonatal Med 2010;15:1–8.

44. Clark RB, Brown MA, Lattin DL. Neostigmine, atropine, and glycopyrrolate: does neostigmine cross the placenta? Anesthesiology 1996;84:4502.

45. Mhyre JM, Riesner MN, Polley LS, et al. A series of anesthesia-related maternal deaths in Michigan, 1985-2003. Anesthesiology 2007;106:1096–104.

46. Wilson RD, Johnson MP, Flake AW, et al. Reproductive outcomes after pregnancy complicated by maternal-fetal surgery. Am J Obstet Gynecol 2004;191:1430–6.

47. Roberts D, Neilson JP, Kilby M, et al. Interventions for the treatment of twin-twin transfusion syndrome [review]. Cochrane Database Syst Rev 2008;(1):CD002073.

48. Casella DP, Tomaszewski JJ, Ost MC. Posterior urethral valves: renal failure and prenatal treatment. Int J Nephrol 2012. http://dx.doi.org/10.1155/2012/351067.

49. Tworetzky W, Wilkins-Haug L, Jennings RW, et al. Balloon dilation of severe aortic stenosis in the fetus: potential for prevention of hypoplastic left heart syndrome: candidate selection, technique, and results of successful intervention. Circulation 2004;110:2125–31.

50. Marshall AC, Van der Velde ME, Tworetzky W, et al. Creation of an atrial septal defect in utero for fetuses with hypoplastic left heart syndrome and intact or highly restrictive atrial septum. Circulation 2004;110:253–8.

51. Deprest J, Nicolaides K, Doné E, et al. Technical aspects of fetal endoscopic tracheal occlusion for congenital diaphragmatic hernia. J Pediatr Surg 2011;46:22–32.

52. Kohl T, Tchatcheva K, Merz W, et al. Percutaneous fetoscopic patch closure of human spina bifida aperta: advances in fetal surgcial techniques may obviate the need for early postnatal neurosurgical intervention. Surg Endosc 2009;23: 890–5.
53. Lee H, Wagner AJ, Sy E, et al. Efficacy of radiofrequency ablation for twin-reversed arterial perfusion sequence. Am J Obstet Gynecol 2007;196:459.e1–4.
54. Tran KM. Anesthesia for fetal surgery. Semin Fetal Neonatal Med 2010;15:40–5.
55. Van de Velde M, De Buck F, Van Mieghem T, et al. Fetal anaesthesia: is this necessary for fetoscopic therapy? Fetal Matern Med Rev 2010;21:24.
56. Van de Velde M, Van Schoubroeck D, Lewi LE, et al. Remifentanil for fetal immobilization and maternal sedation during fetoscopic surgery: a randomized, double-blind comparison with diazepam. Anesth Analg 2005;101:251–8.
57. Leveque C, Murat I, Toubas F, et al. Fetal neuromuscular blockade with vecuronium bromide: studies during intravascular intrauterine transfusion in isoimmunized pregnancies. Anesthesiology 1992;76:642–4.
58. Hirose S, Farmer DL, Lee H, et al. The ex utero intrapartum treatment procedure: looking back at the EXIT. J Pediatr Surg 2004;39:375–80.
59. Butwick A, Aleshi P, Yamout I. Obstetric hemorrhage during an EXIT procedure for severe fetal airway obstruction. Can J Anaesth 2009;56:437–42.
60. Marwan A, Crombleholme TM. The EXIT procedure: principles, pitfalls, and progress. Semin Pediatr Surg 2006;15:107–15.
61. Noah MM, Norton ME, Sandberg P, et al. Short-term maternal outcomes that are associated with the EXIT procedure, as compared with cesarean delivery. Am J Obstet Gynecol 2002;186:773–7.
62. Simpson JL, Greene MF. Fetal surgery for myelomeningocele? N Engl J Med 2011;11:1076–7.

Fetal Anesthesia and Pain Management for Intrauterine Therapy

Roland Brusseau, MD*, Arielle Mizrahi-Arnaud, MD

KEYWORDS

- Fetal anesthesia • Fetal access • Fetal drug delivery • Fetal monitoring
- Fetal resuscitation

KEY POINTS

- There is a range of fetal interventions that are undertaken; the nature of procedure, as well as its ramifications for maternal and fetal nociception, will dictate the nature of the fetal anesthetic.
- Fetal access may be limited, often requiring combined modalities of drug delivery (eg, transplacental and intramuscular).
- Fetal monitoring is often limited to fetal heart rate monitoring, requiring an understanding of fetal cardiovascular physiology and how medications and interventions may affect fetal well-being and how these are revealed by the fetal heart rate.
- Fetal cardiovascular collapse can be sudden, requiring that there be a fetal resuscitation plan in place before beginning an intervention.

A RANGE OF POSSIBLE FETAL INTERVENTIONS

As experience with fetal intervention has grown,[1] so too has the knowledge about fetal anesthesia and analgesia. With some endoscopic procedures, the site of surgical intervention is not innervated; thus, the fetus may not sense a noxious stimulus, and its anesthetic requirements may be minimal. Nevertheless, fetal immobility remains essential to procedural safety and success. Other interventions may require that a needle be inserted into the fetus, which may elicit a noxious stimulus and possibly even cause pain. Open procedures can produce significant noxious stimuli.

In addition to surgical demands, each mother and fetus exhibits a unique physiologic, pharmacologic, and pathophysiologic profile. Both fetal and maternal hemodynamic stability, as well as uteroplacental integrity, must be assured; given that fetal

Department of Anesthesia, Perioperative and Pain Medicine, Boston Children's Hospital, 300 Longwood Avenue, Boston, MA 02115, USA
* Corresponding author.
E-mail address: roland.brusseau@childrens.harvard.edu

Clin Perinatol 40 (2013) 429–442
http://dx.doi.org/10.1016/j.clp.2013.05.006
0095-5108/13/$ – see front matter © 2013 Elsevier Inc. All rights reserved.

perinatology.theclinics.com

hemodynamic collapse can be sudden and dramatic, a plan to resuscitate the fetus must be developed.

Fetal interventions may be roughly divided into 3 categories (**Table 1**). Open midgestational (or hysterotomy-based) procedures are generally performed between 18 and 26 weeks and typically involve exteriorization of the fetus (or affected fetal body part) with subsequent replacement in the uterus, allowing further maturation. Such procedures are generally performed on fetuses with well-defined lesions and for whom there is the expectation of preterm demise or significant postpartum morbidity or mortality without intervention.

Ex utero intrapartum therapy (EXIT) procedures, also known as operations on placental support, are generally performed on term or near-term fetuses with significant airway obstruction or pulmonary insufficiency. In such cases, surgical intervention is performed with intact uteroplacental function before cord clamping. EXIT-to-extracorporeal membrane oxygenation (ECMO) cases similarly depend on intact placental function before ECMO cannulation and initiation.

Finally, there are an ever-increasing variety of techniques for minimally invasive fetal procedures. Fetoscopic, ultrasound-guided, and fetal transesophageal echocardiographically assisted procedures may be undertaken at nearly any gestational age for the ligation or ablation of aberrant fetoplacental vessels, the placement of shunts

Table 1
Diseases eligible for fetal intervention

Disease	Intervention Types
CCAM	EXIT, EXIT-to-ECMO (if significant airway obstruction)
CDH	EXIT, EXIT-to-ECMO, or minimally invasive (ultrasound- or fetoscopically guided tracheal plug placement and removal)
Cervical teratoma	EXIT, EXIT-to-ECMO (if significant airway obstruction)
CHAOS	EXIT, EXIT-to-ECMO (if significant airway obstruction)
Congenital goiter	EXIT, EXIT-to-ECMO (if significant airway obstruction)
Cystic hygroma	EXIT, EXIT-to-ECMO (if significant airway obstruction or high-output cardiac failure)
HLHS	Minimally invasive (ultrasound-guided percutaneous aortic valve dilation)
Hydronephrosis and bladder outlet obstruction	Minimally invasive (ultrasound- or fetoscopically guided shunt placement)
MMC	EXIT, minimally invasive (fetoscopic patch application)
Pulmonary sequestration, bronchogenic cysts, and mixed or hybrid pulmonary lesions	EXIT
SCT	EXIT, EXIT-to-ECMO (for high-output cardiac failure)
TRAP	Minimally invasive (fetoscopic laser/photoablation of aberrant vasculature)
TTTS	Minimally invasive (fetoscopic laser/photoablation of aberrant vasculature)

Abbreviations: CCAM, cystic adenomatoid malformation; CDH, congenital diaphragmatic hernia; CHAOS, congenital high airway obstruction syndrome; ECMO, extracorporeal membrane oxygenation; EXIT, ex utero intrapartum therapy; HLHS, hypoplastic left heart syndrome; MMC, myelomeningocele; SCT, sacrococcygeal teratoma; TRAP, twin reversed arterial perfusion sequence; TTTS, twin-twin transfusion syndrome.

or plugs, or modification of cardiac anatomy. Such techniques are typically used in situations when severe morbidity will result and other therapeutic options (typically medical) have failed.

Because maternal anesthesia for fetal surgery is discussed in detail elsewhere in this volume by Dr Sviggum, this article largely addresses the fetal considerations for anesthesia and pain management during intrauterine therapy. Nevertheless, the choice of maternal anesthetic has significant ramifications not only for the fetus but also for the selection of fetal anesthetic and analgesic techniques and merits at least a passing discussion.

More specifically, this article emphasizes the challenges facing the anesthetist during interventions that occur *without maternal general anesthetics,* at which time fetal access is limited, direct delivery of medications to the fetus is indicated, and monitoring is often unreliable. Particular attention is paid to the principles of fetal circulation and oxygenation and their ramifications for fetal resuscitation techniques.

A RANGE OF ANESTHETIC OPTIONS FOR MOTHER AND FETUS
Mother

Local anesthesia
Local anesthesia is almost exclusively used for trocar insertion sites with percutaneous procedures. The most obvious advantage is maternal safety because the mother receives no intravenous medications. The disadvantages of this technique include an increased risk of injury to the nonanesthetized, nonparalyzed fetus as well as the absence of fetal analgesia and uterine relaxation. Patients on tocolytic therapy or those with polyhydramnios and uterine contractions may be at further risk of worsening contractions with this approach.[2]

Monitored anesthesia care
Intravenous sedation involves the maternal administration of benzodiazepines, opioids, and occasionally low-dose induction agents. The advantages include the possible provision of anesthesia and analgesia to the fetus via the transplacental transfer of agents and decreased maternal anxiety and pain. Depending on the amount and effect of the drugs administered, this sedation may increase the mother's risk of aspiration caused by an unprotected airway. This technique also provides no uterine relaxation.

Regional neuraxial blockade
Neuraxial techniques with or without sedation (spinal, epidural, or combined spinal and epidural anesthesia) have been used with fetoscopic techniques and, on occasion, without an adjunct general anesthetic, for open techniques. A T4 sensory level blockade is required for most surgical uterine manipulations. Pure neuraxial techniques provide no uterine relaxation and they do not provide fetal analgesia/anesthesia. Neuraxial anesthesia is associated with an increased maternal risk (failed block, high spinal, total spinal, intravascular injection of local anesthetic).[3]

General anesthesia
General anesthesia with inhalational anesthetics provides both maternal and fetal anesthesia and dose-dependent uterine relaxation even in patients who have received tocolytic therapy for preoperative uterine premature contractions.[4]

Combined regional and general anesthesia
A combined regional and general anesthetic technique is often used for open procedures and for patients with anterior placentas in whom laparotomy with or without

externalization of the uterus for safe trocar insertion is anticipated. In addition to providing the advantages of both the regional and the general anesthetic techniques listed previously, this method allows for planned postoperative pain control.

Fetus

The proliferation of minimally invasive fetal interventions and the apparent lack of a requirement for maternal general anesthetics in such cases have called into question the need for fetal anesthesia and analgesia. However, a significant body of evidence has grown to suggest the importance of mitigating the fetal stress response to enhance fetal outcome and possibly limit preterm labor.[2,5]

It is clear that the fetus is capable of mounting a physiochemical stress response to noxious stimuli as early as 18 weeks' gestation. Given the state of current knowledge, it is impossible to know exactly when the fetus first becomes capable of experiencing pain, although most agree that the gestational age range in which this occurs is between 20 and 30 weeks. It so happens that this range coincides with the gestational ages during which most fetal interventions occur.[6]

For these reasons, most practitioners provide fetal anesthesia or analgesia of some sort during both open and minimally invasive procedures. However, because access to the fetus is limited in the latter cases, alternative routes of administration are frequently required. Potential methods include transplacental, direct intramuscular, direct intravascular, and intra-amniotic administration; each route of administration has advantages and disadvantages that can have a direct impact on the overall outcome (**Table 2**).

Transplacental access

Many fetal interventions (open or endoscopic) rely on transplacental drug administration to provide anesthesia and analgesia for both the mother and fetus (**Table 3**).

Table 2
Routes for fetal drug delivery

Route	Disadvantages	Notes
Transplacental	Delayed delivery; significantly higher maternal levels required to achieve therapeutic fetal concentrations	Fetal isoflurane levels reach 70% of maternal isoflurane levels in 60 min; most commonly used induction agents rapidly cross the placenta.
IM	Variable absorption, bleeding, tissue damage	Fentanyl (20–50 mcg/kg) and pancuronium (200 mcg/kg) may be given for open procedures and with ultrasound guidance during minimally invasive procedures.
IV	Very difficult to obtain access, bleeding, vessel thrombosis	Standard neonatal doses may be delivered; blood may be given via this route.
Intracardiac	Difficult to establish, may produce arrhythmias, may lead to pericardial effusion and tamponade	It is best reserved for emergent resuscitation. Dose volumes should be as small as possible, generally between 0.2–0.5 mL.
Intra-amniotic	Experimental; correct dosing currently unknown	It allows for minimally invasive drug deliver; it may be useful for sustained delivery of medications.

Abbreviations: IM, intramuscularly; IV, intravenously.

Table 3 Maternal and fetal anesthetic management		
Procedure Type	**Maternal Anesthesia**	**Fetal Anesthesia[a]**
EXIT, EXIT-to-ECMO	General anesthesia with or without epidural/regional anesthesia	With general anesthesia, fetus is anesthetized transplacentally. This anesthetic may be supplemented by opioids (eg, fentanyl, 10–50 mcg/kg) and muscle relaxants (eg, vecuronium 0.2 mg/kg) delivered IM or IV. Atropine 20 mcg/kg may also be given to support fetal heart rate.
Minimally invasive (*innervated tissues, ie, fetus proper*)	Local or regional anesthesia (spinal, epidural, CSE, or regional block) with or without sedation	Fetal opioid (eg, fentanyl 10–50 mcg/kg) IM or IV Fetal muscle relaxant (eg, vecuronium 0.2 m/kg) IV or IM Atropine 20 mcg/kg IV/IM/IC may also be given in to support fetal heart rate In addition (or substitution) maternal remifentanil 0.1–0.2 mcg/kg/min IV
Minimally invasive (*noninnervated tissues: cord, placenta, and so forth*)	Local or regional anesthesia (spinal, epidural, CSE, or regional block) with or without sedation	Minimal fetal requirement Maternal remifentanil 0.1–0.2 mcg/kg/min IV

Abbreviations: CSE, combined spinal and epidural; IC, intracardiac; IM, intramuscularly; IV, intravenously.

[a] All dosages are based on estimated fetal weight.

Many, but not all, drugs cross the placenta (eg, remifentanil).[7] Lipid solubility, pH of both maternal and fetal blood, degree of ionization, protein binding, perfusion, placental area and thickness, and drug concentration are factors that influence the extent of transplacental drug diffusion.[8] The most obvious disadvantage with this approach is that the mother must be exposed to every drug that the fetus is intended to receive, often at large concentrations to achieve adequate drug concentrations in the fetus. In addition, the uptake of drugs may be impaired if there is reduced placental blood flow. This impairment has implications for successful anesthesia and analgesia both in terms of the delivered fetal dose and the time interval that must be allowed from maternal administration to the start of the fetal intervention.

All inhaled anesthetics cross the placental barrier, but uptake in the fetus is slower than in the mother.[8] However, this is offset by the reduced minimal alveolar concentration for anesthesia in the fetus, resulting in a similar onset of anesthesia as in the mother.[9] Fetal anesthesia is also important to reduce the fetal stress response, which, through catecholamine release, can reduce placental blood flow and exacerbate any hypoxia.[10–13]

Intravascular access

Intravascular fetal drug administration ensures immediate drug levels, and no additional dosing calculations are necessary because placental perfusion does not significantly alter dosing. Intravascular access can be obtained via the umbilical cord (which is not innervated), larger fetal veins (eg, hepatic vein), or intracardiac, as the specific intervention dictates.[14] One advantage of administering drugs via the umbilical vein is the ability to provide analgesia before the surgical insult. Muscle relaxants, analgesics, vagolytic agents, and resuscitation drugs can be given with assurance of immediate access to the fetal circulation.

Establishing intravascular access in the fetus requires inserting a needle in a fetus that is often not sedated from maternally administered agents. The needle may injure the moving fetus, and there is a risk of bleeding from the fetus, umbilical cord, and placenta. Uncontrolled bleeding could impair the surgical view, and it places the fetus and mother in jeopardy because an open hysterotomy may be necessary to control the bleeding. Establishing access via the umbilical cord vessels may also produce vascular spasm, potentially compromising fetal perfusion.

Intramuscular access

Intramuscular injection involves inserting a needle under ultrasound guidance into a fetal extremity or buttock. This route is the most common route of fetal drug administration currently in use for minimally invasive procedures. Unlike umbilical cord injection, the noxious stimulus to the fetus from the intramuscular injection stimulates the fetal stress response. Although the bleeding risk from intramuscular injection is less than that with intravascular injections, there remains a risk of bleeding and injury from the needle itself. Furthermore, if the fetus is already stressed, blood will be diverted away from muscle (the site of drug administration) and toward the fetal heart and brain. In this case, it may be impossible to estimate the time course for the drug to be absorbed from the intramuscular site.

Intra-amniotic access

Intra-amniotic fentanyl, sufentanil, thyroxine, vasopressin, and digoxin have been safely administered in large pregnant animal models, with only minimal drug detected in the mother.[15,16] If the safety and efficacy of this method of drug delivery hold true in human trials, intra-amniotic drug administration may become the preferred method for fetal drug delivery.

FETAL MONITORING

A hysterotomy is not needed for many surgical interventions; thus, the fetus remains within the uterus, making access for direct monitoring often impossible. Even for those fetuses that are partially delivered for an invasive procedure, monitoring is obtainable only intermittently and is frequently unreliable because the fetus must remain within a fluid environment during the procedure, making the direct placement of available monitors difficult.

Current methods for monitoring fetal well-being include fetal heart rate (FHR) monitoring, direct measurement of fetal blood gases, fetal electrocardiography (ECG), fetal pulse oximetry, fetal echocardiography, and Doppler ultrasonography of fetal cerebral blood flow. For purely intrauterine procedures, echocardiography and Doppler ultrasound are the only currently feasible monitoring modalities.

Use of FHR Monitoring and Doppler Ultrasonography for Fetal Interventions

Currently, FHR monitoring with Doppler ultrasonography is the standard for the intrapartum assessment of fetal well-being. FHR monitoring is also used perioperatively during fetal interventions. The FHR is documented before maternal induction of anesthesia to serve as a baseline for comparison and to reassure the perinatologist, surgeon, and anesthesiologist that the fetus is stable. *Ultrasonography, crucially, is also used to establish (if not previously determined) the estimated fetal weight for the calculation of drug dosages.*

The FHR may be continuously monitored intraoperatively by fetal echocardiography and with intermittent palpation of the umbilical cord in open cases. Most induction agents (eg, propofol)[17,18] rapidly cross the placenta, whereas inhaled agents generally take longer to equilibrate between the mother and fetus,[19] yet both induction and volatile agents will rapidly decrease FHR and FHR variability.

Doppler Ultrasonography of Fetal Cerebral Blood Flow

Antepartum Doppler ultrasonography studies of the fetal circulation in cases of intrauterine growth restriction with presumed hypoxia have shown a compensatory redistribution, with an increase in peripheral vascular resistance in the fetal body and placenta and a compensatory reduction in peripheral vascular resistance in the fetal brain, producing a brain-sparing effect.[20] Intrapartum Doppler ultrasonography has verified the brain-sparing response in the presence of intrapartum arterial hypoxemia, as reflected by increased mean flow velocity in the fetal middle cerebral artery.[21]

Preliminary studies of the middle cerebral artery pulsatility index in minimally invasive procedures, such as fetal blood sampling, transfusion, shunt insertion, tissue biopsy, and ovarian cyst aspiration, have demonstrated significant cerebral hemodynamic responses (decreases in the middle cerebral artery pulsatility index) in fetuses that underwent procedures involving transgression of the fetal body. This response was not noted in the fetuses undergoing procedures at the noninnervated placental cord insertion.[22]

The redistribution of the fetal circulation is not a limitless protective mechanism; with persistent cerebral hypoxia, the active vasodilation of the cerebral vessels may fail, leading to disastrous consequences for the fetus.

Fetal ECG and Pulse Oximetry

Although not possible in purely intrauterine procedures, if the fetus must be externalized, fetal ECG and pulse oximetry are possible monitoring modalities. Several groups have used fetal ECG analysis to determine whether changes in the time interval (PR and RR interval) and signal morphology (T to QRS ratio) correlate with fetal or neonatal outcomes. Studies in animals and humans have shown that under normal conditions, there is a negative correlation between the PR interval and the FHR: as the FHR slows, the PR interval lengthens; and as the FHR increases, the PR interval shortens. *The opposite relationship occurs in acidemic infants.*[23,24]

Pulse oximetry is less reliable for multiple reasons. Any fetal condition that decreases vascular pulsations (hypotension, vasoconstriction, shock, strong uterine contractions) can produce inaccurate oximetry readings.[25] Further, because direct contact of the oximeter must be made with the fetal skin surface, anything that interferes with light transmission or skin adhesion (eg, fetal or maternal movement, vernix caseosa, caput succedaneum) can influence the quality and accuracy of the oximeter.[26,27] Oximetry readings also vary in relation to the site of sensor application; several studies have found reduced baseline oxygen saturation values with the use of the oxygen sensor on the fetal buttock compared with the fetal head.[28,29]

Finally, because the normal range of fetal blood oxygen saturation ($FSpO_2$) of 30% to 70% lies in the middle of the oxygen hemoglobin dissociation curve, small changes in pH or Po_2 cause large changes in $FSpO_2$.[30]

Use of Fetal Blood Sampling During Fetal Interventions

In suspected cases of fetal compromise during an open intervention, fetal blood can be obtained from capillary vessels, a peripheral vein, a central vein, or a puncture of the umbilical vessels. The fetus' small size and friable tissue make vascular access difficult. Puncture of the umbilical vessels can lead to cord spasm, hematoma, and even fetal death and, thus, should be reserved for circumstances when no other options are available. During an endoscopic intervention, access to the fetal circulation is possible through the puncture of the umbilical vessels. With most fetal cardiac interventions, a needle and/or catheter is placed directly through the fetal myocardium, allowing access for blood samples; only a very small sample should be withdrawn because of the small circulating fetal blood volume.

KEY ASPECTS OF FETAL CARDIOVASCULAR PHYSIOLOGY
FHR and Cardiac Output

Because monitoring in intrauterine cases is largely limited to transuterine echocardiography, the physiology of the FHR, fetal cardiac output, and what those parameters can reveal about fetal oxygenation are important for fetal anesthetic and resuscitation management.

FHR is maintained more than the intrinsic rate of the sinoatrial node by a combination of vagal and sympathetic inputs as well as circulating catecholamines.[31–33] FHR decreases throughout gestation, accompanied by an increase in stroke volume as the heart grows. Hypoxic stress in late gestation produces a reflex bradycardia, with a normal heart rate or tachycardia developing a few minutes later. The later tachycardia is caused by an increase in plasma catecholamines causing β-adrenergic stimulation.[34] The disproportionately vagal tone of the fetal nervous system and the immaturity of baroreflex mechanisms add a further challenge because fetal distress, including hypoxemia, will often present as a decreased FHR. Direct irritation of the myocardium (as during aortic valve dilations) or other strong vagal stimuli may produce sudden and profound bradycardia.

Cardiac output in the fetus is determined largely by heart rate. The combined ventricular output of the left and right ventricles in the human fetus is 450 mL/kg/min.[35] During development, the ability of the fetus to increase the stroke volume is limited by a reduced proportion of functioning contractile tissue and a limited ability to increase the heart rate because of a relatively reduced β-receptor density and immature sympathetic drive. Thus, if blood volume is reduced by hemorrhage, the heart cannot compensate by increasing stroke volume; or, conversely, if volume is increased, the walls are less able to distend and cardiac efficiency is reduced (although this second effect is reduced substantially by the huge, relatively compliant placental circulation). Therefore, the only way for the fetus to increase cardiac output is to increase the heart rate.

Despite this homeostatic limitation, the fetus is able to withstand significant hemorrhage. Sheep studies have shown that the fetal lamb can restore arterial blood pressure and heart rate very quickly, without any measurable disturbance in acid-base balance after acute loss of 20% of their blood volume.[36] Even after a 40% reduction in blood volume, the ovine fetal blood pressure recovers to normal within 2 minutes and the heart rate within 35 minutes.[37]

However, given that fetal blood volume is approximately 100 to 110 mL/kg, and many patients are less than 1 kg, even a small amount of blood loss can lead to severe hemodynamic compromise. Immature fetal hepatic and hematologic function may lead to impaired hemostasis and enhanced surgical losses. Such coagulopathy may be worsened by fetal cooling during open interventions.

In the setting of hemorrhage, oxygen delivery to the brain and heart is maintained secondary to vascular redistribution (central sparing effect) and blood volume replacement from the placenta and extravascular space, with 40% of the volume loss being corrected within 30 minutes.[37] The development of acidemia indicates that the fetus is not able to compensate; acidosis shifts the oxygen dissociation curve to the right, thereby decreasing fetal hemoglobin oxygen saturation but improving the release of oxygen from hemoglobin. Blood flow during periods of hypoxia increases more than 100% to the brainstem but only 60% to the cerebral hemispheres.[38]

Fetal Oxygenation

The fetus exists in an environment of low oxygen tension, with Po_2 being approximately one-fourth that of the adult. The maximum Po_2 of umbilical venous blood is approximately 30 mm Hg. The hemoglobin oxygen dissociation curve is shifted to the left because of fetal hemoglobin (hemoglobin F), thereby increasing the affinity for oxygen. Thus, for any given Po_2, the fetus has a greater affinity for oxygen than the mother. The Po_2 at which hemoglobin is 50% desaturated is approximately 27 mm Hg for the adult and 20 mm Hg for the fetus.[39-41]

Studies in both animals and humans have demonstrated that maternal hypocapnia may also influence fetal oxygenation via umbilical venous flow. Maternal hypocapnia significantly reduces umbilical venous blood flow and has been shown to produce fetal hypoxia and metabolic acidosis. Conversely, maternal hypercapnia and acidosis have been demonstrated to increase umbilical venous flow and increase fetal arterial Po_2.[42]

Uteroplacental Circulation

Fetal dependence on the placenta for oxygenation, gas, drug, and waste exchange makes maintenance of uteroplacental circulation a highest priority for fetal anesthetic management. Because the fetal pulmonary system is essentially off-line in utero, enhanced umbilical blood flow is the chief determinant of increased fetal oxygenation.[43] Oxygen supply to fetal tissues depends on several factors. First, the mother must be adequately oxygenated. Second, there must be an adequate flow of well-oxygenated blood to the uteroplacental circulation. This blood flow may be reduced from maternal hemorrhage (reduced maternal blood volume) or compression of the inferior vena cava (reduced venous return), which increases uterine venous pressure, thus, reducing uterine perfusion.

Additionally, aortic compression reduces uterine arterial blood flow. Care must be taken to position the mother in such a way as to prevent aortocaval compression. The surgical incision of hysterotomy itself reduces uteroplacental blood flow by as much as 73% in sheep, whereas fetoscopic procedures with uterine entry have no effect.[44] This potential diminution of flow has been shown to result in decreased fetal oxygenation and underlies the recommendation to maintain maternal blood pressure within 10% of the baseline.

Even if the uterine circulation is adequate, the fetus still depends on uteroplacental blood flow and umbilical venous blood flow for tissue oxygenation. Care must be taken to not interrupt umbilical vessel blood flow by manipulation or kinking the cord, which can cause vasospasm. Umbilical vasoconstriction can also occur as part of a fetal stress reaction caused by the release of fetal stress hormones. Increases in amniotic fluid volume increase amniotic pressure and impair uteroplacental perfusion.[45,46]

Placental vascular resistance can be increased, raising fetal cardiac afterload, by the surge in fetal catecholamine production stimulated by surgical stress.[47]

Inhalational anesthetics may cause maternal vasodilatation and, thus, in theory, could cause or exacerbate preexisting fetal hypoxia. Studies of anesthetics in hypoxic ovine fetuses have shown that isoflurane exacerbates preexisting acidosis.[48] It also causes blunting of the usual vascular redistribution response to fetal hypoxia, but owing to a reduction in cerebral oxygen demand, the balance of cerebral oxygen supply and demand is unaffected.

INTRAUTERINE FETAL RESUSCITATION

Given the immaturity of fetal organ function, the fetal disposition to cardiovascular instability and collapse, and the multiple stresses of surgery and its associated anesthetics on fetal compensatory mechanisms, a plan for fetal resuscitation must always be established in advance (**Table 4**).

Both maternal and fetal factors may contribute to fetal decompensation, and both maternal and fetal interventions may contribute to effective fetal resuscitation. Whether or not uteroplacental insufficiency is implicated, measures should be taken to maximize oxygen delivery to the fetus. These maternal measures include left lateral positioning to relieve aortocaval compression, fraction of inspired oxygen of 1.0 (if intubated), or high-flow oxygen administration with a face mask to increase fetal oxygen saturation. A rapid maternal intravenous fluid infusion, possibly including vasopressor administration, may be used to improve uterine blood flow. If there is evidence of uterine contraction, efforts must be taken to enhance uterine relaxation, including tocolysis if necessary.

Limited access to the fetus with hemodynamic decompensation may complicate resuscitation measures. Hemodynamic compromise may result from hypoxemia, acute fetal hemorrhage or routine surgical bleeding, preexisting fetal cardiac disease and/or anemia, electrolyte abnormalities, hypothermia, and other forms of generalized fetal distress. Open procedures lend direct access to the fetus and allow direct cardiac compressions (100–150 compressions per minute), intravascular or

Table 4 Fetal resuscitation interventions		
Intervention	Dose[a]	Notes
Atropine	20 mcg/kg (minimum 0.1 mg)	Useful to counteract significant fetal vagal responses to stress and hypoxemia; useful as prophylaxis before intervention
Epinephrine	10–20 mcg/kg	May be repeated every 3 min; increasing doses may be of limited benefit
Calcium gluconate	100 mg/kg	Calcium chloride may be substituted, 20 mg/kg
Sodium bicarbonate	1–2 mEq/kg	Of unclear benefit; given acidemia inherent to anesthesia with volatile anesthetics, may be reasonable to enhance efficacy of epinephrine
PRBCs	10–15 mL/kg to achieve an Hb increment of 2–3 g/dL	Generally reserved for cute loss >25% estimated blood volume

Abbreviations: Hb, hemoglobin; PRBCs, packed red blood cells.
[a] All doses are based on estimated fetal weight.

intramuscular delivery of routine resuscitation medications (epinephrine, atropine, sodium bicarbonate), and packed red blood cells (PRBCs). When giving PRBCs, consideration should be given to pH correction of the packed cells to limit excess potassium delivery. Calcium gluconate may be needed to limit citrate-induced hypocalcemia. To assure normothermia and prevent umbilical kinking, the fetus should be continuously bathed in warm fluids.

During minimally invasive procedures, similar medications may be given, but delivery is generally limited to intramuscular or intracardiac administration under ultrasound guidance. Even PRBCs may be delivered via an intracardiac route, but, as discussed earlier, special care must be taken to adjust blood pH and temperature and to deliver volume slowly so as not to distend the fetal heart or produce excessively hypoxemic cardiac output (see note about drug volumes for fetal administration). Large pericardial effusions should be drained. If resuscitation fails, maternal transabdominal or transmyometrial compressions may also be considered, although their efficacy may be limited. Consideration should also be given to emergent delivery of viable fetuses, although preparation for such should be a part of preprocedure planning.

Note about drug volumes for fetal administration

Special care must be taken when considering intracardiac delivery of medications or blood because the fetal heart chamber volume is quite small (left ventricular stroke volume 0.3 mL at 20 weeks, 2 mL at 34 weeks[49]) and a large hypoxic (and possibly hypothermic) volume, when delivered to the left ventricle, may result in significant myocardial ischemia when that volume traverses the coronary ostia. Further, blood should be warmed, pH adjusted, and consideration given to the possibility of a large potassium load being delivered.

http://fetalmedicine.com/fmf/2008-29.pdf

In general, volumes for intracardiac or intramuscular injections should be limited (if possible) to approximately 0.2 mL to account for both cardiac chamber size during intracardiac administration and limiting tissue damage following intramuscular administration.

POSTOPERATIVE CONSIDERATIONS

Preterm labor postoperatively poses the greatest risk to the fetus. Maternal and fetal stress, and hysterotomy in particular, greatly increases the risk of preterm delivery, compromising fetal well-being directly via preterm delivery and limiting the maturational efficacy of the intervention. Maternal prophylaxis with tocolytic agents and aggressive pain control are the standard therapy following open interventions.

Fetal assessment is more difficult. FHR analysis in the immediate postoperative period may be useful for determining fetal distress; echocardiography may also reveal the fetus' general cardiovascular state, and cerebral artery pulsatility indices may further help assess fetal well-being. The fetal ductus arteriosus should also be monitored for patency and diameter change following maternal indomethacin exposure.

A LOOK TO THE FUTURE

Clearly, with advances in surgical and anesthetic techniques and technologies, significant progress may be made in midgestation fetal intervention. There is already movement toward expanding treatment to include not only life-threatening fetal pathologies but also preemptive management of fetal disorders that are not necessarily life threatening but have significant, disabling postpartum morbidities.

The particular challenges for anesthesiologists are to develop methods to provide selective fetal anesthesia and analgesia as well as techniques of targeted uterine relaxation such that safer, specifically tailored anesthetics may be provided to all patients involved in the fetal intervention. Enhanced fetal monitoring will help the anesthesiologist provide better care for the fetus both intraprocedurally and in the postoperative period. With such advances, the provision of fetal anesthesia may become a more routine part of pediatric surgical and anesthetic practice, bringing with it new opportunities for practice and research and new problems to be solved.

REFERENCES

1. Deprest JA, Flake AW, Gratacos E, et al. The making of fetal surgery. Prenat Diagn 2010;30:653–67.
2. Van de Velde M, De Buck F, Van Mieghem T, et al. Fetal anaesthesia: is this necessary for fetoscopic therapy? Fetal Matern Med Rev 2010;21:24.
3. Myers LB, Watcha MF. Epidural versus general anesthesia for twin-twin transfusion syndrome requiring fetal surgery. Fetal Diagn Ther 2004;19:286–91.
4. Tran KM. Anesthesia for fetal surgery. Semin Fetal Neonatal Med 2010;15:40–5.
5. Anand KJ, Maze M. Fetuses, fentanyl, and the stress response: signals from the beginnings of pain? Anesthesiology 2001;95:823–5.
6. Lee SJ, Ralston HJ, Drey EA, et al. Fetal pain: a systematic multidisciplinary review of the evidence. JAMA 2005;294:947–54.
7. Kan RE, Hughes SC, Rosen MA, et al. Intravenous remifentanil: placental transfer, maternal and neonatal effects. Anesthesiology 1998;88(6):1467–74.
8. Sibley C, D'Souza S, Glazier J, et al. Mechanisms of solute transfer across the human placenta: effects of intrauterine growth restriction. Fetal Matern Med Rev 1998;10:197–206.
9. Garcia PJ, Olutoye OO, Ivey RT, et al. Case scenario: anesthesia for maternal-fetal surgery: the ex utero intrapartum therapy (EXIT) procedure. Anesthesiology 2011;114:1446–52.
10. Giannakoulopoulos X, Sepulveda W, Kourtis P, et al. Fetal plasma cortisol and beta-endorphin response to intrauterine needling. Lancet 1994;344:77–81.
11. Gitau R, Fisk NM, Teixeira JM, et al. Fetal hypothalamic-pituitary-adrenal stress responses to invasive procedures are independent of maternal responses. J Clin Endocrinol Metab 2001;86:104–9.
12. Fisk NM, Gitau R, Teixeira JM, et al. Effect of direct fetal opioid analgesia on fetal hormonal and hemodynamic stress response to intrauterine needling. Anesthesiology 2001;95:828–35.
13. Giannakoulopoulos X, Teixeira J, Fisk N, et al. Human fetal and maternal noradrenaline responses to invasive procedures. Pediatr Res 1999;45(4 Pt 1): 494–9.
14. Tran KA, Maxwell LG, Cohen DE, et al. Quantification of serum fentanyl concentrations from umbilical cord blood during ex utero intrapartum therapy. Anesth Analg 2012;114(6):1265–7.
15. Hamamoto K, Iwamoto HS, Roman CM, et al. Fetal uptake of intraamniotic digoxin in sheep. Pediatr Res 1990;27:282–5.
16. Strumper D, Durieux ME, Gogarten W, et al. Plasma concentrations after intraamniotic sufentanil in chronically instrumented pregnant sheep. Anesthesiology 2003;98:1400–6.
17. Kosaka Y, Takahashi T, Mark LC. Intravenous thiobarbiturate anesthesia for cesarean section. Anesthesiology 1969;31:489–506.

18. Daillard P, Cockshott ID, Lirzin JD, et al. Intravenous propofol during cesarean section: placental transfer, concentrations in breast milk and neonatal effects: a preliminary study. Anesthesiology 1989;71:827–34.
19. Warren TW, Datta S, Ostheimer GW, et al. Comparison of the maternal and neonatal effects of halothane, enflurane and isoflurane for cesarean delivery. Anesth Analg 1983;62:516–20.
20. Wladimiroff JW, Tonge HM, Stewart PA. Doppler ultrasound assessment of cerebral blood flow in the human fetus. Br J Obstet Gynaecol 1986;93:471–5.
21. Sutterlin MW, Seelbach-Gobel B, Oehler MK, et al. Doppler ultrasonographic evidence of brain-sparing effect in fetuses with low oxygen saturation according to pulse oximetry. Am J Obstet Gynecol 1999;181:216–20.
22. Jeronima MA, Teixeira MD, Glover V, et al. Acute cerebral redistribution in response to invasive procedures in the human fetus. Am J Obstet Gynecol 1999;181:1018–25.
23. Mohajer MP, Sahota DS, Reed NN, et al. Cumulative changes in the fetal electrocardiogram and biochemical indices of fetal hypoxemia. Eur J Obstet Gynecol Reprod Biol 1994;55:63–70.
24. van Wijngaarden WJ, Sahota DS, James DK, et al. Improved intrapartum surveillance with PR interval analysis of the fetal electrocardiogram: a randomized trial showing a reduction in fetal blood sampling. Am J Obstet Gynecol 1996;174:1295–9.
25. Yam J, Chua S, Arulkumaran S. Intrapartum fetal pulse oximetry: II. Clinical application. Obstet Gynecol Surv 2000;55:173–83.
26. Gardosi JO, Damianou D, Schram C. Artifacts in fetal pulse oximetry: incomplete sensor-to-skin contact. Am J Obstet Gynecol 1994;170:1169–70.
27. Reed CA, Baker RS, Lam CT, et al. Application of near-infrared spectroscopy during fetal cardiac surgery. J Surg Res 2011;171:159–63.
28. Gardosi JO, Schram C, Symonds M. Adaptation of pulse oximetry for fetal monitoring during labor. Lancet 1991;337:1265–7.
29. Luttkus AK, Dimer JA, Dudenhausen JW. Are pulse oximetry findings in the breech consistent with fetal physiology? Am J Obstet Gynecol 1998;178:48S.
30. Chua S, Yeong SM, Razvi K, et al. Fetal oxygen saturation during labour. Br J Obstet Gynaecol 1997;104:1080–3.
31. Jones CT, Robinson RO. Plasma catecholamines in foetal and adult sheep. J Physiol 1975;248:15–33.
32. Martin AA, Kapoor R, Scroop GC. Hormonal factors in the control of heart rate in normoxaemic and hypoxaemic fetal, neonatal and adult sheep. J Dev Physiol 1987;9:465–80.
33. Eden RD, Seifert LS, Frese-Gallo J, et al. Effect of gestational age on baseline fetal heart rate during the third trimester of pregnancy. J Reprod Med 1987;32:285–6.
34. Cohn HE, Piasecki GJ, Jackson BT. The effect of beta-adrenergic stimulation on fetal cardiovascular function during hypoxemia. Am J Obstet Gynecol 1982;144:810–6.
35. Gilbert RD. Control of fetal cardiac output during changes in blood volume. Am J Physiol 1980;238:H80–6.
36. Itskovitz J, Goetzman BW, Rudolph AM. Effects of hemorrhage on umbilical venous return and oxygen delivery in fetal lambs. Am J Physiol 1982;242:H543–8.
37. Meyers RL, Paulick RP, Rudolph CD, et al. Cardiovascular responses to acute, severe haemorrhage in fetal sheep. J Dev Physiol 1991;15:189–97.
38. Schenone MH, Mari G, The MC. Doppler and its role in the evaluation of fetal anemia and fetal growth restriction. Clin Perinatol 2011;38:83–102.

39. Motoyama EK, Rivard G, Acheson F, et al. Adverse effect of maternal hyperventilation on the fetus. Lancet 1966;1:286–8.
40. Motoyama EK, Rivard G, Acheson F, et al. The effect of changes in maternal pH and Pco2 on the Po2 of fetal lambs. Anesthesiology 1967;28:891–903.
41. Rivard G, Motoyama E, Acheson F, et al. The relation between maternal and fetal oxygen tensions in sheep. Am J Obstet Gynecol 1967;97:925–30.
42. O'Rourke N, Kodali BS. Laparoscopic surgery during pregnancy. Curr Opin Anaesthesiol 2006;19:254–9.
43. Habib AS. A review of the impact of phenylephrine administration on maternal hemodynamics and maternal and neonatal outcomes in women undergoing cesarean delivery under spinal anesthesia. Anesth Analg 2012;114:377–90.
44. Gaiser RR, Kurth CD. Anesthetic considerations for fetal surgery. Semin Perinatol 1999;23:507–14.
45. Bower SJ, Flack NJ, Sepulveda W, et al. Uterine artery blood flow response to correction of amniotic fluid volume. Am J Obstet Gynecol 1995;173:502–7.
46. Fisk NM, Tannirandorn Y, Nicolini U, et al. Amniotic pressure in disorders of amniotic fluid volume. Obstet Gynecol 1990;76:210–4.
47. Rychik J. Acute cardiovascular effects of fetal surgery in the human. Circulation 2004;110:1549–56.
48. Baker BW, Hughes SC, Shnider SM, et al. Maternal anesthesia and the stressed fetus: effects of isoflurane on the asphyxiated fetal lamb. Anesthesiology 1990;72:65–70.
49. Hamill N, Romero R, Hassan S, et al. Repeatability and reproducibility of fetal cardiac ventricular volume calculations using spatiotemporal image correlation and virtual organ computer aided analysis. J Ultrasound Med 2009;28:1301–11.

Multimodal Postcesarean Delivery Analgesia

Anne Lavoie, MD, FRCPC*, Paloma Toledo, MD, MPH

KEYWORDS

- Acute pain • Cesarean delivery • Chronic pain • Multimodal analgesia
- Neuraxial analgesia • Nonsteroidal antiinflammatory drugs • Opioid analgesia
- Chronic pain

KEY POINTS

- Acute pain after cesarean delivery is common, and some patients may develop chronic postcesarean delivery pain.
- There are multiple options for postcesarean delivery analgesia, including neuraxial anesthesia, peripheral nerve blockade, and various combinations of oral, parenteral, and rectally administered medications.
- Long-acting neuraxial opioid medications provide the best postcesarean delivery analgesia and should be considered as part of a multimodal analgesic regimen.

INTRODUCTION

Avoidance of postoperative pain is a priority for both physicians and patients.[1,2] A prospective observational study that used priority rankings to evaluate obstetric patient preferences found that the 2 most important concerns for parturients were avoidance of intraoperative and postoperative pain.[2] Therefore, the goals of anesthetic care during labor and delivery should include:

- Optimization of peripartum pain management
- Maximizing patient satisfaction
- Minimizing medication-related side effects to the mother and her infant
- Allowing for early return to baseline function
- Preventing a prolonged hospital length of stay.

Cesarean deliveries are known to be associated with acute postoperative pain. However, there is also evidence to suggest that there may be an association with

Disclosures: None.
Conflicts of Interest: None.
Department of Anesthesiology, Northwestern University, Feinberg School of Medicine, 251 East Huron Street, F5-704, Chicago, IL 60611, USA
* Corresponding author.
E-mail address: anne.lavoie@umontreal.ca

Clin Perinatol 40 (2013) 443–455
http://dx.doi.org/10.1016/j.clp.2013.05.008
0095-5108/13/$ – see front matter © 2013 Elsevier Inc. All rights reserved.

the development of chronic postoperative pain as well.[3,4] Pain is multifactorial, and the experience of pain is subjective, with significant interindividual variability. Patient demographics and emotional states are known to influence the experience of pain.[5–7] In addition, select genetic polymorphisms, such as those found on the G118 allele, may be associated with increased postoperative pain, although the results of genetic studies have been conflicting.[8–10] It would be overly simplistic to reduce postcesarean delivery analgesia to a single form of treatment, especially in the context of the emotional surge associated with delivery. Thus, the use of a multimodal analgesic regimen, which uses a combination of drugs with different mechanisms of action, aims to achieve optimal analgesia through additive or synergistic drug actions and minimize associated side effects.[11] Several studies in the postcesarean delivery setting have shown the superiority of multimodal analgesia compared with single-drug therapy alone.[12–14]

Postcesarean delivery analgesia can be achieved through multiple routes: neuraxial anesthesia and analgesia, peripheral nerve blockade, and various combinations of oral, parenteral, and rectally administered medications (**Box 1**). The most common multimodal analgesic regimen includes a combination of neuraxial and systemic opioids and nonsteroidal antiinflammatory medications. In addition to standard pharmacologic treatment options, there are also nonpharmacologic interventions available to practitioners. This article summarizes and reviews the epidemiology, physiology, and treatment options for the management of postcesarean delivery pain.

POSTCESAREAN DELIVERY PAIN

Pain comes from the Old French word *peine, poena* in Latin, which means punishment or penalty. Pain is defined as an unpleasant sensory and emotional experience associated with actual or potential tissue damage; or described in terms of such damage.[15] In the United States, pain is one of the most common symptoms leading patients to seek medical attention, which can significantly interfere with both quality of life and general functioning. Furthermore, national estimates of the cost of pain, which includes lost productivity and treatment costs, range from $560 to $635 billion annually.[16,17]

Approximately 18.5 million cesarean deliveries are performed annually worldwide.[18] In the United States, cesarean deliveries account for 30.5% of all births; a rate that has doubled since the mid-1990s.[19] In a prospective, longitudinal study of 1228 women,[20] 96% of participants reported pain immediately after delivery. Several studies have attempted to estimate the incidence of chronic postcesarean delivery pain (**Fig. 1**). In prospective studies, the prevalence of persistent pain 2 months post partum have been estimated to be approximately 10%.[3] An analysis of pain at 6 months and 1 year after delivery from that cohort revealed low rates of persistent pain, with

---

Box 1
Analgesic options for the management of postcesarean delivery pain

Neuraxial analgesia (spinal, epidural, combined spinal-epidural) with a long-acting opioid

Systemic opioid analgesics (intravenous, intramuscular, oral opioids)

Nonopioid analgesics (nonsteroidal antiinflammatory drugs, acetaminophen)

Peripheral nerve blockade

Nonpharmacologic analgesic options (music therapy, massage)

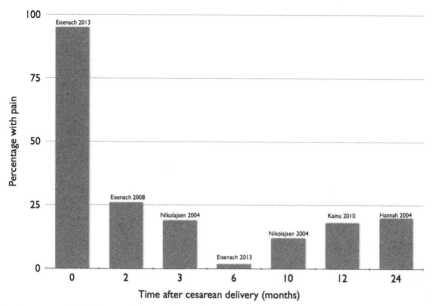

Fig. 1. Reported incidence of pain after cesarean delivery. Each bar represents the percentage of patients reporting pain after cesarean delivery. Time is shown in months. Time 0 represents pain immediately after delivery. The last name of the first author and study year are displayed above each bar.

rates of 1.8% and 0.3%, respectively.[20] In contrast, higher rates of postpartum pain have been obtained through survey-based studies. A survey mailed to 245 women 1 year after delivery found that the incidence of incisional pain at 3 months was approximately 19%, which decreased to 12% at 10 months post partum.[21] A slightly higher estimate of pain at 1 year after delivery was obtained in a Finnish survey (n = 600, response rate 78%), which found the incidence of persistent pain after cesarean delivery to be 18%.[4] At 2 years post partum, the incidence of chronic pain was approximately 20% in women who had elective cesarean deliveries for breech presentation (n = 1,159, 79% response rate).[22] Studies that have attempted to characterize the intensity of persistent postpartum pain have found that a few women have daily severe or excruciating pain.[4,21,22] Although the differences in incidence rates can largely be attributed to differences in study methodology, including varying definitions of chronic pain and data acquisition, most of these studies suggest that pain after childbirth is a significant public health concern.

PHYSIOLOGY OF POSTCESAREAN DELIVERY PAIN

There are 2 primary types of pain: fast (sharp) and slow (throbbing) pain, the latter of which is associated with tissue destruction. Pain receptors are free-nerve endings that respond to 3 types of stimuli: mechanical, thermal, or chemical (inflammatory mediators). Pain impulses are transmitted to the dorsal horn of the spinal cord via the neospinothalamic and the paleospinothalamic tract through fast (Aδ fibers) and slow pain (C fibers). Pain stimulates the release of several neurotransmitters and cellular mediators, including prostaglandins, substance P, glutamate, and calcitonin gene-related peptide. These neurotransmitters bind to receptors on nociceptive fibers, causing further release of neurotransmitters and signal transmission to the central nervous system.

Cesarean delivery pain has 2 primary components: somatic and visceral pain. Somatic pain arises from direct tissue trauma from the surgical incision, whereas visceral pain is caused by inflammation. Somatic pain is transmitted via the anterior division of spinal segmental nerves, whereas visceral uterine nociceptive stimuli return to the central nervous system via afferent nerve fibers that ascend through the inferior hypogastric plexus and enter the spinal cord via the T10-L1 spinal nerves.[23]

Most cesarean deliveries are performed using a Pfannenstiel incision, a technique associated with less blood loss, fewer infections, and less postoperative pain than other incision types.[24] A Pfannenstiel incision usually involves the T11-T12 dermatomes, whereas a vertical incision may extend from the T10-L1 dermatomes. However, operative pain may extend beyond these dermatomes from stretching of the skin or intraperitoneal tissue manipulation.

PHARMACOLOGIC ANALGESIC STRATEGIES
Neuraxial Analgesia

Most cesarean deliveries in the United States are performed using neuraxial anesthetic techniques.[25] The American Society of Anesthesiologist's *Practice Guidelines for Obstetric Anesthesia* recommend the use of neuraxial opioids for postoperative analgesia.[26] The mechanism of opioid action is dependent on both the route of administration (spinal vs epidural) and the lipid solubility of the drug. Intrathecal opioids act primarily at μ receptors located within the dorsal horn of the spinal cord. In contrast, opioids administered in the epidural space act via 3 mechanisms: (1) systemic absorption by the vascular system (ie, supraspinal effect); (2) diffusion into the intrathecal space with subsequent action at the dorsal horn; and (3) rostral spread within the cerebral spinal fluid to the brainstem. Highly lipid-soluble opioids such as fentanyl and sufentanil have a rapid onset of action; however, because they are rapidly absorbed into lipid membranes and epidural veins, they also have a short duration of action. In contrast, hydrophilic opioids such as morphine have a slower onset of action, with a longer duration of analgesia. As a result, combinations of both lipophilic and hydrophilic opioids are often used to decrease intraoperative local anesthetic requirements while providing extended postoperative analgesia.

The decision on which neuraxial technique to use (spinal anesthesia, epidural anesthesia, or combined spinal-epidural anesthesia) for a given patient depends on multiple patient factors (eg, airway examination, obesity, medical comorbidities), surgical factors (eg, anticipated duration of surgery), and fetal factors (eg, presence of fetal distress). Neuraxial opioids may be administered intrathecally, as well as epidurally. A Cochrane review (n = 751)[27] found no differences in intraoperative analgesia, need for intraoperative conversion to general anesthesia, postoperative pain relief, or need for neonatal interventions between spinal and epidural anesthesia. A retrospective cohort study (n = 949),[28] which directly compared the quality of postcesarean delivery analgesic outcomes for patients receiving intrathecal morphine versus epidural morphine versus intravenous patient-controlled analgesia (PCA) morphine, found that patients who received intrathecal or epidural morphine reported lower pain scores at rest and with movement. There were no differences in postoperative analgesia between the 2 neuraxial anesthetic modalities. Therefore, for elective and nonelective cesarean deliveries, the preferred anesthetic technique seems to be spinal anesthesia.[25]

Given its hydrophilic properties, intrathecal morphine provides the longest duration of postcesarean delivery analgesia. The duration of postoperative analgesia ranges from 14 to 36 hours, with a median duration of 27 hours to first request for supplemental analgesia.[29] In contrast, lipophilic opioids such as fentanyl do not confer significant postoperative analgesia with a median time to first request for supplemental analgesia after an intrathecal local anesthetic plus fentanyl mixture of only 4 hours (range 2–13 hours).[29] Therefore, in the absence of contraindications, intrathecal morphine should be considered the gold standard for providing prolonged postoperative analgesia.

The optimal dose of morphine for postcesarean delivery analgesia has also been extensively studied. In a randomized controlled study (n = 108) in which parturients undergoing elective cesarean delivery under spinal anesthesia were randomized to escalating doses of intrathecal morphine ranging from 0 to 0.5 mg,[30] the investigators found no differences in postoperative intravenous PCA morphine use between groups that received greater than 0.075 mg of intrathecal morphine. However, with escalating intrathecal morphine doses there was a dose-dependent increase in pruritus and the need for opioid-related side effect treatment. The investigators concluded that doses of intrathecal morphine greater than 0.1 mg did not significantly improve analgesia; but did increase opioid-related side effects.

If epidural anesthesia is selected for cesarean delivery, epidural morphine also provides excellent postoperative analgesia. It is well established that epidural morphine provides superior postoperative analgesia to intravenous or intramuscularly delivered morphine.[28,31] A prospective dose-finding study (n = 60)[32] randomized patients undergoing cesarean delivery under epidural anesthesia to escalating doses of epidural morphine (0–5 mg) and evaluated the quality of postoperative analgesia and opioid-related side effects. With escalating doses of morphine, there was a linear decrease in intravenous PCA morphine use. However, there also appeared to be a ceiling effect above 3.75 mg epidural morphine. In contrast to intrathecal morphine,[30] opioid-related side effects were not dose dependent with escalating doses of epidural morphine.[32] A systematic review (n = 431) found that the median duration of epidural morphine analgesia was 30 hours (95% confidence interval: 25–24 hours).[33] The efficacy and duration of morphine analgesia are significantly reduced when morphine is administered after 2-chloroprocaine when compared with epidural lidocaine.[34] Although the mechanism for this interaction is not clear, providers may choose to supplement epidural anesthesia with a longer-acting local anesthetic such as bupivacaine or increase the dose of epidural morphine to try to achieve optimal analgesia.

Other long-acting neuraxial opioid options include extended-release morphine and hydromorphone.[35,36] The use of neuraxial meperidine has been described for postoperative analgesia. Although it has been shown to provide 2 to 4 hours of postoperative analgesia, it is associated with an increased incidence of intraoperative nausea and vomiting compared with local anesthetic alone.[37] The use of adjuvant medications such as clonidine and neostigmine has been described to improve the quality of neuraxial anesthesia. However, their use is underexplored within cesarean delivery populations.[23]

Systemic Opioid Analgesic Techniques

There are several choices for opioid analgesia using multiple delivery routes (eg, intravenous bolus administration, intravenous PCA, intramuscular injection). Because there are large interindividual differences in pharmacokinetics with intramuscular injections, and because intramuscular injections are uncomfortable for patients, intravenous options are used more frequently for postoperative analgesia. In patients who have received neuraxial morphine, supplemental opioid analgesia may not be necessary during the first 24 hours, with as-needed medications being prescribed for breakthrough pain. However, for patients who receive general anesthesia, or for those who undergo neuraxial anesthesia without a long-acting neuraxial opioid, systemic opioids are required during the postoperative period.

PCA has been shown to be superior to intermittent bolus injections or intramuscular injections with regard to pain control, patient satisfaction, and adverse effects.[38] The choice of opioid should be made according to the speed of onset, duration of action, efficacy, and side effect profile. The American College of Obstetricians and Gynecologists recommend against the use of meperidine, because it has been associated with normeperidine neurotoxicity in the newborn.[39,40] Regardless of the opioid chosen (ie, morphine, hydromorphone, fentanyl), it is important to adjust the dose and the interval lockout time according to equivalent dosage and the duration of action, respectively. Whether or not to incorporate a continuous basal infusion in addition to the PCA during the first 24 hours postoperatively is controversial. As with neuraxial opioid administration, it is important to monitor for respiratory depression and sedation in patients receiving parenteral opioid analgesia.

Tramadol is a weak μ-opioid receptor agonist. It also induces serotonin release and inhibits the reuptake of norepinephrine. Although there were high expectations for tramadol to confer analgesia with fewer side effects when compared with pure opioid agonists, it has not been shown to be beneficial for postcesarean delivery analgesia. In a randomized controlled trial (n = 204), Mitra and colleagues[41] studied a combination of tramadol and diclofenac compared with acetaminophen and diclofenac for postoperative analgesia after cesarean delivery. Although there were statistically significant differences between the 2 drug regimens, there were no clinically significant differences in pain scores during the first 24 hours after delivery. However, patients in the tramadol/diclofenac group had a 7-fold higher incidence of nausea when compared with control patients.

Codeine is a prodrug that needs to be metabolized to morphine for analgesic efficacy. The enzyme responsible for this conversion is absent within nearly 10% of the white population. These poor metabolizers are not likely to obtain analgesia; however, they are likely to experience undesirable opioid-related side effects such as nausea and vomiting. Furthermore, there are some ultrarapid CYP2D6 metabolizers who are at risk of codeine intoxication. There has been a recent warning by the US Food and Drug Administration on codeine use in nursing mothers after the death of a breastfed 13-day-old neonate believed to have suffered a morphine overdose because his mother was taking codeine. Subsequent investigation revealed that the mother was a CYP2D6 ultrarapid metabolizer.[42,43] Because of these concerns, codeine is not recommended for use during the peripartum period. Tramadol is also influenced by the CYP2D6 genotype, and interactions with any other coadministered medication undergoing CYP2D6 metabolism should be anticipated.

Nonopioid Analgesic Techniques

Nonsteroidal antiinflammatory drugs

Nonsteroidal antiinflammatory drugs (NSAIDs) provide inflammation suppression and inhibition of the cyclooxygenase (COX) enzyme, which converts arachidonic acid to prostaglandins and thromboxane. NSAIDs also inhibit a variety of chemical mediators (eg, bradykinin) that are involved in the inflammatory and nociceptive response of acute pain physiology. NSAIDs have been shown to be effective in reducing postcesarean delivery pain, particularly the visceral component of pain.[23] NSAIDs have also been shown to enhance opioid analgesia and decrease opioid-related side effects through their opioid-sparing effect.[44] NSAIDs are known to have undesirable side effects, such as gastrointestinal and postoperative bleeding caused by nonselective COX-1 inhibition. However, most multimodal analgesic regimens do not require high-dose or prolonged use of these medications for effective analgesia. There has been concern about drug transfer to breast-milk and associated neonatal complications in patients receiving NSAIDs; however, the American Academy of Pediatrics regards this class of drugs to be safe for use in breastfeeding women.[45]

Ketorolac is an NSAID that is available for intravenous administration. After transition to oral intake, patients may be moved to oral NSAIDs. The addition of acetaminophen to NSAID medications has been extensively studied as well. Although most studies have failed to show additional analgesic benefit when acetaminophen was added to an NSAID regimen after cesarean delivery,[11] Munishankar and colleagues[46] reported a reduction in morphine consumption using a combined NSAID-acetaminophen regimen when compared with acetaminophen alone (33.8 mg vs 54.5 mg morphine). These conflicting results may be explained by increased acetaminophen clearance during the third trimester of pregnancy and during the postpartum period.[47] Therefore, most experts agree that NSAIDs, unless contraindicated, should be an important component of any multimodal regimen after cesarean delivery.

Anxiolytics

Anxiety has been associated with increased morphine consumption, obstetric complications, and postpartum depression.[48] High State Trait and Anxiety Inventory scores, reflecting preoperative anxiety, are known predictors of increased analgesic requirements after cesarean delivery.[49] However, unless a patient complains of anxiety, it is unlikely that including an anxiolytic medication as part of a multimodal analgesic regimen confers significant analgesic benefit.

Ketamine

Ketamine is an N-methyl-D-aspartate antagonist that has been used for postcesarean delivery analgesia. Heterogeneity exists among the studies that have evaluated the use of ketamine for postcesarean delivery analgesia, including the type of anesthesia used (ie, general vs neuraxial) as well as the dosing regiments (ie, single fixed dose vs weight-based dosing).[50–52] Ketamine has an opioid-sparing effect when used in combination with general anesthesia but has not been shown to have such an effect when neuraxial anesthesia is used.[52] Because high-dose ketamine is associated with many undesirable side effects, further work is necessary to better define its role during the postpartum period.

Peripheral Nerve Blockade

Transversus abdominis plane (TAP) blockade, ilioinguinal nerve blockade, and local anesthetic infiltration have all been described as adjuvant analgesic techniques for postcesarean delivery analgesia. However, the TAP block seems to be the most commonly used regional block when comparing these 3 techniques.[53–56] The TAP block is a regional anesthesia block in which local anesthetic is deposited within the facial plane between the internal oblique and transversus abdominis muscles in the lumbar triangle of Petit.[57] Nerves located in this fascial plane include the 9th to 11th thoracic intercostal nerves, the subcostal nerve, and the 2 branches of L1, the ilioinguinal nerve, and iliohypogastric nerves.[23,57]

McDonnell and colleagues[53] evaluated the analgesic efficacy of bilateral TAP blocks using 1.5 mL/kg of 0.75% ropivacaine versus an equal volume saline in patients undergoing elective cesarean delivery with a bupivacaine/fentanyl spinal anesthetic technique (n = 50). All patients received a multimodal analgesic regimen during the postoperative period, which included scheduled oral acetaminophen, rectal diclofenac, and patient-controlled intravenous morphine. Patients within the TAP block group had significantly reduced morphine requirements and lower postoperative visual analogue pain scores when compared with placebo controls. These differences persisted for 48 hours into the postoperative period. Subsequent studies, which used TAP blocks in combination with neuraxial morphine, failed to show any incremental benefit in postoperative analgesia.[58]

A randomized controlled study (n = 80) recently compared postoperative analgesia with a 2-mg/kg bilateral bupivacaine TAP block to intrathecal morphine.[59] Patients were randomized to 1 of 4 groups: saline TAP block/intrathecal morphine, saline TAP/intrathecal saline, bupivacaine TAP block/intrathecal morphine, or bupivacaine TAP block/intrathecal saline. All patients received a standardized postoperative analgesic regimen. The patients who received intrathecal morphine had the lowest pain scores with movement and the least morphine consumption. The TAP block did not improve pain with movement or reduce morphine consumption when given in combination with intrathecal morphine. Two recently published meta-analyses have similarly concluded that TAP blocks do not confer incremental analgesic benefit when given in combination with intrathecal morphine. However, TAP blocks are believed to be beneficial in the absence of intrathecal opioids.[60,61] TAP blockade has also been described as a rescue analgesic technique for breakthrough pain after spinal anesthesia with intrathecal morphine.[62] **Box 2** summarizes patients who are candidates for TAP blocks. Because of the large volumes of local anesthetic injected during the regional technique, providers should be aware of the potential for local anesthetic toxicity, because several studies have documented high serum local anesthetic concentrations within 15 minutes after the procedure.[63,64]

NONPHARMACOLOGIC ANALGESIC STRATEGIES
Music

Music can alter emotions by mediating the endorphin system. In the nonobstetric setting, a meta-analysis of 8 randomized controlled trials (n = 712) found that listening to music reduces anxiety and pain during colonoscopies.[65] One randomized controlled study[66] evaluated the effect of music in patients undergoing cesarean delivery under general anesthesia (n = 100). Patients were randomized to listen to either Spanish guitar music from induction to skin incision versus white noise. There were no differences in postoperative pain scores, morphine consumption, or postoperative anxiety scores. In contrast, in another randomized controlled study (n = 60), patients undergoing cesarean delivery who listened to their favorite music for 40 minutes before surgery had less anxiety and lower systolic and diastolic blood pressures than those patients who did not listen to any music before surgery.[67] In a similar randomized controlled trial (n = 60),[68] listening to music for 30 minutes before cesarean delivery was associated with lower anxiety scores and pain scores postoperatively.

Box 2
Patients who are candidates for TAP blockade

Patients who do not receive neuraxial opioids

Patients who undergo general anesthesia for cesarean delivery

Patients with breakthrough pain after neuraxial analgesia

Massage Therapy

Massage therapy may induce excitation of the central analgesia system and trigger the release of endorphins. A recent study[69] randomized patients to receive either 20 minutes of massage (5 minutes on each hand and foot), or no massage after cesarean delivery (n = 40) and evaluated postoperative pain. There was a significant decrease in pain scores, as well as a delay to the first request for rescue analgesia, within the massage therapy group.

Aromatherapy

A limited number of studies have evaluated the effect of aromatherapy, using lavender essence, on postcesarean delivery pain. Lavender is known to have antinociceptive properties.[70] Lavender essence, in addition to a standard analgesic regimen, has been shown to be successful in reducing pain scores after elective cesarean delivery after spinal anesthesia.[71]

Breastfeeding and Skin-to-Skin Contact

In animal studies, oxytocin has been shown to play a role in attachment behaviors, as well as in reducing pain thresholds.[72,73] It is possible that breastfeeding and skin-to-skin contact with the newborn, which are known to release neurotransmitters, endorphins, and oxytocin, may modulate postcesarean delivery analgesia. However, it is possible that the increased oxytocin levels from breastfeeding or skin-to-skin contact may be counteracted by systemic and neuraxial opioids. In animal studies, opioids have been shown to inhibit oxytocin release.[74] No prospective study has evaluated the role of breastfeeding or skin-to-skin contact on postcesarean delivery pain.

DISCUSSION

Pain after cesarean delivery is a multifactorial phenomenon. Because pain is considered the fifth vital sign, adequate pain control is regarded as a basic human right.[75] The Joint Commission recommends that pain be evaluated and treated, as would any other abnormal vital sign.[75] Appropriate treatment of pain allows for an earlier return to baseline function and greater patient satisfaction in addition to several other maternal and infant benefits, including early maternal-infant bonding.[27] There are several options for providing effective analgesia after cesarean delivery. However, a multimodal analgesic approach that includes neuraxial opioids seems to be the gold standard for providing optimal patient outcomes. Future study is needed to refine available and developing analgesic techniques, as well as to explore the possibility of patient-specific therapy that is based on risk-stratification and patient pharmacogenetic profiles to optimize postoperative analgesia.

REFERENCES

1. Macario A, Weinger M, Truong P, et al. Which clinical anesthesia outcomes are both common and important to avoid? The perspective of a panel of expert anesthesiologists. Anesth Analg 1999;88:1085–91.
2. Carvalho B, Cohen SE, Lipman SS, et al. Patient preferences for anesthesia outcomes associated with cesarean delivery. Anesth Analg 2005;101:1182–7.
3. Eisenach JC, Pan PH, Smiley R, et al. Severity of acute pain after childbirth, but not type of delivery, predicts persistent pain and postpartum depression. Pain 2008;140:87–94.

4. Kainu JP, Sarvela J, Tiippana E, et al. Persistent pain after caesarean section and vaginal birth: a cohort study. Int J Obstet Anesth 2010;19:4–9.

5. Lumley MA, Cohen JL, Borszcz GS, et al. Pain and emotion: a biopsychosocial review of recent research. J Clin Psychol 2011;67:942–68.

6. Zatzick DF, Dimsdale JE. Cultural variations in response to painful stimuli. Psychosom Med 1990;52:544–57.

7. Bisgaard T, Klarskov B, Rosenberg J, et al. Characteristics and prediction of early pain after laparoscopic cholecystectomy. Pain 2001;90:261–9.

8. Wong CA, McCarthy RJ, Blouin J, et al. Observational study of the effect of mu-opioid receptor genetic polymorphism on intrathecal opioid labor analgesia and post-cesarean delivery analgesia. Int J Obstet Anesth 2010;19:246–53.

9. Sia AT, Lim Y, Lim EC, et al. A118G single nucleotide polymorphism of human mu-opioid receptor gene influences pain perception and patient-controlled intravenous morphine consumption after intrathecal morphine for postcesarean analgesia. Anesthesiology 2008;109:520–6.

10. Tan EC, Lim EC, Teo YY, et al. Ethnicity and OPRM variant independently predict pain perception and patient-controlled analgesia usage for post-operative pain. Mol Pain 2009;5:32.

11. Siddik SM, Aouad MT, Jalbout MI, et al. Diclofenac and/or propacetamol for postoperative pain management after cesarean delivery in patients receiving patient controlled analgesia morphine. Reg Anesth Pain Med 2001;26:310–5.

12. Dolin SJ, Cashman JN, Bland JM. Effectiveness of acute postoperative pain management: I. Evidence from published data. Br J Anaesth 2002;89:409–23.

13. Apfelbaum JL, Chen C, Mehta SS, et al. Postoperative pain experience: results from a national survey suggest postoperative pain continues to be undermanaged. Anesth Analg 2003;97:534–40.

14. Perkins FM, Kehlet H. Chronic pain as an outcome of surgery. A review of predictive factors. Anesthesiology 2000;93:1123–33.

15. Bonica JJ. The need of a taxonomy. Pain 1979;6:247–8.

16. Breivik H, Borchgrevink PC, Allen SM, et al. Assessment of pain. Br J Anaesth 2008;101:17–24.

17. Gaskin DJ, Richard P. The economic costs of pain in the United States. J Pain 2012;13:715–24.

18. Gibbons L, Belizan JM, Lauer JA, et al. The global numbers and costs of additionally needed and unnecessary caesarean sections performed per year: overuse as a barrier to universal coverage. World Health Report. Background Paper No. 30. Geneva (Switzerland): World Health Organization; 2010.

19. Zhang J, Troendle J, Reddy UM, et al. Contemporary cesarean delivery practice in the United States. Am J Obstet Gynecol 2010;203:326.e1–10.

20. Eisenach JC, Pan P, Smiley RM, et al. Resolution of pain after childbirth. Anesthesiology 2013;118:143–51.

21. Nikolajsen L, Sorensen HC, Jensen TS, et al. Chronic pain following Caesarean section. Acta Anaesthesiol Scand 2004;48:111–6.

22. Hannah ME, Whyte H, Hannah WJ, et al. Maternal outcomes at 2 years after planned cesarean section versus planned vaginal birth for breech presentation at term: the international randomized Term Breech Trial. Am J Obstet Gynecol 2004;191:917–27.

23. McDonnell NJ, Keating ML, Muchatuta NA, et al. Analgesia after caesarean delivery. Anaesth Intensive Care 2009;37:539–51.

24. Dahlke JD, Mendez-Figueroa H, Rouse DJ, et al. Evidence-based surgery for cesarean delivery: an updated systematic review. Am J Obstet Gynecol 2013. [Epub ahead of print].
25. Bucklin BA, Hawkins JL, Anderson JR, et al. Obstetric anesthesia workforce survey: twenty-year update. Anesthesiology 2005;103:645–53.
26. American Society of Anesthesiologists Task Force on Obstetric Anesthesia. Practice guidelines for obstetric anesthesia: an updated report by the American Society of Anesthesiologists Task Force on Obstetric Anesthesia. Anesthesiology 2007;106:843–63.
27. Ng KW, Parsons J, Cyna AM, et al. Spinal versus epidural anaesthesia for caesarean section. Cochrane Database Syst Rev 2004;(2):CD003765.
28. Lim Y, Jha S, Sia AT, et al. Morphine for post-caesarean section analgesia: intrathecal, epidural or intravenous? Singapore Med J 2005;46:392–6.
29. Dahl JB, Jeppesen IS, Jorgensen H, et al. Intraoperative and postoperative analgesic efficacy and adverse effects of intrathecal opioids in patients undergoing cesarean section with spinal anesthesia: a qualitative and quantitative systematic review of randomized controlled trials. Anesthesiology 1999;91:1919–27.
30. Palmer CM, Emerson S, Volgoropolous D, et al. Dose-response relationship of intrathecal morphine for postcesarean analgesia. Anesthesiology 1999;90: 437–44.
31. Eisenach JC, Grice SC, Dewan DM. Patient-controlled analgesia following cesarean section: a comparison with epidural and intramuscular narcotics. Anesthesiology 1988;68:444–8.
32. Palmer CM, Nogami WM, Van Maren G, et al. Postcesarean epidural morphine: a dose-response study. Anesth Analg 2000;90:887–91.
33. Bonnet MP, Mignon A, Mazoit JX, et al. Analgesic efficacy and adverse effects of epidural morphine compared to parenteral opioids after elective caesarean section: a systematic review. Eur J Pain 2010;14(894):e891–9.
34. Toledo P, McCarthy RJ, Ebarvia MJ, et al. The interaction between epidural 2-chloroprocaine and morphine: a randomized controlled trial of the effect of drug administration timing on the efficacy of morphine analgesia. Anesth Analg 2009;109:168–73.
35. Carvalho B, Riley E, Cohen SE, et al. Single-dose, sustained-release epidural morphine in the management of postoperative pain after elective cesarean delivery: results of a multicenter randomized controlled study. Anesth Analg 2005;100:1150–8.
36. Dougherty TB, Baysinger CL, Henenberger JC, et al. Epidural hydromorphone with and without epinephrine for post-operative analgesia after cesarean delivery. Anesth Analg 1989;68:318–22.
37. Yu SC, Ngan Kee WD, Kwan AS. Addition of meperidine to bupivacaine for spinal anaesthesia for Caesarean section. Br J Anaesth 2002;88:379–83.
38. American Society of Anesthesiologists Task Force on Acute Pain Management. Practice guidelines for acute pain management in the perioperative setting: an updated report by the American Society of Anesthesiologists Task Force on Acute Pain Management. Anesthesiology 2004;100:1573–81.
39. Wittels B, Glosten B, Faure EA, et al. Postcesarean analgesia with both epidural morphine and intravenous patient-controlled analgesia: neurobehavioral outcomes among nursing neonates. Anesth Analg 1997;85:600–6.
40. Goetzl LM. ACOG practice bulletin. Clinical management guidelines for obstetrician-gynecologists number 36, July 2002. Obstetric analgesia and anesthesia. Obstet Gynecol 2002;100:177–91.

41. Mitra S, Khandelwal P, Sehgal A. Diclofenac-tramadol vs. diclofenac-acetaminophen combinations for pain relief after caesarean section. Acta Anaesthesiol Scand 2012;56:706–11.

42. Koren G, Cairns J, Chitayat D, et al. Pharmacogenetics of morphine poisoning in a breastfed neonate of a codeine-prescribed mother. Lancet 2006;368:704.

43. Landau R. Pharmacogenetic influences in obstetric anaesthesia. Best Pract Res Clin Obstet Gynaecol 2010;24:277–87.

44. Gadsden J, Hart S, Santos AC. Post-cesarean delivery analgesia. Anesth Analg 2005;101:S62–9.

45. American Academy of Pediatrics Committee on Drugs. Transfer of drugs and other chemicals into human milk. Pediatrics 2001;108:776–89.

46. Munishankar B, Fettes P, Moore C, et al. A double-blind randomised controlled trial of paracetamol, diclofenac or the combination for pain relief after caesarean section. Int J Obstet Anesth 2008;17:9–14.

47. Kulo A, van de Velde M, de Hoon J, et al. Pharmacokinetics of a loading dose of intravenous paracetamol post caesarean delivery. Int J Obstet Anesth 2012;21: 125–8.

48. Jamison RN, Taft K, O'Hara JP, et al. Psychosocial and pharmacologic predictors of satisfaction with intravenous patient-controlled analgesia. Anesth Analg 1993;77:121–5.

49. Pan PH, Coghill R, Houle TT, et al. Multifactorial preoperative predictors for post-cesarean section pain and analgesic requirement. Anesthesiology 2006;104: 417–25.

50. Lavand'homme P. Postcesarean analgesia: effective strategies and association with chronic pain. Curr Opin Anaesthesiol 2006;19:244–8.

51. Bilgen S, Koner O, Ture H, et al. Effect of three different doses of ketamine prior to general anaesthesia on postoperative pain following Caesarean delivery: a prospective randomized study. Minerva Anestesiol 2012;78:442–9.

52. Bauchat JR, Higgins N, Wojciechowski KG, et al. Low-dose ketamine with multimodal postcesarean delivery analgesia: a randomized controlled trial. Int J Obstet Anesth 2011;20:3–9.

53. McDonnell JG, Curley G, Carney J, et al. The analgesic efficacy of transversus abdominis plane block after cesarean delivery: a randomized controlled trial. Anesth Analg 2008;106:186–91.

54. Wolfson A, Lee AJ, Wong RP, et al. Bilateral multi-injection iliohypogastric-ilioinguinal nerve block in conjunction with neuraxial morphine is superior to neuraxial morphine alone for postcesarean analgesia. J Clin Anesth 2012;24:298–303.

55. Carvalho B, Clark DJ, Yeomans DC, et al. Continuous subcutaneous instillation of bupivacaine compared to saline reduces interleukin 10 and increases substance P in surgical wounds after cesarean delivery. Anesth Analg 2010;111: 1452–9.

56. Rackelboom T, Le Strat S, Silvera S, et al. Improving continuous wound infusion effectiveness for postoperative analgesia after cesarean delivery: a randomized controlled trial. Obstet Gynecol 2010;116:893–900.

57. Jankovic ZB, du Feu FM, McConnell P. An anatomical study of the transversus abdominis plane block: location of the lumbar triangle of Petit and adjacent nerves. Anesth Analg 2009;109:981–5.

58. Costello JF, Moore AR, Wieczorek PM, et al. The transversus abdominis plane block, when used as part of a multimodal regimen inclusive of intrathecal morphine, does not improve analgesia after cesarean delivery. Reg Anesth Pain Med 2009;34:586–9.

59. McMorrow RC, Ni Mhuircheartaigh RJ, Ahmed KA, et al. Comparison of trans-versus abdominis plane block vs spinal morphine for pain relief after Caesarean section. Br J Anaesth 2011;106:706–12.

60. Mishriky BM, George RB, Habib AS. Transversus abdominis plane block for analgesia after Cesarean delivery: a systematic review and meta-analysis. Can J Anaesth 2012;59:766–78.

61. Abdallah FW, Halpern SH, Margarido CB. Transversus abdominis plane block for postoperative analgesia after Caesarean delivery performed under spinal anaesthesia? A systematic review and meta-analysis. Br J Anaesth 2012;109: 679–87.

62. Mirza F, Carvalho B. Transversus abdominis plane blocks for rescue analgesia following Cesarean delivery: a case series. Can J Anaesth 2012;60(3):299–303.

63. Griffiths JD, Barron FA, Grant S, et al. Plasma ropivacaine concentrations after ultrasound-guided transversus abdominis plane block. Br J Anaesth 2010;105: 853–6.

64. Griffiths JD, Le NV, Grant S, et al. Symptomatic local anaesthetic toxicity and plasma ropivacaine concentrations after transversus abdominis plane block for Caesarean section. Br J Anaesth 2013;110(6):996–1000.

65. Bechtold ML, Puli SR, Othman MO, et al. Effect of music on patients undergoing colonoscopy: a meta-analysis of randomized controlled trials. Dig Dis Sci 2009; 54:19–24.

66. Reza N, Ali SM, Saeed K, et al. The impact of music on postoperative pain and anxiety following cesarean section. Middle East J Anesthesiol 2007;19:573–86.

67. Kushnir J, Friedman A, Ehrenfeld M, et al. Coping with preoperative anxiety in cesarean section: physiological, cognitive, and emotional effects of listening to favorite music. Birth 2012;39:121–7.

68. Li Y, Dong Y. Preoperative music intervention for patients undergoing cesarean delivery. Int J Gynaecol Obstet 2012;119:81–3.

69. Abbaspoor Z, Akbari M, Najar S. Effect of foot and hand massage in post-cesarean section pain control: a randomized control trial. Pain Manag Nurs 2013. [Epub ahead of print].

70. Woronuk G, Demissie Z, Rheault M, et al. Biosynthesis and therapeutic proper-ties of *Lavandula* essential oil constituents. Planta Med 2011;77:7–15.

71. Hadi N, Hanid AA. Lavender essence for post-cesarean pain. Pak J Biol Sci 2011;14:664–7.

72. Higham JP, Barr CS, Hoffman CL, et al. Mu-opioid receptor (OPRM1) variation, oxytocin levels and maternal attachment in free-ranging rhesus macaques *Macaca mulatta*. Behav Neurosci 2011;125:131–6.

73. Uvnas-Moberg K, Bruzelius G, Alster P, et al. Oxytocin increases and a specific oxytocin antagonist decreases pain threshold in male rats. Acta Physiol Scand 1992;144:487–8.

74. Vuong C, Van Uum SH, O'Dell LE, et al. The effects of opioids and opioid ana-logs on animal and human endocrine systems. Endocr Rev 2010;31:98–132.

75. Lanser P, Gesell S. Pain management: the fifth vital sign. Healthc Benchmarks 2001;8:68–70, 62.

Assessment of Pain in the Neonate

Lynne G. Maxwell, MD[a,b,*], Carrie P. Malavolta, MSN, CRNP[c],
Maria V. Fraga, MD[c,d]

KEYWORDS

- Neonate • Pain • Assessment • Pain scales

KEY POINTS

- Many neonatal pain assessment tools are available.
- Although "brain-oriented" technologies have been explored as more subjective indicators of neonatal pain, none are currently ready for clinical implementation.
- Each NICU should choose a limited number of tools for pain assessment in different populations (full term, preterm) and context and type of pain (procedural, postoperative).
- Nurses should be trained and evaluated for appropriate use of selected tools.
- Standards should be established for triggers for administration of rescue medication.

More than 15 million premature infants are born worldwide each year.[1] These infants, along with term neonates who are born ill, compromised either by congenital abnormalities or by peripartum or intrauterine adverse events, spend their first weeks of life hospitalized in the neonatal intensive care unit (NICU) where they are subjected to multiple invasive procedures that are frequently painful. It has been reported that infants born at 25 to 42 weeks of gestation experienced an average of 14 painful procedures a day during the first 2 weeks of life.[2–4] In addition, many neonates, both premature and term, undergo surgical procedures associated with postoperative pain. Pain is an unpleasant sensory and emotional experience associated with actual or potential tissue damage (International Association for the Study of Pain Subcommittee on Taxonomy [IASP], 1986).[5] It is important to understand that the inability of these neonatal patients to communicate verbally or nonverbally does not mean that an infant is not experiencing pain. As the IASP states, "The inability to communicate verbally does not negate the possibility that an individual is experiencing pain and is in need

[a] Anesthesiology and Critical Care, Perelman School of Medicine, University of Pennsylvania, 3400 Spruce Street, Philadelphia, PA 19104, USA; [b] Department of Anesthesiology and Critical Care Medicine, The Children's Hospital of Philadelphia, 3401 Civic Center Boulevard, Philadelphia, PA 19104, USA; [c] Division of Neonatology, The Children's Hospital of Philadelphia, 3401 Civic Center Boulevard, Philadelphia, PA 19104, USA; [d] Department of Pediatrics, Perelman School of Medicine, University of Pennsylvania, 3401 Civic Center Boulevard, Philadelphia, PA 19104, USA
* Corresponding author. Department of Anesthesiology and Critical Care Medicine, The Children's Hospital of Philadelphia, 3401 Civic Center Boulevard, Philadelphia, PA 19104.
E-mail address: maxwell@email.chop.edu

Clin Perinatol 40 (2013) 457–469
http://dx.doi.org/10.1016/j.clp.2013.05.001   perinatology.theclinics.com
0095-5108/13/$ – see front matter © 2013 Elsevier Inc. All rights reserved.

of appropriate pain-relieving treatment."[5] Indeed, this circumstance requires caregivers to be knowledgeable about and to implement the most valid and reliable pain assessment tools to optimize pain management in this vulnerable population.

NEURODEVELOPMENTAL CONSIDERATIONS FOR PAIN ASSESSMENT

Although neonates were formerly suspected of having blunted, immature responses to pain, it is now clear that premature and full-term newborns have the neuroanatomic pathways from periphery to cortex required for nociception. In fact, by the 24th week of gestation, painful stimuli are associated with physiologic, hormonal, and metabolic markers of the stress response.[6] Indeed, pain perception and the stress response may be greater in preterm infants because of immaturity of descending inhibitory pathways.

Because the still-developing nervous system of immature preterm neonates differs from that of term infants, preterm neonates are particularly vulnerable to the effects of pain and stress. The developmental neurobiology of pain confirms that afferent systems are fully functional at 24 weeks' gestation; however, the self-regulatory autonomic and neuroendocrine systems modulating sensory experience may be immature in preterm babies. Development of descending inhibitory pathways may be delayed in both neurotransmitter-receptor relationships and in neural connections in the dorsal horn.[7] Tactile threshold is lower, so these infants become sensitized to repeated skin breaking and even tactile stimuli, leading to greater sensitivity to pain during and after this vulnerable period.[8] Careful observation of physiologic and behavioral indicators demonstrates that the sensory, distressing, and disruptive impact of pain is evident in this population; however, recognizing pain and distinguishing it from other conditions remain a challenge. This is especially true because although infants born at younger gestational ages clearly perceive pain, perhaps to a heightened degree, at the same time they do not have the capability to display the full spectrum of pain behavior seen in infants born closer to term, therefore requiring modification of assessment tools to take these differences into account.

IMPLICATIONS OF PAIN EXPERIENCED IN THE NEONATAL PERIOD

Although there is still little empiric data specifically related to long-term effects of early physical pain, studies have shown that newborns, especially preterm infants, are vulnerable to long-term effects that may lead to permanent changes in brain processing and impaired brain development,[9,10] including altered pain sensitivity and maladaptive behavior later in life.[11,12] A wide spectrum of developmental, learning, and behavioral problems are prevalent among preterm infants, especially in extremely low birth weight (ELBW, <1000 g) neonates. These outcomes are confounded by multiple factors, and are in part mediated by neonatal illness as well as socioeconomic environment. The view that the NICU environment may be a factor in altered development has been expressed for some time, with early repetitive pain interacting with other stressors in the NICU currently viewed as having the most pervasive potential effects.[13,14] After discharge from the NICU, biobehavioral responsivity to invasive skin damage of former ELBW infants was compared with term-born healthy infants at 4 and 8 months corrected age.[15–17] Pain reactivity of ELBW infants at 4 months corrected age did not appear grossly altered. At 8 months, ELBW infants initially showed greater facial response compared with term-born infants, but only immediately following finger lance. However, the response of the ELBW infants attenuated rapidly, showing more rapid behavioral and physiologic dampening (less facial and autonomic responses) during recovery. Furthermore, the ELBW infants displayed higher basal resting heart rate, suggesting a possible long-term "resetting" of autonomic regulation. Conversely, parent rating of their child's pain sensitivity to everyday bumps at 18 months corrected age showed that ELBW toddlers were significantly less reactive to everyday pain compared with heavier preterm (1000–2500 g) and term-born infants.[18]

Even infants born at term show persistent effects of pain experienced in the neonatal period. Full-term infants who underwent circumcision without analgesia in the newborn period showed increased pain responses to immunization at 4 to 6 months of age when compared with both female infants and infants who had circumcision with analgesia.[19] These healthy infants do not have the confounders that may affect changes in pain perception and development seen in the premature population. In summary, some studies provide a basis for concern that pain response and behavior may be altered in former preterm infants but potentially confounding factors need to be considered carefully in evaluating human responses beyond infancy, because there are multiple sources of stress and impacts on neurologic development other than early pain that may contribute to alteration in neurodevelopment.

PAIN ASSESSMENT METHODOLOGY

The gold standard of pain assessment is self-report, using validated scales, such as a numeric scale, or visual analog scale for individuals who are cognitively intact and older than 8, and tools such as the Faces-Revised or Oucher scale for cognitively intact children ages 4 to 8.[20] Because neonates are nonverbal, physiologic, biobehavioral, and behavioral indicators are used as a surrogate for self-report. Despite considerable research on the assessment of pain in infants undergoing neonatal intensive care, critical methodological issues remain. Pain assessment in infants becomes even more challenging when typical distress behaviors are confounded by mechanical ventilation, pharmacologic interventions, and physical restraint inherent to care in the NICU.

PHYSIOLOGIC INDICATORS OF PAIN

Physiologic indicators of pain that are measured by neonatal pain assessment tools are typically relatively noninvasive measures. These include changes in heart rate, respiratory rate, blood pressure, and oxygen saturation.[21] Without the presence of an indwelling arterial line, blood pressure measurements via a cuff may be difficult to obtain without inducing discomfort. Use of vital signs alone for pain assessment has been demonstrated to be ineffective because of the inability of neonates to mount a sustained autonomic response to pain and the presence of other factors, such as mechanical ventilation and pharmacologic intervention that may impact vital signs.[22] Physiologic measures may be the only method of assessing pain in infants who are pharmacologically paralyzed or who are severely neurologically impaired. However, it has been suggested that the validity and reliability of these measures are questionable, as they are influenced by other physiologic confounders, such as hypovolemia or fever (increased heart rate), or pulmonary parenchymal disease or atelectasis (desaturation, increased work of breathing with grunting).[23]

BEHAVIORAL INDICATORS OF PAIN

Behavioral parameters, such as facial activity, cry, body movements and resting positions, fussiness/consolability, and sleeplessness have been the most studied indicators.[21] The ability to assess behavioral indicators may depend on gestational age, mechanical ventilation, and pharmacologic interventions, including sedation and pharmacologic paralysis.[10] The individual parameters in all pain scales used in preterm infants were originally derived from observations of term-born infants. Although preterm infants respond with facial, motor, and physiologic changes, with patterns similar to those seen in term infants, their responses are of smaller magnitude as gestational age decreases,[9,21] and they may have dampened facial responses to repeated invasive procedures. In addition, they may "shut down" behaviorally to invasive stimuli, leading clinicians to the potentially erroneous conclusion that these infants are not experiencing pain.[24] Furthermore, lack of observation of infants for longer periods of time may fail to capture delayed responses, resulting in underestimation of the need for caregiver intervention.

Currently, no individual physiologic or behavioral indicators reliably and specifically mark the presence of pain in preterm neonates. Moreover, dissociations between physiologic and behavioral responses to painful stimuli are common.[22] For these reasons, reliance on a unidimensional pain index is insufficient.

- Despite awareness of the importance of pain prevention, neonates continue to be exposed to multiple painful procedures daily as part of their routine care
- Currently, no physiologic or behavioral indicators specifically mark the presence of pain in *preterm* neonates
- Preterm neonates are vulnerable to long-term effects that may lead to permanent changes in brain processing, including altered pain sensitivity and maladaptive behavior later in life

PAIN ASSESSMENT

Accurate assessment of pain is vital to ensure optimal effectiveness and safety of pain management therapy in neonates who experience pain during the course of their NICU stay. As discussed previously, neonatal pain assessment is complicated by the fact that neonates are preverbal and must rely completely on caregivers for pain assessment.[25]

PARENTAL INVOLVEMENT IN PAIN ASSESSMENT

In older preverbal or nonverbal children, parents play an essential role in the pain-assessment process, as they know their children better than intermittent care providers in the hospital setting. However, the NICU presents some unique challenges in the integration of parent input for pain assessment. For a variety of reasons, parents may or may not be present in the NICU.[26] To provide the appropriate level of care after birth, a neonate may need to be transferred to a NICU at another hospital while the mother remains at the delivering hospital. Sometimes the circumstances surrounding the birth may have resulted in the mother being critically ill and unable to visit the NICU. During a prolonged NICU stay, parents may need to return to work or visit less frequently because of the need to care for other children. All of these factors may lead to a reduced parental presence in the NICU.[26]

Even when parents are able to be present, there may be several factors that prevent parents from feeling comfortable providing input on their baby's pain. New parents often feel insecure about their babies, and if something unexpected has occurred, such as a premature birth, a term infant with a congenital malformation, or a traumatic birth, parents may feel even further unqualified to assist in providing pain assessment.[27] Parents may feel ambivalent: they simply do not wish to see their baby in pain but not too sedated. The NICU environment includes many painful procedures, as well as infants who respond differently to pain based on gestational age, illness, or medical treatment. All of these things can be very disconcerting and frightening to parents and make it more difficult for them to be active participants in pain assessment. If primary nursing is available for very sick neonates from the onset of care, the primary nurse can assist both in providing an accurate description of the baseline for a given infant and also in educating parents on what to look for and the continuum between adequate analgesia and oversedation.[28]

NEONATAL PAIN ASSESSMENT TOOLS

Because neonates are preverbal, and parents may not be able to provide assistance in pain assessment, nurses and other care providers must be well trained in neonatal pain assessment to ensure adequate pain management.[29] A large variety of validated neonatal pain-assessment tools have been developed. These tools vary in their combination of physiologic and behavioral measures, as well as whether they take gestational age into account. Additionally, tools have been designed and validated for different types of pain, including procedural, postoperative, acute, and chronic pain.[30] Although more than 40 different neonatal pain assessment tools have been developed,[31] only a few are regularly incorporated into use in most NICUs. Because no comprehensive data exist on those used most commonly, one must infer this from tools used in published studies of neonatal pain. **Table 1** summarizes the features of these commonly used scales according to parameters measured, neonatal population, and painful conditions for which they have been validated, and scale metric.[29] Commonly used neonatal pain tools are listed in **Table 1**.

- 2 scales have metric adjustment for prematurity (Premature Infant Pain Profile/ Neonatal Pain, Agitation, and Sedation Scale [PIPP/N-PASS])
- Other scales have been used in premature infants, although developed in full-term infants
- Only 1 scale takes sedation into account (N-PASS)

As previously discussed, gestational age can significantly impact the ability of a neonate to mount or display a response to pain, whether through physiologic or behavioral indicators. Historically, neonates have been stratified into groups according to gestational age, birth weight, or postconceptual age (gestational age plus postnatal age). Most neonatal pain scales that make adjustments for prematurity do so using gestational age. Premature infants of all gestational ages (fewer than 37 weeks) demonstrate a decreased ability to mount a physiologic response to painful stimuli.[22,25] Multiple factors may influence a premature infant's vital signs, and an increase in heart rate and/or respiratory rate may not be an indicator of pain alone. In addition, very premature infants may be completely unable to demonstrate a change in vital signs because of pain, and the ability to sustain this for any prolonged period of time is markedly diminished.[23] Similarly, the lack of energy reserve present in premature infants of any gestational age may result in an absent or muted behavioral response to painful stimuli.[30] Only 2 of the aforementioned commonly used pain scales (PIPP and N-PASS) have a metric adjustment to account for prematurity; however, other scales have demonstrated validity and reliability in the premature population.[29]

In addition to gestational age, scales are tested for validity and reliability based on the type of pain that they are designed to assess. These types of pain include procedural, postoperative, acute, and chronic (or prolonged) pain. Additionally, some scales take sedation into account.[29] The presence of agitation or sedation in a neonate can

Table 1
Summary of neonatal pain assessment tools

Pain Assessment Tool	Gestational Age/Post-conceptional Age	Physiologic Components	Behavioral Components	Type of Pain	Adjusts for Prematurity	Scale Metric
PIPP (Premature Infant Pain Profile)[58]	28–40 wk	Heart rate, oxygen saturation	Alertness, brow bulge, eye squeeze, nasolabial furrow	Procedural and Postoperative	Yes	0 to 21
CRIES (Cries, Requires Oxygen, Increased Vital Signs, Expression, Sleeplessness)[59]	32–56 wk	Blood pressure, heart rate, oxygen saturation	Cry, expression, sleeplessness	Postoperative	No	0 to 10
NIPS (Neonatal Infant Pain Scale)[60]	28–38 wk	Breathing pattern	Facial expression, cry, arms, legs, alertness	Procedural	No	0 to 7
COMFORT (and COMFORTneo)[35,61]	0–3 y (COMFORTneo: 24–42 wk)	Respiratory response, blood pressure, heart rate	Alertness, agitation, physical movements, muscle tone, facial tension	Postoperative (COMFORTneo: prolonged)	No	8 to 40
NFCS (Neonatal Facial Coding System)[62]	25 wk to Term	None	Brow bulge, eye squeeze, nasolabial furrow, open lips, stretch mouth (vertical and horizontal), lip purse, taut tongue, chin quiver	Procedural	No	0 to 10
N-PASS (Neonatal Pain, Agitation, and Sedation Scale)[33]	0–100 d	Heart rate, respiratory rate, blood pressure, oxygen saturation	Crying/irritability, behavior state, facial expression, extremities/tone	Acute and prolonged pain. Also assesses sedation	Yes	Pain: 0 to 10 Sedation −10 to 0
EDIN (Échelle de la Douleur Inconfort Noveau-Né – Neonatal Pain and Discomfort Scale)[32]	25–36 wk	None	Facial activity, body movements, quality of sleep, quality of contact with nurses, consolability	Prolonged	No	0 to 15
BPSN (Bernese Pain Scale for Neonates)[63]	27–41 wk	Respiratory pattern, heart rate, oxygen saturation	Alertness, duration of cry, time to calm, skin color, brow bulge with eye squeeze, posture	Procedural	No	0 to 27

be misinterpreted as pain by those scales that do not take sedation into account.[25] The vast majority of scales were designed for acute pain, either procedural and/or postoperative. The presence of prolonged pain in neonates is much more difficult to assess, as neonates may adapt to the presence of prolonged pain from the standpoint of both physiologic and behavioral measures.[32] Only 2 scales have demonstrated validity and reliability for prolonged pain (N-PASS and EDIN [Échelle Douleur Inconfort Nouveau-Né (Neonatal Pain and Discomfort Scale)]),[32,33] but the COMFORTneo scale, adapted for use in neonates based on the COMFORT scale,[34] has shown promise in measuring prolonged pain in one study.[35]

When choosing specific scales to use for neonatal pain, it is always important to select scales that have been proven validated and reliable, and, if possible, have studies replicating this.[33] There are many challenges to selecting appropriate scales for a given NICU setting. This includes the fact that NICU populations are diverse, often made up of premature and term infants; some sedated, paralyzed, and mechanically ventilated infants; and some surgical infants. If a given scale relies on an audible cry for assessment, then this scale may not be usable for a sizable portion of the given population. As noted previously and in **Table 1**, scales may have demonstrated validity and reliability only for a certain gestational age and a certain type of pain, which makes selecting a single scale for the entire NICU population very difficult.[30] Practical considerations also must be factored into scale choice.

As can be seen in **Table 1**, another major difference among tools is the scale metric (the numerical range of possible scores). Although the most commonly used scales in older infants, children, and adults use a 0 to 10 scale, neonatal scales vary widely, with maximum scores ranging from 7 to 40 and minimum scores from 0 to 8. This variability makes the use of tools with disparate scales problematic in a single NICU and may impair education, as well as attempts to compare outcomes for research purposes.

Choosing the best scale, or scales, for a given NICU population will require close examination of the typical patient population(s) for the unit. Scales should be ultimately considered more useful if they are demonstrated to be valid and reliable, if they account for a broad range of gestational ages, and if they have a long track record of use. Even if a scale is determined to be valid and reliable, the feasibility and practical utility must be examined by those who will be using it.[36] If 2 scales are chosen for use on a unit, care providers must be carefully trained and their performance evaluated on an ongoing basis to ensure that they remain consistent among themselves for individual patients. Units may choose to adapt a scale designed for procedural pain to assess pain in all circumstances, but clinicians must constantly assess what they may be missing by not using a scale designed to monitor postoperative pain or in cases of prolonged pain.

NOVEL PHYSIOLOGIC PAIN ASSESSMENT TOOLS AND BIOMARKERS

Despite the plethora of neonatal pain assessment tools, there is no generally agreed on "gold standard" and there are problems of inconsistency among assessors. Because of the imperfect nature of the various multidimensional neonatal pain assessment tools described previously, more objective, technology-based autonomic, brain, and biohormonal measures have been explored as a possibly more objective indicator of pain level. These tools include autonomic measures, such as heart rate variability,[37] skin conductance, and brain measures, such as electroencephalogram (EEG) or near-infrared spectroscopy (NIRS). In addition, hormonal markers of stress, such as cortisol and plasma parameters of oxidative stress, have been evaluated. Holsti and colleagues[38] have referred to this approach as "brain-oriented."

Slater and colleagues[39] used NIRS to assess hemodynamic activity over the somatosensory cortex during procedural pain (heel lance) and found correlation between cortical hemodynamic and behavioral responses. NIRS works through the differential absorption of infrared light by hemoglobin and cytochrome aa3, with changes in hemoglobin absorption reflecting changes in cerebral blood flow. There were some painful episodes in which hemodynamic changes were observed in the absence of behavioral changes, suggesting the possibility that pain assessment based on more conventional pain assessment tools may underestimate the pain response in neonates. If this is confirmed with further investigation and the technology made easier to use in the clinical setting, NIRS may provide a more objective measurement of pain. Implementation of NIRS is problematic because movement and other environmental factors (drug treatment, hemodynamic changes, and respiratory changes) can interfere with accuracy, making its clinical utility questionable.

EEG monitoring measures cortical neuronal activity, but isolating cortical evoked responses to pain may require complex "time-lock" technology, as demonstrated by Slater and colleagues,[40] which limits its practical implementation at this time. In addition, it may be difficult to distinguish increased cortical somatosensory activity from that related to motor activity, especially in the smallest infants.

Skin conductance, sometimes referred to as galvanic skin resistance (GSR) is related to palm and sole sweating, which reflects increased sympathetic nervous system activity. Changes in frequency and area under the curve have been demonstrated with procedural pain and have been shown to differentiate between pain (heel stick) and stress (alcohol wipe on skin).[41] Gjerstad and colleagues[42] found that increase in the number of skin conductance fluctuations correlated with increase in COMFORT score with tracheal suction in intubated children, but sensitivity was impaired by other sources of stress (postoperative pain in the first 24 hours after surgery) and subject to movement artifact. In the setting of postoperative pain in older children, however, skin conductance was found to have low sensitivity and specificity. In the awake patient, measurement was confounded by non-noxious factors that affect sympathetic activity, casting doubt on its utility for postoperative pain in neonates.[43] Although heart rate and heart rate variability have been proposed as more objective measures of pain, investigators, such as Oberlander and Saul,[37] have found that medical condition confounders interfere with the utility of heart rate alone as a pain measure and suggest further work.

Cortisol level is a biomarker of pain and stress states, which has been used in clinical trial study designs, but it is impractical for real-time pain assessment for treatment decision making, as there is a considerable delay in obtaining the results. Although a further impediment was the need to draw blood for cortisol determination, recent studies have successfully used salivary cortisol levels. Although some studies have found increased serum or salivary cortisol with increased pain and stress, one study has found a downregulation of serum cortisol response to stress in premature infants with higher exposure to procedural pain in the neonatal period.[44,45] Measures of oxidative stress, such as uric acid and malondialdehyde, have been found to increase after a tissue-damaging procedure.[46] This is not a practical real-time measure of pain but might be useful to assess efficacy of pain treatment strategies in a research setting.

These biologic and brain-based measures have been used experimentally and are theoretically attractive and potentially may be more objective measures of pain in neonates and infants than composite pain assessment tools subjectively interpreted by bedside caregivers. However, the lack of standardization and familiarity with these technologies make their use in the clinical setting impractical at this time; therefore, we remain dependent on the pain assessment tools described previously.

PRACTICAL PROBLEMS IN IMPLEMENTATION OF NEONATAL PAIN ASSESSMENT AND ASSESSMENT-BASED TREATMENT

There is no generally agreed on clinical standard for pain score threshold at which analgesic intervention should be administered. Even in the same infant there is poor correlation between pain score and the presence or absence of analgesic intervention. On the other hand, clinical trials of analgesics frequently establish specific numeric thresholds for different pain interventions, as in the recently study of intravenous acetaminophen by Ceelie and colleagues.[47] This study design follows on the work of Allegaert and colleagues,[48] who demonstrated that implementation of systematic evaluation of pain (both surgical and nonsurgical), including specific interventions based on pain scores, led to an increase in both amount and duration of prescribed analgesics. Despite the availability of multiple neonatal pain scores at the time of these studies, these investigators used a pain scale developed at their institution, the Leuven neonatal pain scale. One proposed method of improving the linkage of pain assessment to analgesic intervention involves the incorporation of a pain and discomfort tool (COMFORT) into the computerized order entry (Computerized Provider Order Entry [CPOE]) system, which was then linked to ordering sufentanil for pain or midazolam for sedation for mechanically ventilated premature infants.[49]

Postoperative studies only rarely link pain scores to specific analgesic treatment, as discussed previously. Franck and colleagues compared 4 pain scales (Children's and Infants' Postoperative Pain Scale [CHIPPS]; Cries, Requires Oxygen, Increased Vital Signs, Expression, Sleeplessness [CRIES]; COMFORT; and PIPP) in addition to urinary and plasma cortisol in 81 neonates after cardiac surgery.[50] This was done separately from the clinical care of the patient. In this setting, they found that the COMFORT scale performed best with both physiologic and behavioral parameters playing a role, correlating best with both plasma cortisol levels and opioid dose, although the caregivers did not consistently use pain assessment in determining the necessity for analgesic intervention. These investigators point out that "there is no consistent definition or objective measure of the "need for analgesia," which may cause bias toward the use of behavioral over physiologic measures or vice versa in intubated, paralyzed patients. This is a fundamental problem in the clinical setting, where there is ambiguity in the interface between distress and pain, and ambivalence on the part of the caregiver with regard to the positive and adverse effects of opioid treatment and the tension between avoiding the adverse effects of untreated pain and the negative consequences of overmedication.[51] It is difficult even for trained nurses to accurately differentiate pain from other sources of distress, especially in intubated patients. Although nonpharmacologic measures (sucrose-pacifier, swaddling, kangaroo care) have been shown to be efficacious in the procedural pain setting, their utility in the setting of postoperative pain is less clear.

PAIN CHAMPIONS

Many audits of compliance with institutional/unit standards of pain assessment have revealed poor compliance and lack of fidelity to the way the tool was to be applied.[52,53] Whatever tools are chosen for a given neonatal unit, it is important that the tool be used in the specific manner described. The meticulous training of "pain champions" or pain assessment "superusers" may be helpful in ongoing training and assessment of accuracy in implementation of pain assessment tools.[54] For example, the PIPP requires 2 periods of observation of the infant for 15 seconds before the procedure and for 30 seconds after the painful stimulus. De Oliveira and colleagues[55] showed that there was variability among raters using the PIPP score for procedural pain. Raters had difficulty applying the tool, especially with respect to the time required for observation and confusion about the definitions of the behavioral categories. This study identified these factors as a source of confusion and lack of reproducibility of scoring among untrained raters, differentiating the "real world" clinical from the research setting. Franck and Bruce[56] identified multiple issues of interpersonal dynamics and caregiver decision making that interfere with effective use of clinical pain assessment and its relationship to pain treatment. Brahnam and colleagues[57] proposed using facial recognition technology for assessment of neonatal facial pain expressions because it has been observed that "health professionals are frequently biased and may over- or under-emphasize elements" of the assessment tool in question. Although use of such facial recognition technology may not be practical in the clinical setting, such photographs could be used in training caregivers.

CONCLUSION

Accurate pain assessment in preterm and term neonates in the NICU is of vital importance because of the high prevalence of painful experiences in this population, in the form of both daily procedural pain and postoperative pain. Over 40 tools have been developed to assess pain in neonates, which rely on physiologic parameters, behavioral parameters, or both. Each NICU should choose a limited number of tools for pain assessment in different populations (full term, preterm) and context and type of pain (procedural, postoperative). Nurses should be well-trained in the use of selected neonatal pain assessment tools, and ongoing evaluation and re-education should be implemented to ensure accurate use of these tools. Currently, there is no combination of physiologic and/or behavioral indicators that mark the presence of pain in preterm neonates as reliably and specifically as those validated in full term infants. This can make pain assessment in preterm neonates particularly challenging. Only two pain assessment tools have a metric adjustment to account for prematurity. Preterm neonates are also vulnerable to long-term sequelae of painful experiences, which may lead to permanent changes in brain processing including altered pain sensitivity and maladaptive behavior later in life. In both term and preterm neonates, parents can be valuable participants in the evaluation of their infant's pain, but they may need reinforcement and education from nursing providers. In the future, "brain-oriented" technologies may become available to help objectively assess neonatal pain. Future directions include the development of the these technologies and the need for further studies on the optimization of the use of current and future neonatal pain assessment tools and on other methods with which to objectively measure and form the basis for safe and effective treatment of neonatal pain.

REFERENCES

1. March of Dimes, PMNCH, Save the Children, WHO. Born too soon: the global action report on preterm birth. In: Howson CP, Kinney MV, Lawn JE, editors. Geneva (Switzerland): World Health Organization; 2012.
2. Simons SH, Van Dijk M, Anand KS, et al. Do we still hurt newborn babies? A prospective study of procedural pain and analgesia in neonates. Arch Pediatr Adolesc Med 2003;157:1058–64.
3. Carbajal R, Rousset A, Danan C, et al. Epidemiology and treatment of painful procedures in neonates in intensive care units. JAMA 2008;300:60–70.
4. Johnston C, Barrington KJ, Taddio A, et al. Pain in Canadian NICUs. Have we improved over the past 12 years? Clin J Pain 2011;27:225–32.

5. Available at: http://www.iasp-pain.org/Content/NavigationMenu/GeneralResource Links/PainDefinitions/default.htm. Accessed February 18, 2013.
6. Lee SJ, Ralston HJ, Drey EA, et al. Fetal pain: a systematic multidisciplinary review of the evidence. JAMA 2005;294:947–54.
7. Beggs S, Fitzgerald M. Development of peripheral and spinal nociceptive systems. In: Anand KJ, Stevens BJ, McGrath PJ, editors. Pain in neonates and infants. 3rd edition. Edinburgh (United Kingdom): Elsevier; 2007. p. 11–24.
8. Vinall J, Steven PM, Chau V, et al. Neonatal pain in relation to postnatal growth in infants born very preterm. Pain 2012;153:1374–81.
9. Johnston CC, Stevens BJ. Experience in neonatal intensive care unit affects pain response. Pediatrics 1996;98:925–30.
10. Brummelte S, Grunau RV, Chau V, et al. Procedural pain and brain development in premature infants. Ann Neurol 2012;71:385–96.
11. Anand KJ, Scalzo F. Can adverse neonatal experiences alter brain development and subsequent behavior? Biol Neonate 2000;77:69–82.
12. Taddio A, Katz J. The effects of early pain experience in neonates on pain responses in infancy and childhood. Paediatr Drugs 2005;7:45–57.
13. Anand KJ. Effects of perinatal pain and stress. In: Mayer EA, Saper CB, editors. Progress in brain research, vol. 122. Amsterdam: Elsevier; 2000. p. 117–29.
14. Grunau RV. Long-term consequences of pain in human neonates. In: Anand KJ, Stevens BJ, McGrath PJ, editors. Pain in neonates: pain research and clinical management, vol. 10. Amsterdam: Elsevier; 2000. p. 55–76.
15. Oberlander TF, Grunau RV, Pitfield J, et al. The developmental character of cardiac autonomic responses to an acute noxious event in 4- and 8-month old healthy infants. Pediatr Res 1999;45(4 Pt 1):519–25.
16. Grunau RV, Oberlander TF, Whitfield MF, et al. Pain reactivity in former extremely low birth weight infants at corrected age 8 months compared with term born controls. Infant Behav Dev 2001;24:41–55.
17. Oberlander TF, Grunau RV, Whitfield MF, et al. Biobehavioral pain responses in former extremely low birth weight infants at four months' corrected age. Pediatrics 2000;105:e6.
18. Grunau RV, Whitfield MF, Petrie JH. Pain sensitivity and temperament in extremely low-birth-weight premature toddlers and preterm and full-term controls. Pain 1994;58:341–6.
19. Taddio A, Katz J, Ilersich AL, et al. Effect of neonatal circumcision on pain response during subsequent routine vaccination. Lancet 1997;349(9052):599–603.
20. Gaffney A, McGrath PJ, Dick B. Measuring pain in children: developmental and instrument issues. In: Schechter NL, Berde CB, Yaster M, editors. Pain in infants, children and adolescents. 2nd edition. Philadelphia: Lippincott Williams & Wilkins; 2000. p. 128–41.
21. Craig KD, Whitfield MF, Grunau RV, et al. Pain in the preterm neonate: behavioral and physiological indices. Pain 1993;52:287–99.
22. Morison SJ, Holsti L, Grunau RV. Are there developmentally distinct motor indicators of pain in preterm infants? Early Hum Dev 2003;72:131–46.
23. Raeside L. Physiologic measures of assessing infant pain: a literature review. Br J Nurs 2011;20:1370–6.
24. Stevens BJ, Johnston CC, Grunau RV. Issues of assessment of pain and discomfort in neonates. J Obstet Gynecol Neonatal Nurs 1995;24:849–55.
25. Koeppel R. Assessment and management of acute pain in the newborn. Washington, DC: Association of Women's Health, Obstetric and Neonatal Nurses; 2007. Web Continuing Education Resource.

26. Garten L, Maass E, Schmalisch G, et al. O father, where art thou? Parental NICU visiting patterns during the first 28 days of life of very low-birth-weight infants. J Perinat Neonatal Nurs 2011;25(4):342–8.

27. Axelin A, Lehtonen L, Pelander T, et al. Mothers' different styles of involvement in preterm infant pain care. J Obstet Gynecol Neonatal Nurs 2010;39:415–24.

28. Franck LS, Oulton K, Bruce E. Parental involvement in neonatal pain management: an empirical and conceptual update. J Nurs Scholarsh 2012;44:45–54.

29. American Academy of Pediatrics Committee on Fetus and Newborn, American Academy of Pediatrics Section on Surgery, Canadian Paediatric Society and Fetus and Newborn Committee. Prevention and management of pain in the neonate: an update. Pediatrics 2006;118:2231–41.

30. Walden M, Gibbins S. Pain assessment and management: guideline for practice. 2nd edition. Glenview (IL): National Association of Neonatal Nurses; 2008. p. 1–29.

31. Ranger M, Johnston CC, Anand KJ. Current controversies regarding pain assessment in neonates. Semin Perinatol 2007;31:283–8.

32. Debillon T, Zupan V, Ravault N, et al. Development and initial validation of the EDIN scale, a new tool for assessing prolonged pain in preterm infants. Arch Dis Child Fetal Neonatal Ed 2001;85:F36–41.

33. Hummel P, Puchalski M, Creech SD, et al. Clinical reliability and validity of the N-PASS: Neonatal Pain, Agitation and Sedation Scale with prolonged pain. J Perinatol 2008;28:55–60.

34. Ambuel B, Hamlett KW, Marx CM, et al. Assessing distress in pediatric intensive care environments: the COMFORT scale. J Ped Psychol 1992;17:95–109.

35. van Dijk M, Roofthooft DW, Anand KJ, et al. Taking up the challenge of measuring prolonged pain in (premature) neonates: the COMFORTneo scale seems promising. Clin J Pain 2009;25:607–16.

36. Duhn LJ, Medves JM. A systematic integrative review of infant pain assessment tools. Adv Neonatal Care 2004;4:126–40.

37. Oberlander T, Saul JP. Methodological considerations for the use of heart rate variability as a measure of pain reactivity in vulnerable infants. Clin Perinatol 2002;29:427–43.

38. Holsti L, Grunau RE, Shany E. Assessing pain in preterm infants in the neonatal intensive care unit: moving to a "brain-oriented" approach. Pain Manag 2011;1: 171–9.

39. Slater R, Cantarella A, Franck L, et al. How well do clinical pain assessment tools reflect pain in infants. PLOS Med 2008;5:928–33.

40. Slater R, Worley A, Fabrizi L, et al. Evoked potentials generated by noxious stimulation in the human infant brain. Eur J Pain 2010;14:321–6.

41. de Jesus JA, Tristao RM, Storm H, et al. Heart rate, oxygen saturation, and skin conductance: a comparison study of acute pain in Brazilian newborns. Conf Proc IEEE Eng Med Biol Soc 2011;2011:1875–9.

42. Gjerstad AC, Wagner K, Henrichsen T, et al. Skin conductance versus the modified COMFORT sedation score as a measure of discomfort in artificially ventilated children. Pediatrics 2008;122:e848–53.

43. Choo EK, Magruder W, Montgomery CJ, et al. Skin conductance fluctuations correlate poorly with postoperative self-report pain measures in school-aged children. Anesthesiology 2010;113:175–82.

44. Cong X, Ludington-Hoe SM, Walsh S. Randomized crossover trial of kangaroo care to reduce biobehavioral pain responses in preterm infants. Biol Res Nurs 2011;13:204–16.

45. Grunau RE, Holsti L, Haley DW, et al. Neonatal procedural pain exposure predicts lower cortisol and behavioral reactivity in preterm infants in the NICU. Pain 2005;113:293–300.

46. Slater L, Asmerom Y, Boskovic DS, et al. Procedural pain and oxidative stress in premature neonates. J Pain 2012;13:590–7.

47. Ceelie I, de Wildt SN, van Dijk M, et al. Effect of intravenous paracetamol on postoperative morphine requirements in neonates and infants undergoing major noncardiac surgery: a randomized controlled trial. JAMA 2013;309:149–54.

48. Allegaert K, Tibboel D, Naulaers G, et al. Systematic evaluation of pain in neonates: effect on the number of intravenous analgesics prescribed. Eur J Clin Pharmacol 2003;59:87–90.

49. Mazars N, Milesi C, Carbajal R, et al. Implementation of a neonatal pain management module in the computerized physician order entry system. Ann Intensive Care 2012;2:38.

50. Franck LS, Ridout D, Howard R, et al. A comparison of pain measures in newborn infants after cardiac surgery. Pain 2011;152:1758–65.

51. Riddell RP, Racine N. Assessing pain in infancy: the caregiver context. Pain Res Manag 2009;14:27–32.

52. Gradin M, Eriksson M. Neonatal pain assessment in Sweden—a fifteen-year follow up. Acta Paediatr 2010;100:204–8.

53. Akuma AO, Jordan S. Pain management in neonates: a survey of nurses and doctors. J Adv Nurs 2011;68:1288–301.

54. Spence K, Henderson-Smart D. Closing the evidence-practice gap for newborn pain using clinical networks. J Paediatr Child Health 2011;47:92–8.

55. de Oliveira MV, de Jesus JA, Tristao RM. Psychophysical parameters of a multidimensional pain scale in newborns. Physiol Meas 2012;33:39–49.

56. Franck LS, Bruce E. Putting pain assessment into practice: why is it so painful? Pain Res Manag 2009;14:13–20.

57. Brahnam S, Chuang CF, Sexton RS, et al. Machine assessment of neonatal facial expressions of acute pain. Decis Support Syst 2007;43:1242–54.

58. Stevens B, Johnston C, Petryshen P, et al. Premature infant pain profile: development and initial validation. Clin J Pain 1996;12:13–22.

59. Krechel SW, Bildner J. CRIES: a new neonatal postoperative pain measurement score. Initial testing of validity and reliability. Paediatr Anaesth 1995;5:53–61.

60. Lawrence J, Alcock D, McGrath P, et al. The development of a tool to assess neonatal pain. Neonatal Netw 1993;12:59–66.

61. van Dijk M, de Boer JB, Koot HM, et al. The reliability and validity of the COMFORT scale as a postoperative pain instrument in 0 to 3-year-old infants. Pain 2000;84:367–77.

62. Grunau RV, Craig KD. Facial activity as a measure of neonatal pain expression. Adv Pain Res Ther 1990;15:147–55.

63. Cignacco E, Mueller R, Hamers JP, et al. Pain assessment in the neonate using the Bernese Pain Scale for Neonates. Early Hum Dev 2004;78:125–31.

Biological and Neurodevelopmental Implications of Neonatal Pain

Suellen M. Walker, MBBS, MMed, MSc, PhD, FANZCA, FFPMANZCA

KEYWORDS

- Pain • Neonate • Postnatal development • Analgesia • Sensory processing

KEY POINTS

- Nociceptive pathways are functional after birth, and pain produces significant physiologic and behavioral responses in both preterm and term-born neonates.
- Clinical evidence for adverse impacts on neurodevelopmental outcome and subsequent pain response is increasing.
- Evaluating the impact of early life pain and/or analgesia requires consideration of intercurrent illness and stress, particularly in preterm-born neonates requiring prolonged intensive care treatment; genetic and environmental factors; and subsequent social and family factors that can modulate behavioral responses.
- Persistent alterations in sensory function have been shown in a range of preclinical models of early injury, and allow evaluation of underlying mechanisms and potential preventive interventions.
- Adequate management of pain is a goal of care at all ages, but specific evaluation of efficacy and effects in early life are required because responses in the developing nervous system may differ from those seen at older ages.

INTRODUCTION

Nociceptive pathways are functional following birth, and neonates who require major surgery or intensive care management are exposed to significant painful stimuli at a time when the developing nervous system is sensitive to changes in sensory experience.[1] Up to 9% of newborns are admitted to neonatal intensive care units (NICUs)[2,3] and the odds of NICU admission increase with preterm birth.[3] Preterm birth is a leading public health problem.[4] Although definitions can vary, more than 12% of babies

Disclosures: The author has no conflicts of interest or relationship with commercial companies. Current research is funded by a British Journal of Anaesthesia/Royal College of Anaesthetists UK project grant and Suellen Walker currently holds a Macintosh Professorship from the Royal College of Anaesthetists.

Portex Unit: Pain Research, UCL Institute of Child Health, Great Ormond St Hospital for Children NHS Foundation Trust, 30 Guilford Street, London WC1N1EH, UK

E-mail address: suellen.walker@ucl.ac.uk

were born preterm in the United States in 2008,[5] and UK statistics reported that 7.7% of all live births were preterm ($\leq$36 weeks' gestational age [GA]) and 0.6% were very preterm ($\leq$27 weeks GA; UK Office for National Statistics; www.www.ons.gov.uk/ons/publications/). Repeated procedural interventions (often >10 per day and several hundred throughout admission[6]) are an essential part of intensive care management, but increase activity in spinal and cortical nociceptive circuits in even the most preterm neonate,[7] and progressively increase hyperalgesia.[8] Major surgery may also be required to treat complications of prematurity or correct congenital anomalies, frequently with staged repairs throughout childhood. The beneficial impact of adequate neonatal anesthesia and analgesia on acute perioperative morbidity has long been recognized.[9]

As awareness of the plasticity of infant pain mechanisms has increased, an important question has arisen regarding the potential for developmentally regulated responses to injury that mediate permanent alterations in pain sensitivity, which are not seen following the same injury at older ages.[1] There is increasing clinical evidence that pain in early life is associated with adverse effects on neurodevelopment and the response to future pain. However, it is difficult to adequately quantify the degree or total load of neonatal pain experience and the efficacy of analgesia throughout NICU admissions and/or the perioperative period, and multiple confounding factors (intercurrent illness, duration of care, and gestational age) make it difficult to determine the specific contribution of pain, tissue injury, or different analgesic interventions in clinical cohorts. Translational laboratory studies facilitate evaluation of potential contributory factors, identify underlying mechanisms, and allow comparison of the relative impacts of different analgesic interventions using both behavioral outcomes and tissue analysis.

ACUTE RESPONSE TO NOXIOUS STIMULI IN NEONATES

Changes in physiologic parameters and behavioral response to acute noxious stimuli are evident following birth and form the basis of multidimensional observer pain assessment tools (**Box 1**).[10,11] Responses are observed in even the most preterm neonates, although the nature, degree, and latency may vary. There may also be divergence between behavioral and physiologic responses,[10] particularly because physiologic responses are influenced by intercurrent illness or medications. Changes in hormonal indices have been used as proxy markers of pain-related stress in research studies[12,13] and as an outcome measure when assessing potential alterations in hypothalamic-pituitary-adrenal (HPA) axis function following NICU.[14–16] Neurophysiologic and imaging measures are increasingly being used in clinical research studies to assess:

1. The function and selectivity of nociceptive pathway at different ages
   i. Near infrared spectroscopy (NIRS). Changes in oxyhemoglobin levels are used as an indicator of increased cerebral blood flow in response to neural activity. Increases in the contralateral somatosensory cortex following heel lance suggest that the cortex is activated by noxious stimuli, but not by touch, even in preterm-born neonates.[17,18]
   ii. Electroencephalography (EEG). Although different forms of analysis may be used, and there is the potential for confounding by motor responses,[19] a nociceptive-specific potential has been reported in central electrodes following heel lance when using a "time-locked stimulus" (ie, release of the stylet for heel lance was accurately detected by an accelerometer and event-marked the EEG record) that allows differentiation of short latency EEG potentials evoked by both noxious and innocuous stimuli, and a late component specific to a noxious

---

Box 1
Acute physiologic response to noxious stimuli

Behavioral response

- Facial response: brow bulge, eye squeeze, nasolabial furrow, horizontal mouth stretch, taut tongue
- Body movement: reflex withdrawal, arching
- Increased muscle tone
- Cry: presence, duration, pitch

Cardiorespiratory

- Increased heart rate and blood pressure
- Decrease in heart rate variability (autonomic modulation)
- Tachypnea
- Desaturation

Neurophysiology

- Near-infrared spectroscopy: increased blood flow in somatosensory cortex
- Electroencephalography: age-specific and modality-specific changes in activity
- Functional magnetic resonance imaging: cortical response to peripheral stimuli

Hormonal

- Increased cortisol
- Altered catecholamine levels

---

stimulus.[20] In addition, the pattern of EEG changes as postnatal age increases (28–45 weeks' gestation), with more modality-specific and localized evoked potentials and better discrimination between touch and noxious stimuli.[21]

   iii. Functional magnetic resonance imaging (fMRI). Passive movement of the hand during chloral hydrate sedation produced activation in the contralateral somatosensory cortex in preterm (median 34 weeks) and term neonates, with a trend of reduced time to positive peak and increased amplitude with age.[22]

2. Quantify pain response and evaluate correlations with other measures
   i. NIRS measures show a correlation between cortical response and observer pain scores using the Premature Infant Pain Profile (PIPP) tool, which was better for facial expression than the physiologic components of the tool. A proportion of neonates lacked any facial response, suggesting that the response to a noxious stimulus may be underestimated by observers in this group.[23] In addition, the latency to facial response was longer in younger neonates (<32 weeks postmenstrual age [PMA]) and those receiving morphine at the time of heel lance.[24]
   ii. At the same PMA (39.2 ± 1.2 weeks), the EEG response to heel lance was greater in neonates born preterm (24–32 weeks) compared with term-born neonates.[25]
   iii. Sucrose reduced the behavioral response and PIPP score following heel lance, but did not suppress associated lower limb reflex or cortical EEG responses.[7]

Developmental changes in structure and function may affect these measures; for example, changes in cerebral blood flow and cerebral metabolic rate may alter NIRS readings and age-related changes influence EEG patterns.[26] Because changing levels of neural activity may affect functional connectivity and structural brain development (discussed later), there is increasing awareness of the need not only to reduce behavioral responses but also to protect the brain from damaging effects of excess activity.[1,10] Further studies are required to determine whether measures of cortical activity can detect dose-dependent effects of analgesic and sedative interventions, and whether modulating these parameters has an impact on subsequent outcome.

NEURODEVELOPMENTAL IMPACT OF NEONATAL PAIN AND INJURY

Many studies have demonstrated adverse neurodevelopmental outcomes following neonatal intensive care, particularly in preterm-born infants. However, the specific contribution of pain, injury, and analgesia are difficult to determine, and different statistical methodologies have been used to correct for confounding factors such as intercurrent illness, other treatments, and gestational age.[27–29] Significant age-related changes in brain development in terms of structure (eg, cortical folding)[30] and connectivity[31] occur during the third trimester and neonatal period. Comparisons between preterm-born and age-equivalent healthy term controls have identified additional structural deficits (decreased white matter volume and periventricular leukomalacia, decreases in cortical gray and deep gray matter, smaller corpus callosal areas, ventricular hypertrophy).[30,32] Other factors, particularly respiratory disease[33] and hypotension,[27] have been shown to make independent contributions. Advanced imaging techniques are increasingly used. Blood oxygen level–dependent fMRI and fMRI connectivity indicate changes associated with functional activity, resting state activity,[31] and connectivity in the brain.[30] Diffusion tension imaging and fractional anisotropy improve resolution of structural changes in white matter, axonal development, and structural connectivity; and the degree of white matter damage at term has been shown to be predictive of neurocognitive outcome at 4 to 6 years of age.[34] These techniques and results are summarized in recent reviews.[30,35,36] However, the impact of pain or surgical injury is either not discussed or it is acknowledged that specific contributions are difficult to determine from current data. Greater structural change (smaller brain volume, increased white matter damage) and impaired neurodevelopment (Motor Development Index on Bayley Scales) has been noted in ex-preterms who also required surgery, but there were no specific data about analgesia or pain experience. In addition, the surgical group were younger (gestational age at birth), smaller (more likely to have in utero growth retardation), and had increased respiratory morbidity, thus emphasizing the potential impact of non–pain-related confounding factors.[37]

Recent studies have used the number of skin-breaking procedures as a measure of pain experience throughout the NICU and found associations between higher overall pain exposure and adverse outcomes, such as:

1. Lower scores on motor (Mental Development Index) and psychomotor (Psychomotor Developmental Index) indices of Bayley Scales of Infant Development at 8 and 18 months.[38] The number of days on mechanical ventilation also had an impact. Greater exposure to morphine was associated with worse motor (but not cognitive) development at 8 but not 18 months, although administration was not controlled and the indications were not detailed (ie, dose and duration; use for sedation, procedural or postoperative pain).[38]
2. Impairments of growth if large numbers of painful procedures were required before 32 weeks postconceptional age (PCA) (accounting for 21% of variance in early body growth and 12% of variance in early head growth/circumference). Other factors, such as infection, and hydrocortisone exposure, had greater impacts at later stages (up to 40 weeks PCA).[39]

3. Reduced white matter and subcortical gray matter maturation (assessed by functional anisotropy and subcortical gray matter N-acetylaspartate/choline ratios). Surgery had a similar effect, but to a lesser degree.[27]
4. Slower increase in fractional anisotropy of the corticospinal tract. Greater illness severity in the first 24 hours of life, independent of gestational age, was associated with impaired development of this motor pathway.[40]

LONG-TERM IMPACT ON SENSORY PROCESSING AND FUTURE PAIN RESPONSE: CLINICAL STUDIES

Clinical evidence for persistent changes in sensory processing and/or the response to future pain following early life pain and injury is increasing. However, the reported effects of neonatal pain vary in degree, direction (increase or decrease in pain sensitivity), and functional impact because they are influenced by multiple factors related to study design and use of different outcomes (**Box 2**). Many studies have been conducted following neonatal intensive care and, as with developmental outcomes, they are influenced by intercurrent confounders (gender, gestational age, illness severity and so forth). Neonates requiring intensive care are subject to a large number of procedural interventions,[6] but it is difficult to provide adequate analgesia for brief intense stimuli,[41] and there is variable implementation of analgesic guidelines.[42,43] In addition, clinical management may be influenced by other contextual factors, such as the carer's perceptions about the invasiveness of the procedure and the infant's clinical or neurologic status: non-pharmacological interventions are used more often than pharmacological interventions; use of both increased for more invasive procedures; in infants at highest risk of neurological impairment (eg. severe intrapartum asphyxia or Grade 3 or 4 intraventicular haemorrhage) greater reliance on physiological than behavioural indicators of pain, were more likely to be managed with behavioural interventions irrespective of the type of procedure, and less likely to receive pharmacological treatments.[44] Stratifying results from NICU cohorts is hampered because:

- There are difficulties in quantifying the pain experience across extended periods in intensive care
- The relative impact of skin-breaking procedures versus interventions such as endotracheal suctioning or handling is unclear
- A proportion of neonates also require one or more surgical procedures to treat complications of prematurity or correct congenital anomalies
- The provision and efficacy of analgesia may not be well documented
- The cumulative effects of repeated stress (ie, allostatic load) from multiple interventions is only in part related to pain,[45] but has a significant impact on outcome.

Reported long-term effects following early pain and injury include:

1. Changes in pain-related behavioral outcomes
   Alterations in pain-related behavior or perceptions have been noted in ex-NICU patients, but vary with age.[45,46] Parents reported that somatization (functional pain complaints with no medical explanation) was more common in young preterm children at age 5 years,[47] but this was not apparent at older ages.[48] Effects may be confounded by the behavioral impairments reported in large cohorts of preterm-born infants.[49–51]
   Long-term behavioral responses are also influenced by child coping style, and family and social context.[45] Although the frequency or severity of recurrent pain did not differ, the degree to which pain interfered with activity was higher in a cohort of preterm-born children compared with an age-matched term-born

---

Box 2
Factors influencing reported long-term impact of neonatal pain

Source/type of initial pain and injury

- NICU: procedures ± surgery
- Repeated blood tests (infant of diabetic mother)
- Surgery
- Circumcision

Timing

- Age at time of insult
- Interval before assessment
- Age at time of follow-up

Subsequent test stimulus

- Baseline thermal/mechanical detection or pain thresholds
- Noxious experimental stimulus (eg, prolonged heat, cold pressor test, pressure algometry)
- Procedure (eg, immunization, blood test)

Outcome

- Behavioral response (eg, duration of cry)
- Self-report pain rating
- Perioperative analgesic requirement

Potential confounding factors at initial injury

- Developmental stage
- Sex
- Intercurrent illness
- Stress
- Immune challenge
- Social factors (eg, parental response)
- Dose and type of analgesia

Potential confounding factors at follow-up assessment

- Sensitivity/specificity of outcome
- Observer reliability
- Cognitive and behavioral deficit (eg, ex-preterm)
- Social factors (eg, parental response)
- Psychological state, coping style
- Dose and type of analgesia

---

control group.[52] Higher levels of pain-related catastrophizing were similarly reported in preterm-born children following NICU, and mothers were more likely to engage in solicitous pain-related behavior.[53]

2. Alterations in sensory processing

The reported impact of early life pain and injury on sensory processing is critically dependent on the method of evaluation, and is influenced by the intensity of the stimulus (baseline sensory thresholds vs noxious stimulus), and the time interval between injury and assessment.

i. In infants with unilateral hydronephrosis, the threshold of the ipsilateral abdominal skin reflex was reduced (suggesting referred visceral hyperalgesia) for several months following birth, and did not follow the normal developmental pattern of increasing threshold with increasing postnatal age.[54]

ii. Baseline sensitivity to thermal stimuli was reduced in children from 9 to 12 years old following NICU,[52,55] and changes were more marked in those born preterm[55] and those who also required surgery.[52]

iii. Although baseline thermal thresholds were higher (ie, reduced sensitivity), a prolonged heat stimulus at pain threshold[55] or repeated trials[56] unmasked enhanced perceptual sensitization in preterm-born children.

iv. Mechanical touch detection thresholds around neonatal thoracotomy wounds were reduced 10 to 12 years following surgery[57] and changes were more marked than with smaller scars related to chest drain insertions.[52]

v. Increased sensitivity to a noxious mechanical stimulus (reduced pressure pain threshold) and an increased number of tender points was found in adolescents 12 to 18 years following NICU.[58]

3. Response to future painful stimuli

Sensitivity to subsequent pain has been assessed at variable intervals following different levels of neonatal pain experience.

i. Full-term babies born to diabetic mothers did not react differently to an intramuscular injection at birth, but following repeated heel lances for glucose measurements they displayed an increased behavioral response to a venipuncture some days later (compared with age-matched babies of nondiabetic mothers).[59]

ii. Cortical EEG recordings following heel lance at 39 weeks PMA showed enhanced noxious-evoked potentials in preterm-born neonates (born 24–32 weeks PMA) compared with an age-matched term-born group.[25]

iii. Behavioral responses to immunization (facial response, cry duration) at 4 to 6 months of age were higher in boys circumcised as neonates without analgesia.[60,61] Although facial and heart rate responses to immunization did not differ, stress regulation (lower cortisol concentrations) was altered in preterm versus term-born infants.[62]

iv. Infants who had surgery during the first 3 months of life had increased norepinephrine levels, higher pain scores, and increased perioperative analgesic requirements when subsequent surgery was performed in the same dermatome.[63] Because effects following surgery at different ages have not been compared, it is not possible to confirm that this is a developmentally regulated phenomenon and not just a consequence of repeated surgery that would be seen at any age.

v. Comparison of fMRI responses to moderate pain intensity tonic heat stimuli in children (11–16 years old) found higher activations in primary somatosensory cortex, anterior cingulate cortex, and insula in preterm but not term-born neonates who required NICU, compared with full-term children without early hospitalization.[56]

4. Modulation by analgesia

The extent to which the impact of early pain can be modified by analgesia at the time of the initial insult cannot be fully determined from the current clinical literature. Few studies have been conducted, and data regarding analgesic use and efficacy are not well-reported in ex-NICU cohorts. Further research is required to evaluate the ability of different analgesic regimens to modulate or prevent long-term changes in sensory function and responses to pain, but reported beneficial effects include:

   i. The enhanced behavioral response to immunization following neonatal circumcision was reduced if topical local anesthesia was used before the initial surgery.[61]

   ii. Infants who had undergone surgery in the neonatal period with perioperative morphine did not show any increase in later response to immunization compared with infants without significant previous pain experience.[64]

5. Prevalence of recurrent or chronic pain in later life

Few if any differences in the prevalence of recurrent pains in childhood have been reported in ex-NICU cohorts compared with age-matched controls born at term without health problems.[52,65,66] There has been limited detailed follow-up and, because recurrent pain is prevalent in children,[67] a large sample size would be required to confirm significant differences.

With increasing time since the initial event, multiple other factors may influence or modulate reported associations between early life experience and current pain, as noted in discussions regarding a link between gastric suction at birth and functional abdominal pain in childhood.[68–71] Children who required surgery for pyloric stenosis as neonates have been reported to have an increased likelihood of functional abdominal pain when assessed at 6 to 9 years of age.[72] As shown in follow-up of cohorts with functional abdominal pain in childhood, sensory, psychological, and social factors all influence reported chronic pain in later life.[73,74]

Evaluating long-term effects in clinical studies requires evaluation after a prolonged time during which there have been significant changes in medical care. Follow-up of a large prospective birth cohort in the United Kingdom (n = 18,558) found that preterm birth was associated with a 26% increase in the risk of chronic widespread pain at 42 years of age, but the difference was not statistically significant.[75] It is difficult to predict whether changes in neonatal care and preterm survival rates, when relating current care to that received when this cohort was born in 1958, will have increased or decreased the risk of persistent pain in later life.

PRECLINICAL EVALUATION OF LONG-TERM IMPACT ON SENSORY PROCESSING AND FUTURE RESPONSE TO NOXIOUS STIMULI

Acute behavioral and physiologic responses to a wide range of noxious stimuli have been documented in preclinical research studies across multiple species and stages of postnatal mammalian development. The potential for persistent noxious afferent input to alter the level of sensitivity of nociceptive pathways in the adult nervous system (eg, development of peripheral and central sensitization) is well established,[76,77] but the developing nervous system is particularly susceptible to alterations in neural activity. As a result, early tissue injury may produce effects not seen following the same input at older ages, leading to persistent changes in somatosensory processing and altered sensitivity to future noxious stimuli.[1]

Preclinical studies have been extensively used to evaluate the long-term consequences of early pain and injury.[1] Specific advantages include:

1. The impact of different types and severity of early injury can be evaluated. The degree and duration of inflammation varies with the type and volume of hindpaw injectate; for example, large volumes of complete Freund's adjuvant (CFA) on the

first postnatal day (P1)[78] produce chronic inflammation rather than a specific neonatal insult.[79,80] Persistent effects following formalin are similarly influenced by the concentration and frequency of the initial injections.[81–84] Some studies aim to more closely reproduce clinical stimuli, such as repeated needle injection[85,86] to model procedural pain in NICU, or laparotomy[87] and hindpaw incision[88,89] to investigate surgical injury.

2. Responses at different developmental stages can determine whether there are critical periods during which injury-related alterations in neural activity produce long-term effects. Many studies are performed in the neonatal rodent, which has the advantage of being born at an immature stage, and rapid maturation facilitates following the pattern of change through to adulthood (6–8 weeks of age).[90] To confirm a specific developmentally regulated response, the same injury should be performed across several postnatal ages, and, for accurate comparison, the same intensity of stimulus is delivered. For example, the volume of an inflammatory or chemical stimulus may be adjusted according to body weight,[91] hindpaw size,[92] or degree of local response[93]; or anatomic landmarks may be used to produce incision of the same relative length at different ages.[89]

3. Structural and functional changes in nociceptive pathways and mechanisms underlying persistent sensory changes can be evaluated using a wide range of behavioral and neurophysiologic measures, tissue analysis, and imaging techniques. In addition, the impact on behavioral and tissue outcomes of inhibitors of specific signaling pathways, pharmacologic agonist or antagonist interventions, or genetic modifications can also identify important mechanisms and potential analgesic targets.

Box 3
Laboratory models of neonatal injury

Inflammation: hindpaw injection of age-appropriate volume of inflammatory agent

- CFA: inactivated mycobacteria emulsified in mineral oil
- Carrageenan: polysaccharides extracted from seaweeds

Chemical nociceptive stimuli: injection, application, instillation of noxious chemicals

- Hindpaw formalin (0.2%–15%) produces nociceptive behaviors such as licking, flicking, paw elevation
- Hindpaw capsaicin and mustard oil activate C-fibers via TRPV1 and TRPA1 receptors respectively to produce primary hyperalgesia
- Low pH intramuscular injection

Repeat needle injury: insertion of needle (25 gauge) into or through one or more paws on multiple occasions (eg, 4 times daily from P0 to P7)

Full-thickness skin wound: removal of small full-thickness skin flap from dorsum of hindpaw

Plantar hindpaw incision: midline incision through plantar skin with elevation and longitudinal incision in underlying plantaris muscle; skin closure with suture

Visceral injury: bladder or bowel; chemical stimuli or mechanical distension.

Peripheral nerve injury: trauma to sciatic nerve

- Spared nerve injury, transection of common peroneal and tibial, but not sural, branch
- Chronic constriction injury, ligature around nerve
- Spinal nerve ligation, transection of nerve root, usually L5

Table 1
Long-term effects of neonatal injury in laboratory models

	Changes in Sensory Thresholds and Spinal Cord Function	Mechanisms and Impact of Neonatal Analgesia	Response to Repeat Injury in Adult	Developmental Profile/Critical Period
Severe inflammation 25 µL CFA at P0–1	Sensory thresholds • No change[78–80] • Reduction (ie, increased sensitivity)[98,99] Dorsal horn • Increased spontaneous and evoked firing (adult)[78,100]	Periphery • Chronic inflammation[79,80] • No cell death or change in cell number in DRG[79] • Brief (3–6 d) alterations in mRNA expression in DRG[101] Dorsal horn • Expanded sciatic terminal field (not seen with less severe inflammation)[78,79] • Increase density CGRP[78]	Repeat CFA • Increased behavioral hyperalgesia[78,80] • Increased Fos in dorsal horn[102] Formalin[78] • Earlier onset second phase Capsaicin[103] • Increased thermal and mechanical hyperalgesia • Increased Fos expression in dorsal horn[80] Nerve injury • No change[80]	Inflammation at P0 but no effect at P14 in rats[78,103] and mice[99] Response to capsaicin enhanced if inflammation at P0 not P14[103]
Mild inflammation 1 µL/g (8–10 g) 0.25%–1% carrageenan	Sensory thresholds • Increased thermal and mechanical threshold all paws[91,97,104–107] • Emerges at P34[91] • Reduced baseline and stress-induced neuroendocrine response[97] Dorsal horn • No persistent change in receptive field size or spontaneous or evoked activity[108]	Dorsal horn • Altered gene expression at baseline and differing pattern with reinflammation[109] Brainstem • Increased 5HT receptor expression in PAG[97] • Altered opioid-mediated response in PAG[107] • Enhanced inhibition from the RVM[110] Impact of analgesia • Reduced by morphine[111,112]	CFA[91] • Increased mechanical and thermal hyperalgesia • Present at all time points after injection • No contralateral effect Hindpaw incision[113] • Enhanced hyperalgesia • No contralateral effect • Increased Fos in dorsal horn[104] Colonic distension[104] • Decreased response • Greater response following colonic inflammation	Inflammation in first postnatal week (P0, P1, P3, P5) but not P8 or older[91] Gene changes following inflammation at P3 differ from P12[109] Visceral effects (colon) after inflammation at P3 not P14[104] Altered anxiety trait after P3 but not P12[97]

	Sensory thresholds		Impact of analgesia	
Formalin 5–10 μL of 0.2%–10%	Sensory thresholds • Increased thermal latency following 5 μL 10% formalin multiple paws at P1 to P7[114] or 5 μL of 4% multiple paws P1 to P4[81,82] • No change in thermal sensitivity following 10 μL 0.2%–0.4% in hindpaws P3 to P14[83] or 10 μL of 4% into right paws on P1[84]	Formalin • Increased area under the behavioral response curve[83]	Impact of analgesia • Reduced by morphine[114] • Ketamine reduced hypoalgesia in adult female but not male rodents[81]	Variable concentration and frequency of administration with no direct comparisons at different developmental ages Prolonged effects on microglial activation in cord shown in adults[115]
Full-thickness skin wound on dorsal hindpaw	Sensory thresholds • Persistent mechanical hyperalgesia[116–119] Dorsal horn • Increased receptive field size at 3 and 6 wk[108]	Not evaluated	Periphery • Hyperinnervation (up to 12 wk)[116,120] • Downregulation of inhibitory ephrin-A4[121] • Increased neurotrophic factors, including NGF and NT-3[122–124] Dorsal horn • Ablation of NK-1-expressing neurons reduces impact[118] Impact of analgesia • Single sciatic block with bupivacaine did not prevent persistent hyperalgesia or hyperinnervation[119]	Effect if wound at P0 or P7, but not at P14 or P21[116]
Laparotomy (mice) P0	Sensory thresholds • Hypoalgesia to thermal and mechanical stimuli[87]	Acetic acid AC[87] • Decreased response • Thermal tail latency and AC effects prevented by postprocedure morphine	Morphine prevented long-term sensory changes	Laparotomy only performed at P0 No comparison with surgery at older ages

(continued on next page)

Table 1
(continued)

	Changes in Sensory Thresholds and Spinal Cord Function	Mechanisms and Impact of Neonatal Analgesia	Response to Repeat Injury in Adult	Developmental Profile/Critical Period
Plantar hindpaw/ midthigh incision	Sensory thresholds • Increased thermal and mechanical threshold all paws[125]	Periphery and impact of analgesia • Activity dependent; prevented by sciatic nerve blockade (>6 h)[89,126] Dorsal horn • Priming of neuroimmune response[125] • Enhanced excitatory (glutamatergic) signaling[126]	Repeat plantar incision[125] • Enhanced degree and duration of hyperalgesia • Enhanced microglial reactivity	Incision at P3 or P6 alters future response; no effect if initial injury at P10, P21, P40[89] Midthigh incision at P3 but not P17 enhanced excitatory signaling[126]
Repeat needle stick	Sensory thresholds • Thermal sensitivity at P16, P22, but not at P65[85] • No effect[127,128]	—	Plantar incision • Enhanced degree and duration of hyperalgesia[128]	Repeat needle stick P0 to P7 No comparison with same injury at older ages
Intramuscular injection pH 4 (gastrocnemius daily P12–20)	Periphery[86] • pH 4: increased sensitivity to deep muscle pinch • pH 7: no effect Dorsal horn • Increased spontaneous activity and increased response to colonic distension	Periphery[86] • No detectable changes in muscle histology	Colonic distension[86] • Enhanced response	Effect if injections P12–20, but not in adult[86]

Colonic irritation (mechanical or mustard oil)	Dorsal horn[129] • Increased neuronal firing	Periphery[129] • No detectable changes in bowel histology	Colonic distension[129] • Enhanced response	Effect if repeat injury from P8 to P20 No effect if repeat injury from P21 to P42[129]
Bladder inflammation (intravesical zymosan)	Increased spontaneous micturition frequency[130]	—	Reinflammation of bladder[130] • Increased response to distension • Increased extravasation	Effect if injury P14-16 No effect if injury P28-30[130]
Peripheral nerve injury	Reduced/absent acute mechanical allodynia if injury in first 3 postnatal weeks[131,132] or at P10[133,134]	Dorsal root ganglion (acute response)[135] • Altered expression immune-related genes • Reduced activation of macrophages Spinal cord (acute response) • Reduced initial microglial response[133] • Reduced T-cell infiltration[134]	Delayed-onset hyperalgesia and microglial reactivity[136]	Injury in first 3 postnatal weeks does not produce the acute mechanical allodynia seen following adult injury

Abbreviations: AC, abdominal constriction; CGRP, calcitonin gene–related protein; DRG, dorsal root ganglion; 5HT, 5-hydroxytryptamine; NGF, nerve growth factor; NK-1, neurokinin 1; NT-3, neurotrophin-3; P, postnatal day; PAG, periaqueductal gray; RVM, rostroventral medulla.

4. The degree of modulation by different doses, durations, and types of analgesic intervention on both the acute response and persistent effects of injury can be directly compared.
5. The effect of a single injury or intervention can be assessed in the presence or absence of potential confounders to evaluate individual contributions. Additional factors shown to influence nociceptive processing include exposure to an immune challenge in early life,[94] and neonatal stress,[95] either of which may also be experienced within the clinical context of NICU.

However, interpretation of laboratory studies also has some limitations related to:

1. Extrapolation of developmental stages and periods of susceptibility across species. Direct translation of developmental age from rodents to humans, and the specific timing of events after birth, continues to be debated, but the sequence of development of sensory and reflex systems in rodents correlate with those of human infants.[96]
2. Effect size. The potential clinical impact of statistically significant differences in laboratory studies can be difficult to predict (**Box 3, Table 1**), which may be particularly important when effects of early stimuli on non–pain-related outcomes are assessed. For example, neonatal insults have been associated with alterations in alcohol preference in adult rodents, and both decreases[97] and increases in anxiety-related behavior[81,82,84,98] have been reported following differing types of neonatal noxious stimuli.
3. Nonspecific effects caused by maternal separation, handling, and neonatal stress. These effects can be assessed by inclusion of appropriate control groups.

SUMMARY

- Nociceptive pathways are functional after birth, and pain produces significant physiologic and behavioral responses in both preterm and term neonates.
- Clinical evidence for adverse impacts on neurodevelopmental outcome and subsequent pain response is increasing.
- Evaluating the impact of early life pain and/or analgesia requires consideration of intercurrent illness and stress, particularly in preterm-born neonates requiring prolonged intensive care treatment. In addition, genetic and environmental factors, and social and family factors can modulate subsequent behavioral responses.
- Persistent alterations in sensory function have been shown in a range of preclinical models of early pain and injury, and allow evaluation of underlying mechanisms and potential preventive interventions.
- Adequate management of pain is a goal of care at all ages, but specific evaluation of efficacy and effects in early life are required because responses in the developing nervous system may differ from those seen at older ages.

REFERENCES

1. Fitzgerald M, Walker SM. Infant pain management: a developmental neurobiological approach. Nat Clin Pract Neurol 2009;5:35–50.
2. Sandal G, Erdeve O, Oguz SS, et al. The admission rate in neonatal intensive care units of newborns born to adolescent mothers. J Matern Fetal Neonatal Med 2011;24:1019–21.
3. Tracy SK, Tracy MB, Sullivan E. Admission of term infants to neonatal intensive care: a population-based study. Birth 2007;34:301–7.

4. Institute of Medicine (US) Committee on Understanding Premature Birth and Assuring Healthy Outcomes. Preterm birth: causes, consequences, and prevention. Washington, DC: National Academies Press (US); 2007.

5. Martin J, Osterman MJ, Sutton PD. Are preterm births on the decline in the United States? Recent data from the National Vital Statistics System. Hyattsville (MD): National Center for Health Statistics; 2010. p. 1–8.

6. Carbajal R, Rousset A, Danan C, et al. Epidemiology and treatment of painful procedures in neonates in intensive care units. JAMA 2008;300:60–70.

7. Slater R, Cornelissen L, Fabrizi L, et al. Oral sucrose as an analgesic drug for procedural pain in newborn infants: a randomised controlled trial. Lancet 2010;376:1225–32.

8. Fitzgerald M, Millard C, MacIntosh N. Hyperalgesia in premature infants. Lancet 1988;1:292.

9. Anand KJ, Sippell WG, Aynsley-Green A. Randomised trial of fentanyl anaesthesia in preterm babies undergoing surgery: effects on the stress response. Lancet 1987;1:62–6.

10. Holsti L, Grunau RE, Shany E. Assessing pain in preterm infants in the neonatal intensive care unit: moving to a 'brain-oriented' approach. Pain Manag 2011;1:171–9.

11. Howard RF, Carter B, Curry J, et al. Good practice in postoperative and procedural pain. A guideline from the Association of Paediatric Anaesthetists of Great Britain and Ireland. Pediatr Anaesth 2012;22:1–79.

12. Oberlander TF, Jacobson SW, Weinberg J, et al. Prenatal alcohol exposure alters biobehavioral reactivity to pain in newborns. Alcohol Clin Exp Res 2010; 34:681–92.

13. Guinsburg R, Kopelman BI, Anand KJ, et al. Physiological, hormonal, and behavioral responses to a single fentanyl dose in intubated and ventilated preterm neonates. J Pediatr 1998;132:954–9.

14. Brummelte S, Grunau RE, Zaidman-Zait A, et al. Cortisol levels in relation to maternal interaction and child internalizing behavior in preterm and full-term children at 18 months corrected age. Dev Psychobiol 2011;53:184–95.

15. Grunau RE, Haley DW, Whitfield MF, et al. Altered basal cortisol levels at 3, 6, 8 and 18 months in infants born at extremely low gestational age. J Pediatr 2007; 150:151–6.

16. Grunau RE, Holsti L, Haley DW, et al. Neonatal procedural pain exposure predicts lower cortisol and behavioral reactivity in preterm infants in the NICU. Pain 2005;113:293–300.

17. Slater R, Cantarella A, Gallella S, et al. Cortical pain responses in human infants. J Neurosci 2006;26:3662–6.

18. Bartocci M, Bergqvist LL, Lagercrantz H, et al. Pain activates cortical areas in the preterm newborn brain. Pain 2006;122:109–17.

19. Norman E, Rosen I, Vanhatalo S, et al. Electroencephalographic response to procedural pain in healthy term newborn infants. Pediatr Res 2008;64:429–34.

20. Slater R, Worley A, Fabrizi L, et al. Evoked potentials generated by noxious stimulation in the human infant brain. Eur J Pain 2010;14:321–6.

21. Fabrizi L, Slater R, Worley A, et al. A shift in sensory processing that enables the developing human brain to discriminate touch from pain. Curr Biol 2011;21: 1552–8.

22. Arichi T, Fagiolo G, Varela M, et al. Development of BOLD signal hemodynamic responses in the human brain. Neuroimage 2012;63:663–73.

23. Slater R, Cantarella A, Franck L, et al. How well do clinical pain assessment tools reflect pain in infants? PLoS Med 2008;5:e129.

24. Slater R, Cantarella A, Yoxen J, et al. Latency to facial expression change following noxious stimulation in infants is dependent on postmenstrual age. Pain 2009;146:177–82.

25. Slater R, Fabrizi L, Worley A, et al. Premature infants display increased noxious-evoked neuronal activity in the brain compared to healthy age-matched term-born infants. Neuroimage 2010;52(2):583–9.

26. McKeever S, Johnston L, Davidson A. A review of the utility of EEG depth of anaesthesia monitors in the paediatric intensive care environment. Intensive Crit Care Nurs 2012;28:294–303.

27. Brummelte S, Grunau RE, Chau V, et al. Procedural pain and brain development in premature newborns. Ann Neurol 2012;71:385–96.

28. Roze JC, Denizot S, Carbajal R, et al. Prolonged sedation and/or analgesia and 5-year neurodevelopment outcome in very preterm infants: results from the EPI-PAGE cohort. Arch Pediatr Adolesc Med 2008;162:728–33.

29. Bellu R, de Waal KA, Zanini R. Opioids for neonates receiving mechanical ventilation. Cochrane Database Syst Rev 2008;(1):CD004212.

30. Ment LR, Hirtz D, Huppi PS. Imaging biomarkers of outcome in the developing preterm brain. Lancet Neurol 2009;8:1042–55.

31. Doria V, Beckmann CF, Arichi T, et al. Emergence of resting state networks in the preterm human brain. Proc Natl Acad Sci U S A 2010;107:20015–20.

32. Ball G, Boardman JP, Rueckert D, et al. The effect of preterm birth on thalamic and cortical development. Cereb Cortex 2012;22:1016–24.

33. Anjari M, Counsell SJ, Srinivasan L, et al. The association of lung disease with cerebral white matter abnormalities in preterm infants. Pediatrics 2009;124:268–76.

34. Woodward LJ, Clark CA, Bora S, et al. Neonatal white matter abnormalities an important predictor of neurocognitive outcome for very preterm children. PLoS One 2012;7:e51879.

35. Panigrahy A, Wisnowski JL, Furtado A, et al. Neuroimaging biomarkers of preterm brain injury: toward developing the preterm connectome. Pediatr Radiol 2012;42(Suppl 1):S33–61.

36. Keunen K, Kersbergen KJ, Groenendaal F, et al. Brain tissue volumes in preterm infants: prematurity, perinatal risk factors and neurodevelopmental outcome: a systematic review. J Matern Fetal Neonatal Med 2012;25(Suppl 1):89–100.

37. Filan PM, Hunt RW, Anderson PJ, et al. Neurologic outcomes in very preterm infants undergoing surgery. J Pediatr 2012;160:409–14.

38. Grunau RE, Whitfield MF, Petrie-Thomas J, et al. Neonatal pain, parenting stress and interaction, in relation to cognitive and motor development at 8 and 18 months in preterm infants. Pain 2009;143:138–46.

39. Vinall J, Miller SP, Chau V, et al. Neonatal pain in relation to postnatal growth in infants born very preterm. Pain 2012;153:1374–81.

40. Zwicker JG, Grunau RE, Adams E, et al. Score for neonatal acute physiology-II and neonatal pain predict corticospinal tract development in premature newborns. Pediatr Neurol 2013;48:123–9.e1.

41. Walker SM. Management of procedural pain in NICUs remains problematic. Paediatr Anaesth 2005;15:909–12.

42. Johnston C, Barrington KJ, Taddio A, et al. Pain in Canadian NICUs: have we improved over the past 12 years? Clin J Pain 2011;27:225–32.

43. Lago P, Garetti E, Boccuzzo G, et al. Procedural pain in neonates: the state of the art in the implementation of national guidelines in Italy. Paediatr Anaesth 2013;23(5):407–14.

44. Stevens B, McGrath P, Ballantyne M, et al. Influence of risk of neurological impairment and procedure invasiveness on health professionals' management of procedural pain in neonates. Eur J Pain 2010;14:735–41.

45. Grunau RE, Holsti L, Peters JW. Long-term consequences of pain in human neonates. Semin Fetal Neonatal Med 2006;11:268–75.

46. Grunau RE, Whitfield MF, Petrie J. Children's judgements about pain at age 8-10 years: do extremely low birthweight (< or = 1000 g) children differ from full birth-weight peers? J Child Psychol Psychiatry 1998;39:587–94.

47. Grunau RV, Whitfield MF, Petrie JH, et al. Early pain experience, child and family factors, as precursors of somatization: a prospective study of extremely premature and fullterm children. Pain 1994;56:353–9.

48. Grunau RE, Whitfield MF, Fay TB. Psychosocial and academic characteristics of extremely low birth weight (< or = 800 g) adolescents who are free of major impairment compared with term-born control subjects. Pediatrics 2004;114: e725–32.

49. Marlow N, Wolke D, Bracewell MA, et al. Neurologic and developmental disability at six years of age after extremely preterm birth. N Engl J Med 2005;352:9–19.

50. Bhutta AT, Cleves MA, Casey PH, et al. Cognitive and behavioral outcomes of school-aged children who were born preterm: a meta-analysis. JAMA 2002; 288:728–37.

51. Porter FL, Grunau RE, Anand KJ. Long-term effects of pain in infants. J Dev Behav Pediatr 1999;20:253–61.

52. Walker SM, Franck LS, Fitzgerald M, et al. Long-term impact of neonatal intensive care and surgery on somatosensory perception in children born extremely preterm. Pain 2009;141:79–87.

53. Hohmeister J, Demirakca S, Zohsel K, et al. Responses to pain in school-aged children with experience in a neonatal intensive care unit: cognitive aspects and maternal influences. Eur J Pain 2009;13:94–101.

54. Andrews KA, Desai D, Dhillon HK, et al. Abdominal sensitivity in the first year of life: comparison of infants with and without prenatally diagnosed unilateral hydronephrosis. Pain 2002;100:35–46.

55. Hermann C, Hohmeister J, Demirakca S, et al. Long-term alteration of pain sensitivity in school-aged children with early pain experiences. Pain 2006;125:278–85.

56. Hohmeister J, Kroll A, Wollgarten-Hadamek I, et al. Cerebral processing of pain in school-aged children with neonatal nociceptive input: an exploratory fMRI study. Pain 2010;150:257–67.

57. Schmelzle-Lubiecki BM, Campbell KA, Howard RH, et al. Long-term consequences of early infant injury and trauma upon somatosensory processing. Eur J Pain 2007;11:799–809.

58. Buskila D, Neumann L, Zmora E, et al. Pain sensitivity in prematurely born adolescents. Arch Pediatr Adolesc Med 2003;157:1079–82.

59. Taddio A, Shah V, Gilbert-MacLeod C, et al. Conditioning and hyperalgesia in newborns exposed to repeated heel lances. JAMA 2002;288:857–61.

60. Taddio A, Goldbach M, Ipp M, et al. Effect of neonatal circumcision on pain responses during vaccination in boys. Lancet 1995;345:291–2.

61. Taddio A, Katz J, Ilersich AL, et al. Effect of neonatal circumcision on pain response during subsequent routine vaccination. Lancet 1997;349:599–603.

62. Grunau RE, Tu MT, Whitfield MF, et al. Cortisol, behavior, and heart rate reactivity to immunization pain at 4 months corrected age in infants born very preterm. Clin J Pain 2010;26:698–704.

63. Peters JW, Schouw R, Anand KJ, et al. Does neonatal surgery lead to increased pain sensitivity in later childhood? Pain 2005;114:444–54.

64. Peters JW, Koot HM, de Boer JB, et al. Major surgery within the first 3 months of life and subsequent biobehavioral pain responses to immunization at later age: a case comparison study. Pediatrics 2003;111:129–35.

65. Saigal S, Feeny D, Rosenbaum P, et al. Self-perceived health status and health-related quality of life of extremely low-birth-weight infants at adolescence. JAMA 1996;276:453–9.

66. Saigal S, Stoskopf B, Pinelli J, et al. Self-perceived health-related quality of life of former extremely low birth weight infants at young adulthood. Pediatrics 2006; 118:1140–8.

67. Perquin CW, Hazebroek-Kampschreur AA, Hunfeld JA, et al. Pain in children and adolescents: a common experience. Pain 2000;87:51–8.

68. Anand KJ, Jacobson B, Hall RW. Gastric suction at birth: not an innocent bystander. J Pediatr 2004;145:714 [author reply: 715].

69. Anand KJ, Runeson B, Jacobson B. Gastric suction at birth associated with long-term risk for functional intestinal disorders in later life. J Pediatr 2004; 144:449–54.

70. Di Lorenzo C, Saps M. Gastric suction in newborns: guilty as charged or innocent bystander? J Pediatr 2004;144:417–20.

71. Saps M, Di Lorenzo C. Reply. J Pediatr 2004;145:715.

72. Saps M, Bonilla S. Early life events: infants with pyloric stenosis have a higher risk of developing chronic abdominal pain in childhood. J Pediatr 2011;159: 551–4.e1.

73. Walker LS, Sherman AL, Bruehl S, et al. Functional abdominal pain patient subtypes in childhood predict functional gastrointestinal disorders with chronic pain and psychiatric comorbidities in adolescence and adulthood. Pain 2012;153: 1798–806.

74. Walker LS, Dengler-Crish CM, Rippel S, et al. Functional abdominal pain in childhood and adolescence increases risk for chronic pain in adulthood. Pain 2010;150:568–72.

75. Littlejohn C, Pang D, Power C, et al. Is there an association between preterm birth or low birthweight and chronic widespread pain? Results from the 1958 Birth Cohort Study. Eur J Pain 2012;16:134–9.

76. Petho G, Reeh PW. Sensory and signaling mechanisms of bradykinin, eicosanoids, platelet-activating factor, and nitric oxide in peripheral nociceptors. Physiol Rev 2012;92:1699–775.

77. Woolf CJ. Central sensitization: implications for the diagnosis and treatment of pain. Pain 2011;152:S2–15.

78. Ruda MA, Ling QD, Hohmann AG, et al. Altered nociceptive neuronal circuits after neonatal peripheral inflammation. Science 2000;289:628–31.

79. Walker SM, Meredith-Middleton J, Cooke-Yarborough C, et al. Neonatal inflammation and primary afferent terminal plasticity in the rat dorsal horn. Pain 2003; 105:185–95.

80. Lim EJ, Back SK, Kim MA, et al. Long-lasting neonatal inflammation enhances pain responses to subsequent inflammation, but not peripheral nerve injury in adult rats. Int J Dev Neurosci 2009;27:215–22.

81. Anand KJ, Garg S, Rovnaghi CR, et al. Ketamine reduces the cell death following inflammatory pain in newborn rat brain. Pediatr Res 2007;62: 283–90.

82. Rovnaghi CR, Garg S, Hall RW, et al. Ketamine analgesia for inflammatory pain in neonatal rats: a factorial randomized trial examining long-term effects. Behav Brain Funct 2008;4:35.
83. Walker CD, Xu Z, Rochford J, et al. Naturally occurring variations in maternal care modulate the effects of repeated neonatal pain on behavioral sensitivity to thermal pain in the adult offspring. Pain 2008;140:167–76.
84. Negrigo A, Medeiros M, Guinsburg R, et al. Long-term gender behavioral vulnerability after nociceptive neonatal formalin stimulation in rats. Neurosci Lett 2011;490:196–9.
85. Anand KJ, Coskun V, Thrivikraman KV, et al. Long-term behavioral effects of re-petitive pain in neonatal rat pups. Physiol Behav 1999;66:627–37.
86. Miranda A, Peles S, Shaker R, et al. Neonatal nociceptive somatic stimulation differentially modifies the activity of spinal neurons in rats and results in altered somatic and visceral sensation. J Physiol 2006;572:775–87.
87. Sternberg WF, Scorr L, Smith LD, et al. Long-term effects of neonatal surgery on adulthood pain behavior. Pain 2005;113:347–53.
88. Ririe DG, Vernon TL, Tobin JR, et al. Age-dependent responses to thermal hyperalgesia and mechanical allodynia in a rat model of acute postoperative pain. Anesthesiology 2003;99:443–8.
89. Walker SM, Tochiki KK, Fitzgerald M. Hindpaw incision in early life increases the hyperalgesic response to repeat surgical injury: critical period and dependence on initial afferent activity. Pain 2009;147:99–106.
90. McCutcheon JE, Marinelli M. Age matters. Eur J Neurosci 2009;29:997–1014.
91. Ren K, Anseloni V, Zou SP, et al. Characterization of basal and re-inflammation-associated long-term alteration in pain responsivity following short-lasting neonatal local inflammatory insult. Pain 2004;110:588–96.
92. Jiang MC, Gebhart GF. Development of mustard oil-induced hyperalgesia in rats. Pain 1998;77:305–13.
93. Walker SM, Meredith-Middleton J, Lickiss T, et al. Primary and secondary hyper-algesia can be differentiated by postnatal age and ERK activation in the spinal dorsal horn of the rat pup. Pain 2007;128:157–68.
94. Boisse L, Spencer SJ, Mouihate A, et al. Neonatal immune challenge alters nociception in the adult rat. Pain 2005;119:133–41.
95. Green PG, Chen X, Alvarez P, et al. Early-life stress produces muscle hyperal-gesia and nociceptor sensitization in the adult rat. Pain 2011;152:2549–56.
96. Wood SL, Beyer BK, Cappon GD. Species comparison of postnatal CNS development: functional measures. Birth Defects Res B Dev Reprod Toxicol 2003;68: 391–407.
97. Anseloni VC, He F, Novikova SI, et al. Alterations in stress-associated behaviors and neurochemical markers in adult rats after neonatal short-lasting local inflammatory insult. Neuroscience 2005;131:635–45.
98. Roizenblatt S, Andersen ML, Bignotto M, et al. Neonatal arthritis disturbs sleep and behaviour of adult rat offspring and their dams. Eur J Pain 2010;14:985–91.
99. Blom JM, Benatti C, Alboni S, et al. Early postnatal chronic inflammation produces long-term changes in pain behavior and N-methyl-D-aspartate receptor subtype gene expression in the central nervous system of adult mice. J Neurosci Res 2006;84:1789–98.
100. Peng YB, Ling QD, Ruda MA, et al. Electrophysiological changes in adult rat dorsal horn neurons after neonatal peripheral inflammation. J Neurophysiol 2003;90:73–80.

101. Chien CC, Fu WM, Huang HI, et al. Expression of neurotrophic factors in neonatal rats after peripheral inflammation. J Pain 2007;8:161–7.
102. Tachibana T, Ling QD, Ruda MA. Increased Fos induction in adult rats that experienced neonatal peripheral inflammation. Neuroreport 2001;12:925–7.
103. Hohmann AG, Neely MH, Pina J, et al. Neonatal chronic hind paw inflammation alters sensitization to intradermal capsaicin in adult rats: a behavioral and immunocytochemical study. J Pain 2005;6:798–808.
104. Wang G, Ji Y, Lidow MS, et al. Neonatal hind paw injury alters processing of visceral and somatic nociceptive stimuli in the adult rat. J Pain 2004;5:440–9.
105. Lidow MS, Song ZM, Ren K. Long-term effects of short-lasting early local inflammatory insult. Neuroreport 2001;12:399–403.
106. LaPrairie JL, Murphy AZ. Female rats are more vulnerable to the long-term consequences of neonatal inflammatory injury. Pain 2007;132(Suppl 1):S124–33.
107. Laprairie JL, Murphy AZ. Neonatal injury alters adult pain sensitivity by increasing opioid tone in the periaqueductal gray. Front Behav Neurosci 2009; 3:31.
108. Torsney C, Fitzgerald M. Spinal dorsal horn cell receptive field size is increased in adult rats following neonatal hindpaw skin injury. J Physiol 2003; 550:255–61.
109. Ren K, Novikova SI, He F, et al. Neonatal local noxious insult affects gene expression in the spinal dorsal horn of adult rats. Mol Pain 2005;1:27.
110. Zhang YH, Wang XM, Ennis M. Effects of neonatal inflammation on descending modulation from the rostroventromedial medulla. Brain Res Bull 2010;83: 16–22.
111. Laprairie JL, Johns ME, Murphy AZ. Preemptive morphine analgesia attenuates the long-term consequences of neonatal inflammation in male and female rats. Pediatr Res 2008;64:625–30.
112. Rahman W, Fitzgerald M, Aynsley-Green A, et al. The effects of neonatal exposure to inflammation and/or morphine on neuronal responses and morphine analgesia in adult rats. In: Jensen TS, Turner JA, Wiesenfeld-Hallin Z, editors. Proceedings of the 8th World Congress on Pain Progress in Pain Research and Management, vol. 8. Seattle (WA): IASP Press; 1997. p. 783–94.
113. Chu YC, Chan KH, Tsou MY, et al. Mechanical pain hypersensitivity after incisional surgery is enhanced in rats subjected to neonatal peripheral inflammation: effects of N-methyl-D-aspartate receptor antagonists. Anesthesiology 2007;106:1204–12.
114. Bhutta AT, Rovnaghi C, Simpson PM, et al. Interactions of inflammatory pain and morphine in infant rats: long-term behavioral effects. Physiol Behav 2001;73: 51–8.
115. Li K, Lin T, Cao Y, et al. Peripheral formalin injury induces 2 stages of microglial activation in the spinal cord. J Pain 2010;11:1056–65.
116. Reynolds ML, Fitzgerald M. Long-term sensory hyperinnervation following neonatal skin wounds. J Comp Neurol 1995;358:487–98.
117. Alvares D, Torsney C, Beland B, et al. Modelling the prolonged effects of neonatal pain. Prog Brain Res 2000;129:365–73.
118. Young EE, Baumbauer KM, Hillyer JE, et al. The neonatal injury-induced spinal learning deficit in adult rats: central mechanisms. Behav Neurosci 2008;122: 589–600.
119. De Lima J, Alvares D, Hatch DJ, et al. Sensory hyperinnervation after neonatal skin wounding: effect of bupivacaine sciatic nerve block. Br J Anaesth 1999;83: 662–4.

120. Alvares D, Fitzgerald M. Building blocks of pain: the regulation of key molecules in spinal sensory neurones during development and following peripheral axotomy. Pain 1999;(Suppl 6):S71–85.

121. Moss A, Alvares D, Meredith-Middleton J, et al. Ephrin-A4 inhibits sensory neurite outgrowth and is regulated by neonatal skin wounding. Eur J Neurosci 2005; 22:2413–21.

122. Constantinou J, Reynolds ML, Woolf CJ, et al. Nerve growth factor levels in developing rat skin: upregulation following skin wounding. Neuroreport 1994; 5:2281–4.

123. Reynolds M, Alvares D, Middleton J, et al. Neonatally wounded skin induces NGF-independent sensory neurite outgrowth in vitro. Brain Res Dev Brain Res 1997;102:275–83.

124. Beggs S, Alvares D, Moss A, et al. A role for NT-3 in the hyperinnervation of neonatally wounded skin. Pain 2012;153:2133–9.

125. Beggs S, Currie G, Salter MW, et al. Priming of adult pain responses by neonatal pain experience: maintenance by central neuroimmune activity. Brain 2012;135: 404–17.

126. Li J, Walker SM, Fitzgerald M, et al. Activity-dependent modulation of glutamatergic signaling in the developing rat dorsal horn by early tissue injury. J Neurophysiol 2009;102:2208–19.

127. Knaepen L, Patijn J, Tibboel D, et al. Sex differences in inflammatory mechanical hypersensitivity in later life of rats exposed to repetitive needle pricking as neonates. Neurosci Lett 2012;516:285–9.

128. Knaepen L, Patijn J, van Kleef M, et al. Neonatal repetitive needle pricking: plasticity of the spinal nociceptive circuit and extended postoperative pain in later life. Dev Neurobiol 2013;73:85–97.

129. Al-Chaer ED, Kawasaki M, Pasricha PJ. A new model of chronic visceral hypersensitivity in adult rats induced by colon irritation during postnatal development. Gastroenterology 2000;119:1276–85.

130. Randich A, Uzzell T, DeBerry JJ, et al. Neonatal urinary bladder inflammation produces adult bladder hypersensitivity. J Pain 2006;7:469–79.

131. Howard RF, Walker SM, Mota PM, et al. The ontogeny of neuropathic pain: postnatal onset of mechanical allodynia in rat spared nerve injury (SNI) and chronic constriction injury (CCI) models. Pain 2005;115:382–9.

132. Ririe DG, Eisenach JC. Age-dependent responses to nerve injury-induced mechanical allodynia. Anesthesiology 2006;104:344–50.

133. Moss A, Beggs S, Vega-Avelaira D, et al. Spinal microglia and neuropathic pain in young rats. Pain 2007;128:215–24.

134. Costigan M, Moss A, Latremoliere A, et al. T-cell infiltration and signaling in the adult dorsal spinal cord is a major contributor to neuropathic pain-like hypersensitivity. J Neurosci 2009;29:14415–22.

135. Vega-Avelaira D, Geranton SM, Fitzgerald M. Differential regulation of immune responses and macrophage/neuron interactions in the dorsal root ganglion in young and adult rats following nerve injury. Mol Pain 2009;5:70.

136. Vega-Avelaira D, McKelvey R, Hathway G, et al. The emergence of adolescent onset pain hypersensitivity following neonatal nerve injury. Mol Pain 2012;8:30.

Nonpharmacological Management of Pain During Common Needle Puncture Procedures in Infants

Current Research Evidence and Practical Considerations

Carol McNair, RN(EC), MN, NP-Pediatrics, NNP-BC[a,b],
Marsha Campbell Yeo, RN, PhD, NNP-BC[c,d],
Celeste Johnston, RN, DEd, FCAHS[e,f], Anna Taddio, MSc, PhD[b,g,*]

KEYWORDS

- Needle puncture procedures • Nonpharmacologic pain management • Infants
- Needle-related pain

KEY POINTS

- Needle-related pain is a common experience for infants.
- It behooves us to use all possible strategies to mitigate or prevent that pain and its negative consequences.
- Current research evidence suggests that nonpharmacologic interventions may be used to help ameliorate needle pain.

INTRODUCTION

Medical procedures involving needle puncture are ubiquitous in contemporary health care; they are used to diagnose, treat, and monitor medical conditions. Healthy infants undergo about a dozen punctures in their first year of life alone. These procedures routinely include (1) intramuscular injection of vitamin K to prevent hemorrhagic

[a] Nursing, The Hospital for Sick Children, Toronto, Ontario, Canada; [b] Child Health Evaluative Sciences, The Hospital for Sick Children, 555 University Avenue, Toronto, Ontario, M5G 1X8, Canada; [c] School of Nursing, Faculty of Health Professions, Dalhousie University, Halifax, Nova Scotia, Canada; [d] Department of Pediatrics, IWK Health Centre, Halifax, Nova Scotia, B3K 6R8, Canada; [e] Ingram School of Nursing, McGill University, 3506 University Street, Montreal, Quebec, H3A 2A7, Canada; [f] IWK Health Centre, Halifax, Nova Scotia, Canada; [g] Clinical, Social, and Administrative Pharmacy, Leslie Dan Faculty of Pharmacy, University of Toronto, 144 College Street, Toronto, Ontario M5S 3M2, Canada
* Corresponding author. Leslie Dan Faculty of Pharmacy, University of Toronto, 144 College Street, Toronto, Ontario M5S 3M2, Canada.
E-mail address: anna.taddio@utoronto.ca

Clin Perinatol 40 (2013) 493–508
http://dx.doi.org/10.1016/j.clp.2013.05.003
0095-5108/13/$ – see front matter © 2013 Elsevier Inc. All rights reserved.
perinatology.theclinics.com

disease; (2) intramuscular and subcutaneous injections of immunizations for vaccine-preventable diseases; and (3) heel lance and/or venipuncture for screening of conditions, such as phenylketonuria, hyperbilirubinemia, and hypothyroidism. In approximately 10% to 15% of infants hospitalized for medical conditions, such as prematurity, congenital anomalies, jaundice, and infection, additional needle puncture procedures are undertaken, such as venous cannulation, to enable the administration of nutrition and medication. A list of common needle procedures undertaken in hospitalized infants is displayed in **Box 1**.

Numerous studies have quantified the burden of pain from needle puncture procedures undertaken in hospitalized infants (**Table 1**). Although estimates vary from study to study, recent data involving neonatal intensive care units (NICUs) in France and Canada show neonates routinely experience dozens of procedures per week.[1,2] Cumulatively, infants can be exposed to hundreds of needle procedures over the duration of hospitalization.

It is important to treat needle pain in infants, not only to reduce acute distress and suffering but to also reduce any potential long-term negative impact on brain development and functioning.[6,7] For the most part, pain from needle punctures undertaken in infants is undertreated. Nonpharmacologic interventions represent a relatively new option to traditional pharmacologic approaches for managing needle pain in infants.

The past 2 decades have witnessed a surge of research investigating the effectiveness of nonpharmacologic methods of pain relief. Recent audits of analgesic practices in hospitalized neonates demonstrate that use of nonpharmacologic interventions surpasses analgesic drugs. In one study, the use rate for nonpharmacologic interventions was 18% compared with 2% for pharmacologic interventions.[1] In another study, procedures were more commonly treated with sucrose (14.3%) or other nonpharmacologic interventions (33.0%) compared with pharmacologic interventions (16.0%).[2]

This article is an overview of the current evidence from systematic reviews for the effectiveness of nonpharmacologic interventions for the management of pain in infants undergoing needle procedures, including swaddling/containment, pacifier, rocking/holding, breast-feeding, skin-to-skin care, and sweet-tasting solutions. In addition, implementation considerations and areas for future research are reviewed.

Box 1
Needle procedures undertaken in hospitalized infants

Intramuscular injection

Subcutaneous injection

Heel lance

Venipuncture

Venous cannulation

Central line insertion

Arterial puncture

Arterial cannulation

Lumbar puncture

Suprapubic aspiration

Table 1			
Epidemiology of procedural pain in infants in intensive care			
Number of Painful Procedures	**Period of Time**	**Total Percentage that Were Needle Punctures (%)**	
60.8 per patient	Total stay	70.0	Barker & Rutter,[3] 1995
2–10 per day	First 7 d	90.0	Johnston et al,[4] 1997
14 per day	First 14 d	15.6	Simons et al,[5] 2003
12–16 per day	First 14 d	25.6	Carbajal et al,[1] 2008
0.8 per day	7 d	94.0	Johnston et al,[2] 2011

SWADDLING AND CONTAINMENT

Swaddling and containment are interventions that aim to limit the infant's boundaries, promote self-regulation, and attenuate physiologic and behavioral stress caused by acute pain.[8,9] These interventions are normally differentiated in that swaddling involves wrapping the infant in a sheet or blanket with the limbs flexed; the head, shoulders, and hips neutral, without rotation; and the hands accessible for exploration[10]; however, containment refers to restricting the infant's motions by holding or using an arm to place the neonate's arms and legs near the trunk to maintain a flexed in utero posture, with limbs placed in body midline.[8] Containment can be achieved using accessories, such as rolled blankets or commercially sold neonatal boundaries. Containment provided by a care provider or parent in which they use their hands to hold the infant in a side-lying, flexed, fetal-type position is referred to as *facilitated tucking*.[11] In nonpain conditions, facilitated tucking has been associated with improved duration of sleep, neuromuscular development, and motor organization and reduction in physiologic distress.[12]

Evidence Summary

The effects of swaddling/containment have been examined in both preterm and full-term infants undergoing commonly performed tissue-breaking procedures in the NICU. Collectively, 9 studies including neonates born at less than 37 weeks and 1 study examining the response of term infants up to 1 month were reported in a recent systematic review examining the effect of swaddling or tucking on pain-related distress, pain reactivity, and pain regulation.[9] Additionally, a small meta-analysis of 4 studies conducted in Thailand reports a larger effect of swaddling compared with no intervention on pain scores during heel stick in term infants than in preterm infants.[13] No studies examining the effect of swaddling or containment were reported in older infants. Although there is sufficient evidence to support the use of swaddling/tucking as an efficacious intervention for reducing pain-related distress reactivity and immediate pain-related regulation in preterm infants, its effectiveness in term neonates and older infants is less certain.

Implementation Considerations

Both containment and swaddling keep the infant in a flexed position and restrain the infant's limbs, reducing the stress caused by motor disorganization, which is triggered by strong stimuli. It is a simple and feasible intervention that should be provided to neonates as an intervention for puncture-related procedural pain. The most limiting factors impacting the clinical utility of swaddling relate to (1) the inability to adequately visualize an acutely ill infant, (2) interference with the control of overhead warmers, and

(3) possible dislodgment of indwelling catheters or tubing. Conversely, the use of containment either with positional supports or by touch is a feasible option in these circumstances. There have been some issues raised regarding the cost-benefit ratio for the use of facilitated touch provided by neonatal care providers.[14] Parental involvement dissipates this concern.[15,16] Additionally, the use of parents as active participants in pain relief is associated with diminished parental stress and increased perceived parenting competence.[17] Swaddling or containment is also generally contraindicated for infants with conditions associated with poor skin integrity, such as extreme prematurity or epidermolysis bullosa.

Research Considerations

The relative effectiveness of swaddling/containment in infants of different gestational ages requires additional investigation given the lack of studies conducted in full-term infants and older infants. There is some evidence that the effect of swaddling may be very beneficial for infants with a higher gestational age. Swaddled infants with a post-conceptional age of 31 to 36 weeks seemed to recover physiologic parameters, specifically elevation in arterial oxygen saturation and reduction in heart rate, faster than infants with a postconceptional age of 27 to 31 weeks.[18] To date, no studies have examined the effect of this intervention in older infants up to a year or the sustained effectiveness of swaddling/containment over ongoing procedures or across varied procedures. Future research is recommended to fill these knowledge gaps.

PACIFIER/NONNUTRITIVE SUCKING
Evidence Summary

In the absence of breast milk or supplemental infant formula, nonnutritive sucking (NNS), generally referred to as the placement of a pacifier in the infant's mouth to stimulate a sucking response, has been well studied and reviewed in a recent meta-analysis.[6] The systematic review consisted of the combined effect of 6 studies conducted in preterm neonates, 7 in full-term neonates, and 1 in infants older than 1 month of age. The investigators concluded that there is sufficient evidence that sucking is efficacious in reducing pain-related distress reactivity in preterm neonates and improving immediate pain-related regulation in preterm and term neonates up to 1 month of age.[6]

The mechanism underlying the calming effect of the orotactile stimulation of NNS is unknown. Given the immediate onset of the action and rapid decrease in effect that seems to be associated solely with the action of sucking, it is unlikely to be opioid mediated.[19] It may simply be that sensory stimulation derived from sucking blocks the perception of pain or provides distraction. The most likely hypothesis is that sucking enhances the infants' ability to self-regulate their behavioral pain response.[20] Others have found that lower heart rate is associated with NNS[19] and that less parasympathetic withdrawal occurs following nipple feeding in nonpain conditions.[20,21]

Implementation Considerations

For the most part, NNS is a feasible strategy. However, limitations to its use do exist, primarily related to initiation and sustainability of breast-feeding success and feasibility. Although somewhat less of an issue in some acute settings, this concern is especially apparent for healthy breast-feeding newborns and neonates being cared for in developing countries. With the increasing movement in the Baby Friendly[22] and Neo Baby Friendly hospital initiatives,[23] further controversies regarding the use of NNS may ensue worldwide. Another consideration with NNS is the need for additional support for care providers to ensure that the pacifier stays in place in the neonate's mouth. This aspect is of primary concern in sick and younger newborns. However, increased parental involvement in pain management provides a means to combat this concern.

Research Considerations

Despite the high quality of studies examining the effectiveness of NNS and pain relief, many questions regarding its use remain unanswered. Although some evidence exists to suggest that longer sucking times (ie, greater than 3 minutes) may be more advantageous, there is insufficient data to confirm or refute this hypothesis.[9] Additionally, as with many nonpharmacologic measures, there is a paucity of literature regarding the effectiveness of NNS in older infants or the sustained effect across repeated and various tissue breaking and procedures. Sucking-related benefits may be particularly beneficial in older infants during routine immunization injections. Lastly, very little is known regarding the impact of using NNS for repeated procedural pain on breast-feeding success or the development of oral aversion. Further research is recommended to examine these issues.

ROCKING/HOLDING
Evidence Summary

Rocking is considered a gentle back-and-forth motion that stimulates a vestibular response. This rocking can be accomplished via simulated means; but in the case of pain relief, the effectiveness is great if provided by another person. Holding is defined as the holding of a clothed infant by either a parent or care provider. The research evidence for rocking and holding demonstrates some support for the effectiveness of this intervention as a pain-relieving strategy. In a recent meta-analysis,[9] 2 studies investigated the effect of holding on the pain-related distress and pain reactivity of neonates following a painful procedure.[24,25] Although rocking/holding without skin contact was not pain relieving, there did seem to be sufficient evidence to recommend its use to enhance pain-related regulation.[25–27] Separately, in a meta-analysis including infants undergoing immunization, there was some evidence for the effectiveness of holding on reducing injection-related pain and distress.[27]

Research and Implementation Considerations

Given the small number of studies evaluating rocking and holding and high heterogeneity among them, further investigation is warranted across all age groups. Future studies should attempt to determine the mechanisms underlying the effects of this intervention, specifically with respect to skin contact and familiar presence during holding, which seem to be salient pain-relieving factors. Also, the extreme importance of understanding better ways to enhance parental involvement as active participants in pain management for their infants cannot be overstated.

BREAST-FEEDING OR BREAST MILK
Evidence Summary

There is clear evidence that breast-feeding when compared with placebo or no intervention control effectively reduces pain associated with common needle-puncture procedures in infants.[28,29] Results from a recent update of a systematic review conducted by Shah and colleagues[28] that included 20 randomized trials, 10 pertaining to breast-feeding and 10 investigating supplemental breast milk, demonstrated that pain scores derived from unidimensional and composite pain assessment tools were generally lower in breast-feeding groups compared with placebo. Supplemental breast milk alone does not seem to be as beneficial as breast-feeding. There seems to be some benefit on heart rate, cry duration, behavioral facial response, and some validated pain assessment tool scores when compared with placebo; however, the cumulative pooled results regarding its pain-relieving effect are inconsistent.[28]

Although the exact mechanism of its pain-relieving effect is unknown, it is most likely related to the combined effects of close proximity of the mother[19]; full ventral skin contact, which may mediate the release of beta endorphins and oxytocin[30]; sucking; and the effects of other chemicals in milk. The act of breast-feeding may also divert the infant's attention from the painful stimulus.[31]

Implementation Considerations

If a mother is breast-feeding, breast-feeding offers a feasible intervention for pain management that also promotes mother-infant bonding and interaction. Limitations to its clinical use include (1) the delayed maturation of the sucking reflex of preterm neonates; (2) impaired sucking ability of very sick or critically ill newborns; (3) acceptability of the staff to perform procedures during breast-feeding, including ergonomic considerations, availability of the mother, and flexibility of the neonatal team to reschedule nonurgent procedures; (4) limitation of use to nursing women; and (5) possible adverse effects.

Little has been reported regarding the adverse effects associated with breast-milk administration in younger or sick neonates. Similarly to sweet-tasting agents, the provision of small amounts of breast milk to a sick or very preterm neonate can be associated with episodes of desaturation or choking that are transient and without long-term effects. There are no reports, however, of choking in infants who were breast-fed during painful procedures. Practice uptake considerations previously described regarding implementation of skin-to-skin contact are also applicable to the utility of breast-feeding.

Research Considerations

Little is known regarding the sustained effect of breast-feeding across time or in combination with other interventions, such as sweet taste, on pain response. As with pacifier use, there are concerns that infants may learn to anticipate breast-feeding with an impending painful procedure. Given that breast-feeding is so frequent and painful procedures uncommon/rare, it is unlikely that infants will learn to associate breast-feeding with pain. Nevertheless, this has not been evaluated to date and is worthy of future study. In addition, breast milk is a naturally occurring agent, and future research should investigate potential ways to optimize the use of expressed breast milk for ill or preterm neonates who are unable to breast-feed and undergoing painful procedures. Studies examining the effectiveness of providing expressed breast milk in combination with other strategies, such as skin-to-skin contact, are also warranted.

KANGAROO CARE
Evidence Summary

Ventral skin-to-skin contact between a baby and its mother is commonly referred to as *kangaroo mother care* because of its similarity to marsupial mother-infant behavior. Because there may be times in which caregivers other than the mother are holding the infant, it is simply known as *kangaroo care*. In this paradigm, the infant, wearing only a diaper and cap, is placed on the mother's bare chest between her breasts, and the two are wrapped together with a small blanket, sheet, or a shawl. Typically, the mother sits at about a 60° angle.

Although this practice of holding the infant skin to skin exists in many cultures, it was specifically used as a facsimile of an incubator in Colombia where there was a shortage of incubators for preterm neonates.[32,33] Because it provided warmth from the mother's body and nutrition from her breasts, it was successful as an incubator replacement for some preterm neonates. Serendipitously, it was noted that infants in kangaroo care were more stable physiologically,[34–41] were in quiet sleep for longer periods of time,[42–45] and had improved breast-feeding outcomes.[45–53] Since the first study to test this intervention for pain in 2000,[54] altogether 18 studies have been included in a recent systematic review of kangaroo care for heel lance or needle insertion in preterm and full-term neonates.[55] Most of the studies (n = 15) were conducted in preterm neonates. To date, kangaroo care has not been evaluated for reducing pain in older infants.

The systematic review demonstrated no clear pattern of effects on physiologic (eg, heart rate) and behavioral (eg, facial action) indicators of pain during painful procedures. However, there was some benefit on composite outcomes, including physiologic and behavioral indicators (eg, Premature Infant Pain Profile, Neonatal Infant Pain Scale). Following painful procedures, kangaroo care was associated with more stable regulation.

Given that kangaroo care is a cost-neutral intervention and that it may facilitate infant regulation and provide warmth and comfort via skin-to-skin contact, it may have a role in neonatal pain management. At present, kangaroo care may be recommended as a nonpharmacologic pain management intervention for common needle procedures.

Implementation Considerations

The implementation of kangaroo care for procedural pain includes challenges in addition to the introduction of change of any kind.[56,57] Some barriers to its implementation are pragmatic: ergonomics of taking blood from the heel while the infant is in kangaroo care and the availability of the mother. The stability of the infant, how it is determined, and the comfort of the staff with putting infants, especially intubated infants with many lines, into kangaroo care as well as the comfort of the staff in doing a procedure in the presence of the parent are issues that involve educational efforts.[58] Unit guidelines that are clear and unambiguous are required to determine which infants are eligible for kangaroo care during painful procedures and strategies for educating staff and parents regarding how to carry out kangaroo care. There are a variety of resources available (eg, educational videos, kangaroo care equipment) to facilitate successful kangaroo care. For example, a low, padded stool, such as an ottoman, can be used for staff to sit on to perform a heel lance. The infant's foot can be gently pulled out from under the wrap around the mother. A more expensive stool with variable height settings will allow for different heights of staff or for different procedures, for example, starting an intravenous on the scalp. Staff members can participate in the choice of a seat and test its settings before actually using it.

Regarding issues of feasibility of kangaroo care, for nonurgent needle procedures, scheduling can often be done to accommodate the mother's availability. Others may substitute if the mother is unavailable.[59–61]

Research Considerations

The unanswered questions that remain regarding the use of kangaroo care for procedural pain management are numerous. Thus far, all studies have been performed for a single painful event. Studies examining the efficacy of kangaroo care over time and over multiple procedures are required to determine if it remains effective or becomes more or less effective over time. The optimal duration of kangaroo care before the painful procedure also warrants further examination. How little is needed and if there are lower and upper limits to the age of effectiveness remain unanswered questions. Although there was a wide range of durations reported in studies included in the review (from 1 to 80 minutes), no direct comparisons were made.[55] The dose may depend on age, and there have been no studies directly comparing infants of different gestational age groups, for example, less than or more than 32 weeks. There have been no studies following infants over the first year of life undergoing common needle procedures, such as immunizations.

SWEET-TASTING SOLUTION
Evidence Summary

Oral sweet-tasting solutions (eg, sucrose in water) are the most widely studied nonpharmacologic intervention for pain management in neonates and have been consistently demonstrated to have analgesic effects in infants. Multiple systematic reviews demonstrate a reduction in pain behaviors in infants given sweet solutions during common needle procedures when compared with placebo water or no intervention,[29,62–64] and sweet-tasting solutions are recommended in consensus statements and clinical practice guidelines.[65–68]

Implementation Considerations

Although a variety of sweet-tasting chemicals have been evaluated, including natural and artificial, the most widely studied and used in clinical practice is sucrose.[62] At present, there are more than 115 randomized controlled trials including sucrose for pain management.[63] Sucrose is a disaccharide comprised of glucose and fructose. Sucrose solutions are administered on the infant's tongue with a pacifier, syringe, or cup. Administration with a pacifier stimulates continuous NNS, which may improve effectiveness.[61,69] There is currently no clear recommendation regarding the optimal dose, and there is a 20-fold variation in the doses that have been used. At present, the usual single dose is 0.5 to 2.0 mL of 12% to 24% strength (weight/volume); however, lower doses are typically used in preterm infants (as little as 0.05 mL of 24%) and larger doses in older infants (as much as 10 mL of 25%).[61,62,64] The onset of action is quick (within seconds); the peak effect occurs at 2 minutes; the duration of action is up to 10 minutes.[69] Calming effects may last considerably longer than the analgesic effects, as demonstrated by a study of reduced behavioral distress responses during a subsequent handling procedure performed up to an hour afterward.[70] Multiple-dose regimens use lower single doses, particularly in preterm infants[62] owing to concerns about potential adverse effects.

The mechanism of action by which sucrose blunts pain responses in infants has not been fully elucidated; however, it has been speculated to involve several pathways. One proposed theory is based on the taste-induced release of endogenous opioids; however, others include dopamine and acetylcholine pathways.[71] In addition, sucrose may induce calming and analgesic effects through NNS and distraction. Of note, a recent study failed to demonstrate an effect on pain-specific brain activity,[72,73] questioning whether sucrose is a *true* analgesic. Behavioral indicators of pain, however, were decreased; at present, the clinical significance of that study is not known.

Sucrose is generally well tolerated by infants; adverse effects are rare and transient, including choking, bradycardia, and oxygen desaturation.[62,74] Data are sparse, however, regarding long-term effects. In 2 multiple-dose studies that examined sucrose use over the first 7 and 28 days of life in preterm infants, no differences were reported in neurologic outcomes during the neonatal period.[75,76] However, one study suggested that increasing sucrose consumption was associated with worse neurobehavioral development scores.[77] A secondary analysis[77] revealed that the cut-off of 10 doses over 24 hours differentiated those with decreased neurobehavioral scores. However, that is the only report of cumulative dose effects, and the significance of this result is unknown.

Key issues to be considered when implementing sucrose analgesia include (1) guidelines for use (including dosing regimen and administration techniques); (2) procedures for ordering, dispensing, and documentation; and (3) methods of evaluation. Increased use success may be observed in the presence of the following: a unit guideline, nurse-led ordering, and inclusion of sucrose as part of admission orders.[78] Some centers use commercially available unit-dose products (eg, Tootsweet, SweetEase), whereas others use pharmacy-compounded bulk preparations. Prepackaged products are more convenient; but individual NICUs should consider their storage capacities, frequency of use and other considersations to determine which product they chose.

Continual monitoring of clinical response is important to document effectiveness and safety and to allow for individualization of dosing (ie, dose-titration to response). Finally, on-going communication, support, and reinforcement of practices with staff are also critical to ensure continued implementation success.[79] The use of sweet-tasting solutions as a soothing technique in nonpain scenarios needs to be discouraged, and staff may need reminders to ensure it is not overused.

Research Considerations

Despite the plethora of research with sucrose, audits of pain management practices demonstrate that sucrose use varies widely among different practice settings.[69,80] The variability in use of sucrose may be caused by important knowledge gaps in its pharmacology, including the exact mechanisms of action; the relationship between dose and response for infants of different ages and for different procedures; and the long-term effects with repeated use, including the potential effects on feeding behaviors. In addition, few trials have evaluated the added benefit of sucrose when coadministered with other nonpharmacologic and pharmacologic analgesics, particularly opioids; and the impact of contextual factors (eg, unit culture, staffing levels).[81] All of these factors may contribute to the suboptimal use of sucrose in the clinical setting. Further study of these issues is recommended to optimize its use in infants undergoing needle procedures.

MUSIC THERAPY
Evidence Summary

There is some evidence that music therapy may be beneficial in relieving procedural pain in both full-term and preterm infants. Results from a recent review that included 9 randomized trials examining the efficacy of music for pain associated with circumcision and heel lance indicated that newborns exposed to music therapy seem to have greater physiologic stability and diminished pain response.[82]

Research and Implementation Considerations

Because of the poor quality of some of the studies, a large variation in reported outcomes, and inconsistent findings across procedures, more rigorous trials are needed to confirm or refute the benefits of music therapy for pain relief associated with needle puncture. Additionally, little is known regarding the optimal type or decibel level of the music or potential differences among various gestational age groups.

SENSORIAL SATURATION
Evidence Summary

Sensorial saturation is defined as a multisensory stimulation consisting of delicate tactile, gustative, auditory, and visual stimuli[82] whereby, during the procedure, the infant's attention is attracted by massaging the face, speaking to the infant gently, and instilling a sweet solution on the infant's tongue. Results from a systematic review of 8 studies examining the effect of sensorial saturation for pain relief during heel lance, intramuscular injection, and endotracheal suctioning demonstrated that pain scores were lower in the group receiving this intervention.[82]

Implementation Considerations

Sensorial interventions are straightforward and easy to implement. From a cost-effective perspective, one may argue whether the known benefits outweigh the added costs associated with the need for a second care provider. As with many nonpharmacologic interventions, the most logical solution to this concern would be to increase parental involvement.

One hypothesis addressing the beneficial effect of sensorial stimulation is derived from the Gate Control Theory proposed by Melzack and Wall.[83] Stimuli traveling ascending pathways inhibit the nociceptive signals from painful stimuli through various endogenous mechanisms located along the spinothalamic tract.[84] The stronger these competing stimuli are, including multiple modalities, the more effective they are in blocking the perception of pain. This theory is in keeping with evidence supporting modalities encompassing multiple stimuli and may help explain why interventions, such as kangaroo care, breastfeeding, or sensorial saturation, that involve tactile, auditory, and olfactory mechanisms are generally more effective than single modalities.

Research Considerations

Many unanswered questions remain related to the mechanism of action for sensorial interventions and what is the optimal dose. Finding the balance between too much and too little stimulation is a challenge as there are potential difference among various gestational age groups. Additionally, future research should focus on ways to educate and enhance parent participation so that parents can lead these interventions.

COMPARISONS AND COMBINATIONS OF NONPHARMACOLOGIC PAIN MANAGEMENT INTERVENTIONS

There has been increasing research comparing individual nonpharmacologic pain management interventions as well as their combined effects. When compared with a sweet-tasting solution (oral sucrose), facilitated tucking alone is not as effective in relieving pain reactivity following a heel lance in very preterm neonates.[14] However, its use as an adjuvant therapy, in combination with oral sucrose and NNS, seems to be beneficial.[14,15] Similarly, NNS when combined with sucrose,[62] 30% glucose,[85] or facilitated tucking[15] seems to be synergistic regarding lower pain scores, less crying, more stable sleep patterns, and physiologic stability. Breast-feeding significantly reduced the heart rate elevation and diminished the proportion of crying time, the duration of the first cry, and the total crying time compared with positioning (swaddled and placed in a cot), maternal holding, placebo, pacifier use, no intervention, or the oral sucrose group.[28] Pain scores derived from unidimensional and composite pain assessment tools were generally lower in breast-feeding groups compared with positioning, placebo, or the oral sucrose

		Breast-	Kangaroo	Facilitated Tucking/	Sweet-Tasting
Table 2 Recommended use of nonpharmacologic measures for puncture procedures in neonates and infants					
Intervention	NNS	Feeding	Care	Swaddling	Solution
Intramuscular injection	X	X	X	X	X
Subcutaneous injection	X	X	X	X	X
Heel lance	X	X	X	X	X
Venipuncture	X	X	X	X	X

group. There is some evidence that when compared with sweet taste, breastfeeding is at least as effective and may be synergistic and potentially superior.[29]

In contrast, although supplemental expressed breast milk provided in the absence of the mother seems to be of some benefit on the heart rate, cry duration, behavioral facial response, and some validated pain assessment tool scores when compared with placebo, this was not the case when compared with sucrose 12.5%, 20.0%, or 25.0%. Increase in heart rate, percentage of time crying, and pain scores were significantly higher in the breast-milk group.[28] Kangaroo care has also been studied in combination with other therapies. There were 5 studies that used other treatment controls with kangaroo care. One compared enhanced kangaroo care that added rocking, singing, and sucking to kangaroo care and found no differences in the Premature Infant Pain Profile (PIPP) or time for the heart rate to recover.[59] One study compared sweet taste and holding (clothed) by female research assistants in full-term neonates during a heel lance.[25] The duration of crying was reduced by both, with an additive effect with the combination; but facial actions were only decreased with holding.

SUMMARY

There is sufficient evidence to support the use of nonpharmacologic interventions, particularly breastfeeding, sweet-tasting solutions, and kangaroo care, for common needle-puncture procedures; they are recommended for managing acute pain and distress in neonates and infants during common needle procedures (**Table 2**). Despite our limited understanding of the underlying mechanisms of actions of nonpharmacologic interventions, there seems to be few documented short-term harms from their use. Similar to pediatric pain management whereby distraction techniques are effective in managing painful procedures,[86] the soothing or calming effects of other nonpharmacologic interventions may only be beneficial in this manner.

Some nonpharmacologic interventions are easily implemented, such as NNS and swaddling/tucking, whereas others need a collaborative effort, such as kangaroo care and sweet-tasting solution. Support from the administration and leadership, both formal and informal, is crucial for the implementation of any of these strategies.[57] Informal leadership is part of the complex concept of unit culture. The culture of the unit must be accepting of this implementation.[87,88]

In summary, needle-related pain is a common experience for infants; as health care professionals, it behooves us to use all possible strategies to mitigate or prevent that pain and its negative consequences. Current research evidence suggests that nonpharmacologic interventions may be used to help ameliorate needle pain.

REFERENCES

1. Carbajal R, Rousset A, Danan C, et al. Epidemiology and treatment of painful procedures in neonates in intensive care units. JAMA 2008;300: 60–70.
2. Johnston CC, Fernandes AM, Campbell-Yeo M. Pain in neonates is different. Pain 2011;152(Suppl 3):S65–73.
3. Barker DP, Rutter N. Exposure to invasive procedures in neonatal intensive care unit admissions. Arch Dis Child Fetal Neonatal Ed 1995;72:F47–8.
4. Johnston CC, Collinge JM, Henderson SJ, et al. A cross-sectional survey of pain and pharmacological analgesia in Canadian neonatal intensive care units. Clin J Pain 1997;13(4):308–12.
5. Simons SH, van Dijk M, Anand KS, et al. Do we still hurt newborn babies? Arch Pediatr Adolesc Med 2003;157:1058–64.
6. Brummelte S, Grunau RE, Chau V, et al. Procedural pain and brain development in premature newborns. Ann Neurol 2012;71(3):385–96.
7. Walker SM, Franck LS, Fitzgerald M, et al. Long-term impact of neonatal intensive care and surgery on somatosensory perception in children born extremely preterm. Pain 2009;141:79–87.
8. Huang CM, Tung WS, Kuo LL, et al. Comparison of pain responses of premature infants to the heel stick between containment and swaddling. J Nurs Res 2004; 12(1):31–40.
9. Pillai Riddell R, Racine N, Turcotte K, et al. Nonpharmacological management of procedural pain in infants and young children: an abridged Cochrane review. Pain Res Manag 2011;16(5):321–30.
10. Aucott S, Donohue PK, Atkins E, et al. Neurodevelopmental care in the NICU. Ment Retard Dev Disabil Res Rev 2002;8(4):298–308.
11. Axelin A, Salantera S, Lehtonen L. "Facilitated tucking by parents" in pain management of preterm infants—a randomized crossover trial. Early Hum Dev 2006; 82(4):241–7.
12. van Sleuwen BE, Engelberts AC, Boere-Boonekamp MM, et al. Swaddling: a systematic review. Pediatrics 2007;120(4):e1097–106.
13. Prasopkittikun T, Tilokskulchai F. Management of pain from heel stick in neonates: an analysis of research conducted in Thailand. J Perinat Neonatal Nurs 2003;17(4):304–12.
14. Cignacco E, Axelin A, Stoffel L, et al. Facilitated tucking as a nonpharmacological intervention for neonatal pain relief: is it clinically feasible? Acta Paediatr 2010;99(12):1763–5.
15. Cignacco EL, Sellam G, Stoffel L, et al. Oral sucrose and "facilitated tucking" for repeated pain relief in preterms: a randomized controlled trial. Pediatrics 2012; 129(2):299–308.
16. Liaw JJ, Yang L, Lee CM, et al. Effects of combined use of non-nutritive sucking, oral sucrose, and facilitated tucking on infant behavioural states across heel-stick procedures: a prospective, randomised controlled trial. Int J Nurs Stud 2013;50(7):883–94.
17. Franck LS, Oulton K, Bruce E. Parental involvement in neonatal pain management: an empirical and conceptual update. J Nurs Scholarsh 2012;44(1): 45–54.
18. Fearon I, Kisilevsky BS, Hains SM, et al. Swaddling after heel lance: age-specific effects on behavioral recovery in preterm infants. J Dev Behav Pediatr 1997;18(4):222–32.

19. Blass EM, Ciaramitaro V. A new look at some old mechanisms in human newborns: taste and tactile determinants of state, affect, and action. Monogr Soc Res Child Dev 1994;59(1):I.

20. Carbajal R, Chauvet X, Couderc S, et al. Randomised trial of analgesic effects of sucrose, glucose, and pacifiers in term neonates. BMJ 1999;319(7222):1393–7.

21. McCain GC, Knupp AM, Fontaine JL, et al. Heart rate variability responses to nipple feeding for preterm infants with bronchopulmonary dysplasia: three case studies. J Pediatr Nurs 2010;25(3):215–20.

22. Semenic S, Childerhose JE, Lauzière J, et al. Barriers, facilitators, and recommendations related to implementing the Baby-Friendly Initiative (BFI): an integrative review [review]. J Hum Lact 2012;28(3):317–34. http://dx.doi.org/10.1177/0890334412445195.

23. Nyqvist KH, Häggkvist AP, Hansen MN, et al. Expansion of the ten steps to successful breastfeeding into neonatal intensive care: expert group recommendations for three guiding principles. J Hum Lact 2012;28(3):289–96.

24. Carbajal R, Veerapen S, Couderc S, et al. Analgesic effect of breast feeding in term neonates: randomised controlled trial. BMJ 2003;326(7379):13.

25. Gormally S, Barr RG, Wertheim L, et al. Contact and nutrient caregiving effects on newborn infant pain responses. Dev Med Child Neurol 2001;43(1):28–38.

26. Campos RG. Soothing pain-elicited distress in infants with swaddling and pacifiers. Child Dev 1989;60(4):781–92.

27. Taddio A, Ilersich AL, Ipp M, et al, HELPinKIDS Team. Physical interventions and injection techniques for reducing injection pain during routine childhood immunizations: systematic review of randomized controlled trials and quasi-randomized controlled trials. Clin Ther 2009;31(2):S48–76.

28. Shah PS, Herbozo C, Aliwalas LL, et al. Breastfeeding or breast milk for procedural pain in neonates. Cochrane Database Syst Rev 2012;(12):CD004950. http://dx.doi.org/10.1002/14651858.CD004950.pub3.

29. Shah V, Taddio A, Rieder MJ, HELPinKIDS Team. Effectiveness and tolerability of pharmacologic and combined interventions for reducing injection pain during routine childhood immunizations: systematic review and meta-analyses. Clin Ther 2009;31(Suppl 2):S104–51.

30. Hofer MA. Hidden regulators in attachment, separation, and loss. Monogr Soc Res Child Dev 1994;59:192–207.

31. Gunnar M. The effects of a pacifying stimulus on behavioural and adrenocortical responses to circumcision in the newborn. J Am Acad Child Psychiatry 1984;23(1):34–8.

32. Charpak N, Ruiz-Pelaez JG, Charpak Y, et al. Kangaroo mother program: an alternative way of caring for low birth weight infants? One year mortality in a two cohort study [see comment]. Pediatrics 1994;94(6 Pt 1):804–10.

33. Whitelaw A, Sleath K. Myth of the marsupial mother: home care of the very low birth weight babies in Bogota, Colombia. Lancet 1985;1:1206–8.

34. deLeeuw R, Colin EM, Dunnebier EA, et al. Physiologic effects of kangaroo care in very small preterm infants. Biol Neonate 1991;59:149–55.

35. Bosque EM, Brady JP, Affonso DD, et al. Physiologic measures of kangaroo versus incubator care in a tertiary-level nursery. J Obstet Gynecol Neonatal Nurs 1995;24(3):219–26.

36. Bauer K, Uhrig C, Sperling P, et al. Body temperatures and oxygen consumption during skin-to-skin (kangaroo) care in stable preterm infants weighing less than 1500 grams. J Pediatr 1997;130(2):240–4.

37. Ludington-Hoe SM, Anderson GC, Simpson S, et al. Birth-related fatigue in 34-36-week preterm neonates: rapid recovery with very early kangaroo (skin-to-skin) care. J Obstet Gynecol Neonatal Nurs 1999;28(1):94–103.

38. Gazzolo D, Masetti P, Meli M. Kangaroo care improves post-extubation cardio-respiratory parameters in infants after open heart surgery. Acta Paediatr 2000; 89(6):728–9.

39. Ludington-Hoe SM, Nguyen N, Swinth JY, et al. Kangaroo care compared to in-cubators in maintaining body warmth in preterm infants. Biol Res Nurs 2000; 2(1):60–73.

40. Bohnhorst B, Heyne T, Peter CS, et al. Skin-to-skin (kangaroo) care, respiratory control, and thermoregulation. J Pediatr 2001;138(2):193–7.

41. Ibe OE, Austin T, Sullivan K, et al. A comparison of kangaroo mother care and conventional incubator care for thermal regulation of infants <2000 g in Nigeria using continuous ambulatory temperature monitoring. Ann Trop Paediatr 2004; 24(3):245–51.

42. Messmer PR, Rodriguez S, Adams J, et al. Effect of kangaroo care on sleep time for neonates [review]. Pediatr Nurs 1997;23(4):408–14.

43. Chwo MJ, Anderson GC, Good M, et al. A randomized controlled trial of early kangaroo care for preterm infants: effects on temperature, weight, behavior, and acuity. J Nurs Res 2002;10(2):129–42.

44. Ferber SG, Makhoul IR. The effect of skin-to-skin contact (kangaroo care) shortly after birth on the neurobehavioral responses of the term newborn: a random-ized, controlled trial. Pediatrics 2004;113(4):858–65.

45. Meyer K, Anderson GC. Using kangaroo care in a clinical setting with full-term infants having breastfeeding difficulties. MCN Am J Matern Child Nurs 1999; 24(4):190–2.

46. Furman L, Kennell J. Breastmilk and skin-to-skin kangaroo care for premature infants. Avoiding bonding failure. Acta Paediatr 2000;89(11):1280–3.

47. Ruiz JG, Charpak N, Figuero Z. Predictional need for supplementing breast-feeding in preterm infants under kangaroo mother care. Acta Paediatr 2002; 91(10):1130–4.

48. Johnson AN. The relationship of kangaroo holding to maternal breast milk. J Pediatr Nurs 2006;21(2):137–8.

49. Hake-Brooks SJ, Anderson GC. Kangaroo care and breastfeeding of mother-preterm infant dyads 0-18 months: a randomized, controlled trial. Neonatal Netw 2008;27(3):151–9.

50. Flacking R, Ewald U, Wallin L. Positive effect of kangaroo mother care on long-term breastfeeding in very preterm infants. J Obstet Gynecol Neonatal Nurs 2011;40(2):190–7.

51. Boo NY, Jamli FM. Short duration of skin-to-skin contact: effects on growth and breastfeeding. J Paediatr Child Health 2007;43(12):831–6.

52. Conde-Agudelo A, Belizan JM, Diaz-Rossello J. Kangaroo mother care to reduce morbidity and mortality in low birthweight infants. Cochrane Database Syst Rev 2011;(3):CD002771.

53. Dodd VL. Implications of kangaroo care for growth and development in preterm infants. J Obstet Gynecol Neonatal Nurs 2005;34(2):218–32.

54. Gray L, Watt L, Blass EM. Skin-to-skin contact is analgesic in healthy newborns. Pediatrics 2000;105(1):e14.

55. Johnston C, Campbell-Yeo M, Fernandes A, et al. Skin-to-skin care for proce-dural pain in neonates (under review). Cochrane Database Syst Rev 2012;(3):CD008435. http://dx.doi.org/10.1002/14651858.CD008435.

56. Engler AJ, Ludington-Hoe SM, Cusson RM, et al. Kangaroo care: national survey of practice, knowledge, barriers, and perceptions. MCN Am J Matern Child Nurs 2002;27(3):146–53.
57. Johnson AN. Factors influencing implementation of kangaroo holding in a special care nursery. MCN Am J Matern Child Nurs 2007;32(1):25–9.
58. Chia P, Sellick K, Gan S. The attitudes and practices of neonatal nurses in the use of kangaroo care. Aust J Adv Nurs 2006;23(4):20–7.
59. Johnston CC, Filion F, Campbell-Yeo M, et al. Enhanced kangaroo mother care for heel lance in preterm neonates: a crossover trial. J Perinatol 2009;29(1): 51–6.
60. Johnston CC, Campbell-Yeo M, Filion F. Paternal vs maternal kangaroo care for procedural pain in preterm neonates: a randomized crossover trial. Arch Pediatr Adolesc Med 2011;165(9):792–6.
61. Johnston C, Byron J, Filion F, et al. Alternative female kangaroo care for procedural pain in preterm neonates: a pilot study. Acta Paediatr 2012;101(11): 1147–50.
62. Stevens B, Yamada J, Ohlsson A. Sucrose for analgesia in newborn infants undergoing painful procedures. Cochrane Database Syst Rev 2010;(1): CD001069.
63. Harrison D, Bueno M, Yamada J, et al. Analgesic effects of sweet tasting solutions in infants: current state of equipoise. Pediatrics 2010;126(5): 894–902.
64. Harrison D, Beggs S, Stevens B. Sucrose for procedural pain management in infants. Pediatrics 2012;130:1–8.
65. Anand KJ, Aranda JV, Berde CB, et al. Summary proceedings from the neonatal pain-control group. Pediatrics 2006;117(Suppl 1):S9–22. http://dx.doi.org/10.1542/peds.2005-0620C.
66. Lago P, Garetti E, Merazzi D, et al, on behalf of the Pain Study Group of the Italian Society of Neonatology. Guidelines for procedural pain in the newborn. Acta Paediatr 2009;98(6):932–9.
67. Prevention and management of pain and stress in the neonate. An update. American Academy of Pediatrics. Committee on Fetus and Newborn. Committee on Drugs. Section on Anesthesiology. Section on Surgery. Canadian Pediatric Society. Fetus and Newborn Committee. Pediatrics 2000;105:454–61.
68. Taddio A, Yiu A, Smith RW, et al. Variability in clinical practice guidelines for sweetening agents in newborn infants undergoing painful procedures. Clin J Pain 2009;25(2):153–5.
69. Buscemi N, Vandermeer B, Curtis S. The Cochrane library and procedural pain in children: an overview of reviews. Evid Based Child Health 2008;3:260–79. http://dx.doi.org/10.1002/ebch.225.
70. Taddio A, Shah V, Stephens D, et al. Effect of liposomal lidocaine and sucrose alone and in combination for venipuncture pain in newborns. Pediatrics 2011; 127(4):e940–7.
71. Holsti L, Grunau R. Considerations for using sucrose to reduce procedural pain in preterm infants. Pediatrics 2010;124:1042–7.
72. Slater R, Cornelissen L, Fabrizi L, et al. Oral sucrose as an analgesic drug for procedural pain in newborn infants: a randomized controlled trial. Lancet 2010;376:1225–32.
73. Gibbins S, Stevens B. The influence of gestational age on the efficacy and short-term safety of sucrose for procedural pain relief. Adv Neonatal Care 2003;3(5): 241–9.

74. Taddio A, Shah V, Hancock R, et al. Effectiveness of sucrose analgesia in newborns undergoing painful medical procedures. CMAJ 2008;179(1):37–43.
75. Johnston CC, Filion F, Snider L, et al. Routine sucrose analgesia during the first week of life in neonates younger than 31 weeks' postconceptional age. Pediatrics 2002;110(3):523–8.
76. Stevens B, Yamada J, Beyene J, et al. Consistent management of repeated procedural pain with sucrose in preterm neonates: is it effective and safe for repeated use over time? Clin J Pain 2005;21(6):543–8.
77. Johnston CC, Filion F, Snider L, et al. How much sucrose is too much sucrose? Pediatrics 2007;119(1):226.
78. Lefrak L, Burch K, Caravantes R. Sucrose analgesia: identifying potentially better practices. Pediatrics 2006;118(Suppl 2):S197–202.
79. Johnston C, Barrington KJ, Taddio A, et al. Pain in Canadian NICUs: have we improved over the past 12 years? Clin J Pain 2011;27(3):225–32.
80. Latimer MA, Ritchie JA, Johnston CC. Individual nurse and organizational context considerations for better knowledge use in pain care. J Pediatr Nurs 2010;25(4):274–81.
81. Hartling L, Shaik MS, Tjosvold L, et al. Music for medical indications in the neonatal period: a systematic review of randomised controlled trials. Arch Dis Child Fetal Neonatal Ed 2009;94(5):F349–54.
82. Bellieni CV, Tei M, Coccina F, et al. Sensorial saturation for infants' pain. J Matern Fetal Neonatal Med 2012;25(Suppl 1):79–81.
83. Melzack R, Wall PD. Pain mechanisms: a new theory. Science 1965;150(699):971–9.
84. Quirion R. Pain, nociception and spinal opioid receptors. Prog Neuropsychopharmacol Biol Psychiatry 1984;8(4–6):571–9.
85. Mekkaoui N, Issef I, Kabiri M, et al. Analgesic effect of 30% glucose, milk and non-nutritive sucking in neonates. J Pain Res 2012;5:573–7.
86. Cohen LL. Behavioral approaches to anxiety and pain management for pediatric venous access. Pediatrics 2008;122(Suppl 3):S134–9.
87. Stevens B, Riahi S, Cardoso R, et al. The influence of context on pain practices in the NICU: perceptions of health care professionals. Qual Health Res 2011;21(6):757–70.
88. Kitson A. Recognising relationships: reflections on evidence-based practice. Nurs Inq 2002;9(3):179–86.

Management of Neonatal Abstinence Syndrome from Opioids

Kendra Grim, MD[a], Tracy E. Harrison, MD[a],
Robert T. Wilder, MD, PhD[b],*

KEYWORDS

- Opioids • Neonatal • Abstinence • Withdrawal • Methadone • Buprenorphine

KEY POINTS

- Most infants at risk for neonatal abstinence syndrome have opioid plus another drug exposure; polypharmacy is the rule rather than the exception.
- Scales for the evaluation of neonatal abstinence syndrome are primarily based on opioid withdrawal.
- A standard protocol to treat neonatal abstinence syndrome has not been developed.
- Institute nonpharmacologic strategies for all neonates at risk.
- The American Academy of Pediatrics recommends mechanism-directed therapy (treat opioid withdrawal with an opioid) as the first-line therapy.
- Second-line medications are currently under evaluation.

INTRODUCTION

Neonatal abstinence syndrome (NAS) is defined as a constellation of symptoms typically observed in the newborn of a mother who has received opioids and other medications for a prolonged duration in the antepartum period (**Box 1**).[1] Withdrawal symptoms appear soon after delivery when the newborn is no longer receiving opioids that had been delivered systemically via the placenta. The constellation of behavioral and physiologic signs and symptoms include tremulousness, irritability, inconsolability, as well as feeding intolerance, emesis, watery stools, seizures, tachycardia, and respiratory distress.[2] It has been suggested that affected neonates have an increased propensity for the development of attention-deficit/hyperactivity disorder as they mature.[3]

[a] Department of Anesthesiology, College of Medicine, Mayo Clinic, MB2-860, 200 First Street, Southwest, Rochester, MN 55902, USA; [b] Department of Anesthesiology, College of Medicine, Mayo Clinic, MB2-760, 200 First Street, Southwest, Rochester, MN 55902, USA
* Corresponding author.
E-mail address: wilder.robert@mayo.edu

Clin Perinatol 40 (2013) 509–524
http://dx.doi.org/10.1016/j.clp.2013.05.004   perinatology.theclinics.com
0095-5108/13/$ – see front matter © 2013 Elsevier Inc. All rights reserved.

Box 1
NAS

- A constellation of symptoms observed in the newborn after antenatal or early neonatal exposure to psychotropic medications, for example

  ○ Maternal drug abuse

  ○ Maternal methadone maintenance

  ○ Maternal prescription medication use for chronic pain, including opioids, antidepressants, benzodiazepines, and so forth

  ○ Iatrogenic cause from prolonged neonatal administration of opioids, benzodiazepines, and other psychotropic medications in the setting of critical illness

---

First described in the 1960s, NAS was initially seen in newborns who were delivered to mothers using illicit opioids or taking methadone as part of treatment programs for their opioid addiction.[2] Many of these women are also using other legal and illicit drugs, including alcohol, tobacco, marijuana, cocaine, and others. The affected neonatal population may also include infants born to women being treated for chronic nonmalignant pain with opioids, such as oxycodone, during their pregnancy. As the number of opioid prescriptions is increasing,[4] it is expected that NAS will continue to be an ongoing problem in the neonatal population. Alternatively, NAS may have an iatrogenic cause, observed after attempting to discontinue the administration of opioids and benzodiazepines used in hospitalized critically ill newborns over an extended period. In all settings, the use of a single drug or class of drugs is unusual. Polypharmacy is the rule rather than the exception with infants receiving opioids prenatally and postnatally.

The impact of NAS is concerning because the number of newborns showing symptoms of withdrawal after intrauterine exposure has tripled in the United States between the years of 2000 and 2009.[5] This trend mirrors the rapid increase in abuse and misuse of prescription opioids and translates to one child born every hour who will experience NAS requiring treatment.

Treatment of these neonates can potentially require weeks and extend the hospital length of stay, with the mean cost that may exceed $50,000.[2] The length of stay for those neonates with NAS has not declined during the last decade.[2] This fact may represent the increasing challenges of treatment, particularly of those neonates of mothers who took prescription opioid medications antenatally. Experience with these neonates shows that their abstinence syndrome is more severe, and treatment strategies previously used for babies exposed to methadone are largely ineffective. There currently is no standard protocol for the treatment of NAS specific to prescription medications, although numerous institutions are now enrolling patients in an effort to compare treatment strategies and determine the most effective way to manage these symptoms (**Box 2**).

EVALUATION

Many studies have been aimed to predict severity and treatment plans for infants with NAS. Maternal methadone dose has been evaluated in many studies; however, it does not correlate with the risk of NAS, severity,[6] or management of neonates.[7–13] Limited studies argue that the maternal methadone dose is associated with the duration of NAS, need for treatment, and prolonged hospitalization[14] and recommend the use of the smallest maternal methadone dose as possible.[15] Inadequate maternal

> **Box 2**
> **Concluding NAS points**
>
> - NAS is more severe when related to maternal opioid prescription drugs compared with methadone.
> - In the United States, one child is born every hour necessitating treatment of NAS.
> - The number of infants born with NAS has tripled over the past decade in the United States.
> - Mean hospital cost can approach $50, 000, with Medicaid covering treatment of approximately 78% of neonates.
> - NAS can potentially influence attention and learning as the child develops.
> - Mothers with either prescription or illicit opioid use may have used other drugs in pregnancy that can confound the diagnosis and treatment of the neonate.

methadone dosing, however, may increase the risk of illicit drug use and, thus, may increase overall maternal opioid or polysubstance use. The half-life of the drug (eg, buprenorphine vs methadone) and the timing of the last maternal dose can help predict the onset and severity of NAS.[8,16]

A meconium drug screen can be used to identify neonates at risk; however, it has been shown to be a poor predictor of NAS.[17] Neonatal serum methadone levels are also of minimal benefit for estimating treatment requirements.[18]

NAS occurs in up to 80% of neonates with exposure to methadone,[18,19] and between 30% and 91% of infants with NAS will receive pharmacologic treatment.[8] The onset of NAS is typically 48 to 72 hours, although NAS can be delayed in breast-fed babies.[8] If NAS does not present by the third day of life in neonates exposed to methadone exposure, they are unlikely to require treatment of NAS[20]; however, NAS caused by buprenorphine will usually present later than methadone,[1] with an onset at 40 hours and peak symptoms at 70 hours.[18] If untreated, subacute NAS can be present for weeks to months.[6]

The earliest symptoms are irritability, tremors, high-pitched cry, difficult feeding, and diarrhea.[21] Dysfunction in autonomic regulation, sensory/motor functioning, sleep-wake disturbance, and autonomic dysfunction (sweating, sneezing, fever, nasal stuffiness, yawning, failure to thrive) can follow.[1] More severe dysregulation can also occur, such as mottling, tachypnea, and fever. Myocardial ischemia has even been reported with abrupt cessation of opioids in tolerant infants.[22] These symptoms may be difficult to distinguish from other serious neonatal illnesses, and evaluation for these illnesses may delay the treatment of NAS.[1] Early identification is the key to decrease morbidity.[6] Preterm infants typically have less severe symptoms, present later, and are less likely to require treatment,[8,18] which may be because of the immaturity of the central nervous system (CNS), decreased hepatic/renal metabolism, or decreased transmission of methadone in preterm infants.[9,18] The sex of infants is not a contributing factor for NAS presentation or treatment.[23,24]

Neonates exposed to opioids in pregnancy are at increased risk of sudden infant death syndrome (SIDS). Neonatal insensitivity to carbon dioxide tension can persist for more than 15 days of life.[25] Physicians should counsel families to decrease other risk factors, including smoking, or institute home monitoring.[8]

Scoring/Treatment

The objective of scoring/treatment tools is to recognize drug-exposed infants, monitor the severity of NAS, need for treatment, and response to treatment.[18] Multiple scoring and treatment evaluation tools are clinically available, and many institutions choose their scoring tool depending on their needs.

The Finnegan score (Neonatal Abstinence Score) was an early scale designed to assess NAS.[26] It is the most frequently used score to quantify the severity of symptoms and determine the need for pharmacologic treatment.[1] The Finnegan score is relatively easy and reliable; however, it has potential for bias and subjectivity. Thresholds for treatment may vary by institution, but typically 3 or more scores greater than 8 or a single score greater than 12 recommends pharmacologic treatment.[8,18]

The Lipsitz score is less widely used, but requires less scoring and is therefore less time consuming, and more user friendly.[8] A Lipsitz score of 4 or more typically recommends treatment of NAS.[18]

The NICU Network Neurobehavioral Scale is a specific scale for neonatal stress/abstinence; however, it was not intended to determine treatment thresholds or the response to treatment.[27] A published scoring technique called the 3 score was developed as a screening tool to identify infants at risk for opioid exposure and risk for NAS. The 3 score evaluates for (1) a hyperactive Moro reflex, (2) a mild tremor when undisturbed, and (3) increased muscle tone. Although a useful screening tool, the 3 score is not intended for treatment assessment.[28]

The Withdrawal Assessment Tool-1 (WAT-1)[29,30] was developed for older children withdrawing from opioid infusions in a Pediatric Intensive Care Unit, but has also been used in the Neonatal Intensive Care Unit as a measure of NAS.

Finally, the Sofia Opioid-withdrawal Symptom Scale is a recent scale also designed for infants and children with iatrogenic opioid and benzodiazepine dependence.[31] This scale is primarily designed for older children.

Pupillary dilation has been evaluated to be a potential objective measure of neonatal response to opioids. Pupillary dilation, however, must be used with scoring and treatment tools.[32]

A key feature of all the aforementioned neonatal withdrawal scales is that they are based on symptoms of opioid withdrawal. They tend to be less sensitive to symptoms of withdrawal from other types of medications. The Neonatal Behavioral Scale (**Table 1**) was designed to assess for problems from abrupt selective serotonin reuptake inhibitor (SSRI) withdrawal but is quite nonspecific.[33]

MANAGEMENT
Goals

Neonatal well-being should be pursued, which includes normal eating, feeding, weight gain, and neurocognitive development. As the number of infants with NAS continues to increase, quality care is that which promotes access to cost-effective care.

Nonpharmacologic Strategies

All neonates at risk should be considered for nonpharmacologic strategies for NAS. Multiple interventions are recommended for these infants, and most are simple to perform by medical professionals and easy to teach parents. The most studied and recommended intervention is swaddling.[1,7,8,18,34,35] If the swaddled infant is too warm, a folded blanket across the chest to contain arms can be used instead of swaddling.[35] Environmental stimuli should be minimized,[7,8,18,35] including decreasing light[8,18,34,35] and minimizing noise.[8,18] This practice will also facilitate adequate rest and sleep, which is also very important for NAS treatment.[7] Although comforting touch is beneficial, unnecessary handling should be avoided.[8] Non-nutritive sucking[1] with a pacifier or the infant's hands may also be beneficial.[35]

Table 1
Comparison of neonatal evaluation scales

Modified Finnegan Score[56]		WAT-1[29]		Neonatal Behavioral Syndrome[33]
CNS symptoms		From chart over previous 12 h		Irritability
High-pitched cry	2			
High-pitched cry >2 h	3			
Sleeps <3 h after feeding	1	Any loose/watery stools	1	Jitteriness
Sleeps <2 h after feeding	2	Vomiting/retching/gagging	1	
Sleeps <1 h after feeding	3	Temperature >37.8°C	1	
Mild tremors when disturbed	1	2-min Prestimulus observation		Hypotonia
Marked tremors when disturbed	2			
Mild tremors when undisturbed	3			
Marked tremors when undisturbed	4			
Increased muscle tone	2	Asleep/awake & calm	0	Hypertonia
		Awake & distressed	1	
Excoriation of skin	1	Tremor, none/mild	0	Hyperreflexia
		Moderate/severe	1	
Myoclonic jerks in sleep	3	Any sweating	1	Oxygen requirement
Generalized convulsion	5	Uncoordinated/repetitive movement	1	Apnea
Vegetative symptoms		Yawning or sneezing 0–1	0	Flaring
		≥2	1	
Sweating	1	1-min Stimulus observation		Grunting
Temperature 37.5°C–38.0°C	1			
Temperature >38.0°C	2			
Frequent yawning	1			
Mottling	1			
Nasal stuffiness	2			
Sneezing	1			
Gastrointestinal symptoms		Startle to touch, none/mild	0	Retractions
		Moderate/severe	1	
Frantic sucking	1	Increased muscle tone	1	Vomiting
Poor feeding	2			
Regurgitation	2			
Projectile vomiting	3			
Loose stools	2			
Watery stools	3			
Respiratory symptoms		Poststimulus recovery		Poor feeding
Tachypnea >60/min	1	Time to regain calm <2 min	0	Hypoglycemia
		2–5 min	1	
Tachypnea >60/min with retractions	2	>5 min	2	

(continued on next page)

Table 1 (continued)		
Modified Finnegan Score[56]	**WAT-1[29]**	**Neonatal Behavioral Syndrome[33]**
Total 37; single score >12 or 3 scores >8 considered abnormal	Total 12; scores >3 abnormal	Presence of any 1 item considered positive for neonatal behavioral syndrome secondary to maternal SSRI use

Education of caregivers is very important, especially to provide reassurance and support[1] for mothers who may feel responsible for the infant's suffering. Education of the mother both facilitates treatment of the infants and helps alleviate feelings of maternal guilt.[1] For instance, withdrawal behavior, such as fisting, back arching, and jaw clenching, may be misinterpreted by the mother as dislike of touch.[35] Mothers can be educated to treat these behaviors with soothing techniques (as listed earlier), which also facilitates infant-maternal bonding.[35]

Feeding

Poor feeding with excessive sucking may worsen hunger and NAS symptoms[8]; therefore, appropriate feeding is essential, including the use of high-caloric feeds[7,34,35] and frequent burping by rubbing instead of patting the back.[35] Neonates undergoing treatment of NAS have increased caloric requirements and may develop hyperphagia, with intake of more than 190 mL/kg/d.[21] Hyperphagia can lead to excessive weight gain; therefore, neonates treated for NAS should have careful monitoring of fluid intake and weight gain.[36] Conversely, infants with poor feeding may be considered for gastric feeds because inadequate caloric intake contributes to symptoms of NAS.[8]

Many studies have evaluated the safety and benefit of breast-feeding for infants with in utero opioid exposure. Most studies recommend that breast-feeding be encouraged unless contraindications exist, such as ongoing drug use or human immunodeficiency virus infection.[8] Risk of hepatitis C virus (HCV) transmission to infants is about 10% in HCV RNA–positive mothers,[8] but breast-feeding is not contraindicated.[37] Maternal methadone is found in breast milk, but at low quantities when maternal dose is less than 20 mg/d.[37] Maternal methadone is found in breast milk but at low quantities when maternal dose is less than 20 mg/d.[38] Although breast-feeding may be safe with maternal dosing up to 80 mg/d, neonatal monitoring may be considered for daily doses greater than 20 mg/d.[38] Overall, the American Academy of Pediatrics recommends that maternal methadone consumption not be considered a factor for breast-feeding eligibility.[8,39] Breast-feeding rates in opioid-dependent women are low, however. In one study, only 25% of eligible opioid-dependent mothers breast-fed, and 50% of these quit within 1 week.[40]

Whether breast-feeding is an effective treatment for the prevention of NAS is currently under debate.[18,21] In one study, 26% of breast-fed infants and 78% of formula-fed infants developed NAS.[41] Breast-feeding may be associated with a reduced severity of NAS and a reduction in treatment requirements.[8] Infants have been found to experience NAS with sudden cessation of breast-feeding.[8] The mechanism of this effect is not known because investigators argue the transfer of maternal methadone in breast milk is not sufficient to prevent or treat NAS.[8]

Neonatal weight loss was less profound in exclusively breast-fed infants with the treatment of NAS as compared with formula.[42] Given the other known benefits of breast-feeding, including infant-maternal bonding, breast-feeding should be considered for eligible opioid-dependent mothers. Consider the institution of breast-feeding in a hospital setting and continue supervision of the infant if maternal opioid dose increases, especially with maternal methadone dosing of greater than 20 mg/d.[38]

Pharmacologic Strategies

Although pharmacologic treatment (**Table 2**) for NAS is debated, treatment algorithms have been published (**Table 3**). Most treatment strategies recommend the use of opioids for opioid withdrawal (same pharmacokinetic mechanism) (American Academy of Pediatrics).[1,7,8,18,21] Of note, sedatives are ineffective for the treatment of opioid withdrawal in adults; therefore, many investigators question the efficacy of sedatives for the treatment of NAS.[18] Whether the treatment should be primarily symptom based or weight based is currently debated.[1]

Opioids

Most physicians (94% of UK physicians and 83% of US physicians) use an opioid as the first choice,[7] although the choice of opioid is also debated. Diluted tincture of opium (DTO), also called laudanum, is an alcoholic extract of more than 10 opioid alkaloids.[18] DTO is typically diluted 25 fold but continues to contain alcohol.[6] Despite the presence of alcohol, DTO continues to be recommended by the American Academy of Pediatrics[8] even though oral morphine has been shown to be as effective as DTO and avoids the alcohol exposure of DTO.[34]

Morphine, a pure mu receptor opioid agonist, is preferred by some investigators to the opioid mixture of DTO[34] because it is available in an alcohol-free oral preparation of 0.4 mg/mL.[6] Although morphine has been found to be as effective as DTO for the treatment of NAS,[34] morphine may be associated with an increased duration of hospital stay and need for supportive care.[7] Other studies, however, have shown a trend toward improved weight gain with morphine, with reduced number of days to regain birth weight as compared with DTO.[34] Many treatment protocols for NAS treatment prefer morphine because of the predictable half-life and ease of administration.

Methadone is a mu receptor agonist and N-methyl-d-aspartate antagonist with a long and variable half-life. Studies of neonates show a methadone half-life of 3.8 to 62.0 hours, (mean 19.2 hours [STD 13.6]).[6] Accordingly, methadone can be challenging to titrate for NAS treatment and has been not recommended for this reason in some countries (Australia).[18] Some investigators suggest that methadone dosing (typically 2–3 times per day) facilitates compliance, and the long half-life prevents withdrawal symptoms during weaning. Comparison of methadone and morphine has not shown a difference in outcome between groups, including length of hospital stay.[8,43]

Buprenorphine is a new partial mu opioid agonist and kappa opioid antagonist, with emerging use in neonates undergoing treatment of NAS.[1] The half-life is long, although predictable at 72 hours.[18] Initial use of buprenorphine in neonates has found it to be safe; however, this is based on limited data.[44] Kraft and colleagues[45] published a phase 1 clinical trial with 24 term infants and concluded buprenorphine was safe and effective. Buprenorphine decreased the length of NAS treatment by 40% and length of hospital stay 24% when compared with morphine.

Second-line medications

Phenobarbital is primarily a γ-aminobutyric acid agonist, used widely for the treatment of seizures and is also the most widely used second-line medication by UK and US physicians for the treatment of NAS.[7] Phenobarbital tends to be more liberally used in neonates exposed to multiple substances (including benzodiazepines)[8,46] and

Table 2
Pharmacotherapy

	Mechanism	Side Effects	Advantage	Disadvantage
First line				
Diluted tincture of opium	Mu agonist	Respiratory depression, constipation, sedation	Recommended by American Academy of Pediatrics	Contains alcohol, >10 opioid alkaloids
Morphine	Mu agonist	Respiratory depression, constipation, sedation	Ease of titration	Frequency of dosing (q 3–4 h)
Methadone	Mu agonist, NMDA antagonist	Respiratory depression, constipation, sedation	Ease of dosing (2–3 times daily), half-life facilitates slow taper	Long half-life with unpredictable interpatient variability
Buprenorphine	Partial mu agonist and kappa opioid antagonist	Respiratory depression, constipation, sedation	Long half-life, ease of dosing and taper	Minimal data on use, phase 1 trial formulation contains 30% ethanol
Second line				
Phenobarbital	GABA agonist	Sedation, withdrawal seizures	Reduction in hospital stay and daily opioid use	Sedation, impaired suckling
Clonidine	Alpha 2 agonist	Sedation, bradycardia, hypotension, withdrawal hypertension	Reduced symptoms, length of stay in hospital	
Dexmedetomidine	Alpha 2 agonist	Sedation, bradycardia, hypotension, withdrawal hypertension	8 times more affinity for alpha 2 receptor than clonidine	Limited data for use in neonates, more studies needed

Under Investigation				
Ondansetron	Serotonin (5-HT3) antagonist	Prolonged QT	Reduce symptoms of opioid withdrawal	Efficacy under evaluation
SSRIs	Inhibition of neural uptake of serotonin	Serotonin syndrome	Decreased severity of opioid withdrawal in adults	Limited data in neonates
Maternal vaccine	IgG antibody production against target opioid	Unknown	Prevents transit of target drug across placenta	Noncomplexed IgG antibodies against opioid will cross placenta
Chlorpromazine	Unknown, strong antiadrenergic activity	Tachycardia, thermoregulation problems	Shorter duration of treatment and hospitalization	Very limited data
Not Recommended				
Paregoric	Mixture of opioids, camphor, anise oil, alcohol, benzoic acid	Toxic, contains alcohol		No longer used because of toxicity concerns
Diazepam	Benzodiazepine	Sedation, poor feeding		No longer recommended because of lack of efficacy, adverse effects on feeding
Naloxone	Mu antagonist	Hypertension, acute withdrawal, seizures		Can precipitate acute withdrawal and withdrawal seizures

Abbreviations: GABA, γ-aminobutyric acid; IgG, immunoglobulin G; NMDA, N-methyl-d-aspartate; 5-HT3, 5-hydroxytryptamine type 3 receptor.

Table 3
Sample treatment algorithms

	First-line Medication	Starting Dose	Frequency	Titration	Plateau	Taper	Second-line Medication
Jansson et al,[6] 2009	Morphine	0.02 mg	Every 4 h	Increase by 0.02 mg until symptoms controlled	48 h	Taper by 0.02 mg every 24 h	Consider if dose >0.2 mg morphine every 3 h
Oei & Lui,[18] 2007	Morphine	0.2–0.5 mg/kg/d		Increase 10%–20%	2–3 d		
Kraft & van den Anker,[44] 2012	Morphine	0.4 mg/kg/d	Divided in 6 doses	Increase by 10% per d for NAS >24 on 3 measurements		Taper by 10% daily, discontinue when 0.15 mg/kg/d reached	Phenobarbital when morphine >1 mg/kg/d
Hudak & Tan,[7] 2012	Morphine	0.04 mg/kg	Every 3–4 h	0.04 mg/kg per dose, maximum 0.2 mg/kg per dose			
Ballard,[21] 2002	Morphine	0.08 mg/kg per dose	Every 3–4 h	Day 1: 0.08 mg/kg per dose; Day 2: 0.09 mg/kg per dose; Day 3: 0.1 mg/kg per dose; Day 4: 0.15 mg/kg per dose; Day 5: 0.2 mg/kg per dose (maximum)	F score <8	Taper by 10% daily, discontinue when dose 0.04 mg/kg reached	

Reference	Drug	Dose	Interval	Schedule			
Ballard,[21] 2002	Methadone	0.1 mg/kg	Every 4 h	Day 1: 0.1 mg/kg q 4 h; Day 2: 0.075 mg/kg q 4 h; Day 3: 0.05 mg/kg q 6 h; Day 4: 0.05 mg/kg q 8 h; Day 5: 0.05 mg/kg q 12 h; Day 6: 0.025 mg/kg q 12 h; Day 7: 0.025 mg/kg daily; Day 8: 0.012 mg/kg daily	Patient symptoms	Patient symptoms	
Hudak & Tan,[7] 2012	Methadone	0.05–0.1 mg/kg	Every 6 h	0.05 mg/kg per dose, to effect			
Hudak & Tan,[7] 2012	Clonidine	0.5 mcg/kg	Every 3–6 h		Maximum 1 mcg/kg every 3 h		
Agthe et al,[50] 2009	Clonidine	1 mcg/kg	Every 4 h				
Kraft & van den Anker,[44] 2012	Buprenorphine	15.9 mcg/kg/d	Divided in 3 doses	Increase by 25% for NAS >24 on 3 measurements	3 d	Taper by 10% daily	Phenobarbital

Abbreviation: F score, finnegan neonatal abstinence score.

may have improved efficacy to treat opioid withdrawal seizures.[18,47] Phenobarbital has shown lower rates of treatment failure, reduction in maximal opioid dose, and reduced hospital length of stay.[7] In a study of 20 term infants, the addition of phenobarbital to opioid treatment reduced the severity of symptoms, reduced the amount of opioid required, and decreased the length of hospital stay by 48%.[7,48] Phenobarbital therapy, however, had to be continued for 3.5 months.[7,48] In contrast, the use of morphine alone had an improved outcome in one study, with an average of 10 treatment days as compared with phenobarbital (18 days of therapy).[19]

In a study by Coyle and colleagues,[48] the use of phenobarbital did not cause increased sedation or compromise in feeding or growth; however, concerns about phenobarbital use in the literature include impairment of suckling,[18] adverse effects on the developing brain in long-term therapy,[49] and precipitation of seizures at home during weaning.[34] Langenfeld and colleagues[34] thought it is "unacceptable to administer phenobarbital in high doses as a sedative, for several months" for the treatment of NAS.

Chloroprocaine may decrease NAS symptoms by a reduction in sympathetic tone because it has strong antiadrenergic activity, but the exact mechanism is unknown. There is very limited data available for the safety and efficacy of chlorpromazine for the treatment of NAS.[8] A small study has shown that the duration of treatment and hospitalization may be shorter as compared with morphine.[7]

Clonidine is a central alpha 2 adrenergic receptor agonist that acts at presynaptic receptors in the midbrain and medulla.[50] Clonidine reduces sympathetic outflow by decreasing central catecholamine release,[50] which is thought to palliate symptoms of autonomic overactivity. Clonidine has been shown to reduce median length of treatment in all infants and for infants exposed to methadone. The total morphine dose was approximately 60% lower when combined with clonidine, and the neonates experienced fewer days of drug therapy and hospitalization.[7,50,51] When methadone-exposed infants were given 3 to 4 mcg/kg/d, major withdrawal symptoms were treated.[51] In a study of 14 infants (gestational age of 24.4–40.0 weeks), clonidine 0.5 to 1.0 mcg/kg every 6 hours was used without opioids, for an average treatment duration of 6.8 days with adequate treatment of NAS.[52,53] A study by Agthe and colleagues[50] found that the addition of clonidine to an opioid prevented NAS treatment failure. Adverse side effects of clonidine, including hypotension, bradycardia, or desaturation,[50] were not reported; however, 3 infants in the clonidine group died at home (myocarditis, SIDS, homicide by methadone).[50] The deaths were investigated and not attributed to clonidine. Agthe and colleagues[50] recommended the addition of clonidine for infants undergoing treatment of NAS that requires more than 0.5 mL of DTO or more than 0.2 mg of morphine every 4 hours.

Dexmedetomidine is an alpha 2 agonist with an 8-fold greater affinity for alpha 2 adrenergic receptor than clonidine.[50] Dexmedetomidine is currently approved for short-term sedation in adults; however, it is becoming increasingly popular in children and may be considered in future studies.[50]

Under investigation

Ondansetron is a selective 5-hydroxytryptamine type 3 receptor (5-HT3) antagonist that has been shown to block naloxone precipitated withdrawal in mice and may reduce symptoms of opioid withdrawal in humans.[54] The mechanism is thought to be the modulation of activity of the mesolimbic dopaminergic system by the 5-HT3 receptor.[54]

SSRI medications may decrease the severity of opioid withdrawal in adults[17]; however, safety and efficacy in neonates has yet to be established. Infants of mothers who have been using SSRIs during pregnancy are thought to be at risk for both SSRI withdrawal and serotonin syndrome because both have been reported.[55]

Maternal vaccination to heroin or oxycodone has been proposed. The vaccine would be administered during pregnancy to maintain high antibody titers against the targeted opioid. If exposure to that opioid occurs, the antibody will form a complex with the antigen, preventing the transit of the drug across the blood-brain barrier and placenta. The noncomplexed immunoglobulin G antibodies will cross the placenta into the fetus, which would also make the infant resistant to the targeted drug.[54]

Not recommended

Paregoric was historically used but is no longer recommended because of the toxicity concerns because it contains a mixture of opioids, camphor, anise oil, alcohol, benzoic acid, and other toxic ingredients.[7,8] Naloxone, a mu receptor antagonist, has been reported to provoke acute seizures from NAS when given at birth.[8] Currently, insufficient data exist to support rapid detoxification in neonates.[8] For the treatment of respiratory depression, Ballard[21] recommend supportive measures, including the use mechanical ventilation instead of naloxone. Diazepam, a benzodiazepine, has fallen out of favor because of a lack of efficacy and the adverse effects on feeding.[7,8]

Treatment Location

The optimal setting for treatment needs to be balanced between safety, effective care, and cost. The hospital setting is recommended for many reasons. Aside from treatment of NAS, many of these infants have outstanding medical and social issues that require hospitalization.[18]

Many of the medications for NAS treatment, notably opioids, are potent respiratory depressants.[7] Hospital care facilitates NAS treatment allowing rapid weaning of medications (most in 3 weeks), with close monitoring of the infant and parental care.[8] NAS assessments may be challenging for parents to perform at home, leading to overuse or underuse of medications.[7] A postnatal ward with the mother or primary care giver may be used to provide supervision and has been shown to yield shorter hospitalization than infants admitted to newborn unit.[8]

Outpatient treatment requires initial inpatient stabilization with close multidisciplinary follow-up after discharge.[8] Weaning of medications by 10% to 20% every 2 to 3 days may occur according to weight gain, eating, and sleeping.[18] Physicians may consider weaning by volume to simplify dosage for parents and minimize error. For example, morphine 0.5 mg/mL and phenobarbitone 10 mg/mL can be weaned at 0.1 mL per week regardless of weight.[18] Overall, Jansson and colleagues[6] stated the "optimal treatment for the developing infant with NAS does not necessarily imply the shortest possible hospitalization in the neonatal period."

SUMMARY/DISCUSSION

NAS management is challenging and continues to evolve. The overwhelming consensus is to start with nonpharmacologic strategies for all infants at risk, recognize the need for pharmacologic treatment, and assess the efficacy of treatment frequently. Breast-feeding may be encouraged, especially in the inpatient setting. Opioids are currently considered the first-line therapy, although the type of opioid may be at the discretion of the physician and the comfort of the care team. Second-line therapy has been phenobarbital, although concerns are emerging regarding use of a medication for sedation during opioid withdrawal. Phenobarbital has been effective for the treatment of opioid withdrawal seizures. Clonidine has been shown to be an effective and safe second-line medication for the treatment of NAS symptoms refractory to opioid therapy. The use of new agents, such as buprenorphine, continues to be evaluated.

REFERENCES

1. Jansson LM, Velez M. Neonatal abstinence syndrome. Curr Opin Pediatr 2012; 24(2):252–8.
2. Patrick SW, Schumacher RE, Benneyworth BD, et al. Neonatal abstinence syndrome and associated health care expenditures: United States, 2000-2009. JAMA 2012;307(18):1934–40.
3. Ornoy A, Segal J, Bar-Hamburger R, et al. Developmental outcome of school-age children born to mothers with heroin dependency: importance of environmental factors. Dev Med Child Neurol 2001;43(10):668–75.
4. Manchikanti L, Singh A. Therapeutic opioids: a ten-year perspective on the complexities and complications of the escalating use, abuse, and nonmedical use of opioids. Pain Physician 2008;11(Suppl 2):S63–88.
5. Campo-Flores A. Pain pills' littlest victims. The Wall Street Journal 2012;A3.
6. Jansson LM, Velez M, Harrow C. The opioid-exposed newborn: assessment and pharmacologic management. J Opioid Manag 2009;5(1):47–55.
7. Hudak ML, Tan RC. Neonatal drug withdrawal. Pediatrics 2012;129(2):e540–60.
8. Kuschel C. Managing drug withdrawal in the newborn infant. Semin Fetal Neonatal Med 2007;12(2):127–33.
9. Seligman NS, Salva N, Hayes EJ, et al. Predicting length of treatment for neonatal abstinence syndrome in methadone-exposed neonates. Am J Obstet Gynecol 2008;199(4):396.e1–7.
10. Cleary BJ, Donnelly J, Strawbridge J, et al. Methadone dose and neonatal abstinence syndrome-systematic review and meta-analysis. Addiction 2010;105(12): 2071–84.
11. Seligman NS, Almario CV, Hayes EJ, et al. Relationship between maternal methadone dose at delivery and neonatal abstinence syndrome. J Pediatr 2010; 157(3):428–33, 433.e1.
12. Pizarro D, Habli M, Grier M, et al. Higher maternal doses of methadone does not increase neonatal abstinence syndrome. J Subst Abuse Treat 2011;40(3):295–8.
13. Thajam D, Atkinson DE, Sibley CP, et al. Is neonatal abstinence syndrome related to the amount of opiate used? J Obstet Gynecol Neonatal Nurs 2010; 39(5):503–9.
14. Dashe JS, Sheffield JS, Olscher DA, et al. Relationship between maternal methadone dosage and neonatal withdrawal. Obstet Gynecol 2002;100(6):1244–9.
15. Isemann B, Meinzen-Derr J, Akinbi H. Maternal and neonatal factors impacting response to methadone therapy in infants treated for neonatal abstinence syndrome. J Perinatol 2011;31(1):25–9.
16. Liu AJ, Jones MP, Murray H, et al. Perinatal risk factors for the neonatal abstinence syndrome in infants born to women on methadone maintenance therapy. Aust N Z J Obstet Gynaecol 2010;50(3):253–8.
17. Gray TR, Choo RE, Concheiro M, et al. Prenatal methadone exposure, meconium biomarker concentrations and neonatal abstinence syndrome. Addiction 2010;105(12):2151–9.
18. Oei J, Lui K. Management of the newborn infant affected by maternal opiates and other drugs of dependency. J Paediatr Child Health 2007;43(1–2):9–18.
19. Ebner N, Rohrmeister K, Winklbaur B, et al. Management of neonatal abstinence syndrome in neonates born to opioid maintained women. Drug Alcohol Depend 2007;87(2–3):131–8.
20. Serane VT, Kurian O. Neonatal abstinence syndrome. Indian J Pediatr 2008; 75(9):911–4.

21. Ballard JL. Treatment of neonatal abstinence syndrome with breast milk containing methadone. J Perinat Neonatal Nurs 2002;15(4):76–85.
22. Biswas AK, Feldman BL, Davis DH, et al. Myocardial ischemia as a result of severe benzodiazepine and opioid withdrawal. Clin Toxicol 2005;43(3):207–9.
23. Holbrook A, Kaltenbach K. Gender and NAS: does sex matter? Drug Alcohol Depend 2010;112(1–2):156–9.
24. Unger A, Jagsch R, Bawert A, et al. Are male neonates more vulnerable to neonatal abstinence syndrome than female neonates? Gend Med 2011;8(6): 355–64.
25. Olsen GD, Lees MH. Ventilatory response to carbon dioxide of infants following chronic prenatal methadone exposure. Journal of Pediatrics 1980;96(6):983–9.
26. Finnegan L, Kron R, Connaughton J, et al. Assessment and treatment of abstinence in the infant of the drug-dependent mother. Int J Clin Pharmacol Biopharm 1975;12:19–32.
27. Tronick E, Lester B. The NICU Network Neurobehavioral Scale: a comprehensive instrument to assess substance-exposed and high-risk infants. NIDA Res Monogr 1996;166:198–204.
28. Jones HE, Kaltenbach K, Heil SH, et al. Neonatal abstinence syndrome after methadone or buprenorphine exposure. N Engl J Med 2010;363(24):2320–31.
29. Franck LS, Harris SK, Soetenga DJ, et al. The Withdrawal Assessment Tool-1 (WAT-1): an assessment instrument for monitoring opioid and benzodiazepine withdrawal symptoms in pediatric patients. Pediatr Crit Care Med 2008;9(6): 573–80.
30. Franck LS, Scoppettuolo LA, Wypij D, et al. Validity and generalizability of the Withdrawal Assessment Tool-1 (WAT-1) for monitoring iatrogenic withdrawal syndrome in pediatric patients. Pain 2012;153(1):142–8.
31. Ista E, van Dijk M, de Hoog M, et al. Construction of the Sophia Observation withdrawal Symptoms-scale (SOS) for critically ill children. Intensive Care Med 2009;35(6):1075–81.
32. Heil SH, Gaalema DE, Johnston AM, et al. Infant pupillary response to methadone administration during treatment for neonatal abstinence syndrome: a feasibility study. Drug Alcohol Depend 2012;126(1–2):268–71.
33. Jordan AE, Jackson GL, Deardorff D, et al. Serotonin reuptake inhibitor use in pregnancy and the neonatal behavioral syndrome. J Matern Fetal Neonatal Med 2008;21(10):745–51.
34. Langenfeld S, Birkenfeld L, Herkenrath P, et al. Therapy of the neonatal abstinence syndrome with tincture of opium or morphine drops. Drug Alcohol Depend 2005;77(1):31–6.
35. Velez M, Jansson LM. The opioid dependent mother and newborn dyad: nonpharmacologic care. J Addict Med 2008;2(3):113–20.
36. Shephard R, Greenough A, Johnson K, et al. Hyperphagia, weight gain and neonatal drug withdrawal. Acta Paediatr 2002;91(9):951–3.
37. McQueen KA, Murphy-Oikonen J, Gerlach K, et al. The impact of infant feeding method on neonatal abstinence scores of methadone-exposed infants. Adv Neonatal Care 2011;11(4):282–90.
38. Ito S. Drug therapy for breast-feeding women. N Engl J Med 2000;343(2): 118–26.
39. Bogen DL, Perel JM, Helsel JC, et al. Estimated infant exposure to enantiomer-specific methadone levels in breastmilk. Breastfeed Med 2011;6(6):377–84.
40. Wachman EM, Byun J, Philipp BL. Breastfeeding rates among mothers of infants with neonatal abstinence syndrome. Breastfeed Med 2010;5(4):159–64.

41. Arlettaz R, Kashiwagi M, Das-Kundu S, et al. Methadone maintenance program in pregnancy in a Swiss perinatal center (II): neonatal outcome and social resources. Acta Obstet Gynecol Scand 2005;84(2):145–50.

42. Dryden C, Young D, Campbell N, et al. Postnatal weight loss in substitute methadone-exposed infants: implications for the management of breast feeding. Archives of disease in childhood. Arch Dis Child Fetal Neonatal Ed 2012;97(3):F214–6.

43. Lainwala S, Brown ER, Weinschenk NP, et al. A retrospective study of length of hospital stay in infants treated for neonatal abstinence syndrome with methadone versus oral morphine preparations. Adv Neonatal Care 2005;5(5):265–72.

44. Kraft WK, van den Anker JN. Pharmacologic management of the opioid neonatal abstinence syndrome. Pediatr Clin North Am 2012;59(5):1147–65.

45. Kraft WK, Dysart K, Greenspan JS, et al. Revised dose schema of sublingual buprenorphine in the treatment of the neonatal opioid abstinence syndrome. Addiction 2011;106(3):574–80.

46. Osborn DA, Jeffery HE, Cole MJ. Sedatives for opiate withdrawal in newborn infants. Cochrane Database Syst Rev 2005;(3):CD002053.

47. Sarkar S, Donn SM. Management of neonatal abstinence syndrome in neonatal intensive care units: a national survey. J Perinatol 2006;26(1):15–7.

48. Coyle MG, Ferguson A, Lagasse L, et al. Diluted tincture of opium (DTO) and phenobarbital versus DTO alone for neonatal opiate withdrawal in term infants. J Pediatr 2002;140(5):561–4.

49. Raol Y, Zhang G, Budreck E, et al. Long-term effects of diazepam and phenobarbital treatment during development on GABA receptors, transporters and glutamic acid decarboxylase. Neuroscience 2005;132(2):399–407.

50. Agthe AG, Kim GR, Mathias KB, et al. Clonidine as an adjunct therapy to opioids for neonatal abstinence syndrome: a randomized, controlled trial. Pediatrics 2009;123(5):e849–56.

51. Hoder EL, Leckman JF, Ehrenkranz R, et al. Clonidine in neonatal narcotic-abstinence syndrome. N Engl J Med 1981;305(21):1284.

52. Leikin JB, Mackendrick WP, Maloney GE, et al. Use of clonidine in the prevention and management of neonatal abstinence syndrome. Clin Toxicol 2009;47(6):551–5.

53. O'Mara K, Gal P, Davanzo C. Treatment of neonatal withdrawal with clonidine after long-term, high-dose maternal use of tramadol. Ann Pharmacother 2010;44(7–8):1342–4.

54. McLemore GL, Lewis T, Jones CH, et al. Novel pharmacotherapeutic strategies for treatment of opioid-induced neonatal abstinence syndrome. Semin Fetal Neonatal Med 2013;18(1):35–41.

55. Bot P, Semmekrot BA, van der Stappen J. Neonatal effects of exposure to selective serotonin reuptake inhibitors during pregnancy. Archives of disease in childhood. Arch Dis Child Fetal Neonatal Ed 2006;91(2):F153.

56. Zimmermann-Baer U, Notzli U, Rentsch K, et al. Finnegan neonatal abstinence scoring system: normal values for first 3 days and weeks 5-6 in non-addicted infants. Addiction 2010;105(3):524–8.

Regional Anesthesia in Neonates and Infants

Adrian Bosenberg, MB, ChB, FFA(SA)[a], Randall P. Flick, MD, MPH[b],*

KEYWORDS

- Neonatal care • Regional anesthesia • Ultrasound • Epidural anesthesia
- Caudal block • Brachial plexus blockade • Femoral nerve blockade
- Sciatic nerve blockade

KEY POINTS

- The economic benefits of regional anesthesia include reduction in the anesthetic costs, fewer days in the neonatal intensive care, earlier discharge, and more efficient use of the floor nurse's time.
- Although the benefits of regional anesthesia are significant, safety should remain our primary concern.
- Although most regional anesthetic techniques are simple to perform, they should never be considered routine because of the potential risks involved.
- Continuous infusions and nerve blocks have limited duration; it is prudent to plan subsequent analgesia as part of a multimodal approach.
- Epidural anesthesia should be performed by, or under the guidance of, an experienced practitioner.

INTRODUCTION

Elimination of pain, especially procedural pain, should be the goal of all care providers.[1] Effective pain relief is not only humane but may play a role in the surgical outcome. Pain accompanies major neonatal surgery, which invariably needs to be performed within the first few days of life, a time when critical physiologic transitions are taking place. The challenge is to provide safe and effective analgesia.[1,2] Traditionally, morphine or other opiates are used for pain management; but to completely eliminate pain, ventilatory support and close monitoring in a neonatal intensive care unit (NICU) or similar high-care unit is usually mandated.

Disclosure Statement.

[a] Department of Anesthesiology and Pain Management, Faculty Health Sciences, Seattle Children's Hospital, University Washington, 4800 Sandpoint Way Northeast, Seattle, WA 98105, USA; [b] Anesthesiology and Pediatrics, Mayo Clinic Children's Center, Mayo Clinic, 200 First Street Southwest, Rochester, MN 55905, USA
* Corresponding author.
E-mail address: flick.randall@mayo.edu

Clin Perinatol 40 (2013) 525–538
http://dx.doi.org/10.1016/j.clp.2013.05.011   perinatology.theclinics.com
0095-5108/13/$ – see front matter © 2013 Elsevier Inc. All rights reserved.

Regional anesthesia (the percutaneous introduction of local anesthetics adjacent to a central or peripheral nerve to reduce or eliminate the sensation of pain from a region of the body) was first performed by August Bier[3] before the turn of the previous century. Spinal anesthesia was introduced into the anesthetic care of neonates and infants in 1901 by Bainbridge[4] and was considered the standard of care for lower extremity procedures for at least the next 50 years because general anesthesia for this age group was thought to be unsafe.

Although technically challenging in neonates, proponents of regional anesthesia cite superior pain relief as sufficient evidence to justify its use in this age group.[1] Regional anesthesia has significant benefits and comes closest to achieving the goal of complete analgesia in both ventilated and spontaneously breathing neonates.[1,2,5-7] Most regional blocks are placed under general anesthesia to ensure an immobile patient. Major surgery requires general anesthesia, and regional blockade can be used to reduce the amount of anesthetic needed. The residual effects of general anesthesia can, thus, be reduced.[5-9] In certain situations, spinals,[10] epidurals,[9,11] caudal catheters,[12] and peripheral nerve blocks[13,14] can be performed in awake neonates for procedures (chest drain, peripherally inserted central catheter [PICC] line) or minor surgery (inguinal hernia, circumcision, anoplasty).

The advancement in ultrasound technology has facilitated the placement of nerve blocks in children of all ages.[9] A lack of ossification in the vertebral column of neonates also allows the spinal cord anatomy to be evaluated before neuraxial blockade. The placement of local anesthetic around the relevant peripheral nerve under direct vision allows smaller doses to be used.

DETRIMENTAL EFFECTS OF SURGICALLY INDUCED PAIN

Surgery produces a spectrum of autonomic, hormonal, metabolic, immunologic, and inflammatory effects and neurobehavioral consequences, although pain itself has several deleterious effects on the developing neonate. In the late 1980s, Anand and colleagues[15] first demonstrated that neonates, including premature infants, have the ability to mount a hormonal and metabolic stress response to surgery. The stress response varies in direct proportion to the surgical stimulus[2,16] and is even present after minor surgery. Extreme catecholamine responses seem to be associated with the worst outcomes.[2,7,16] Inhibition of the stress response, therefore, seems logical. Evidence suggests that regional anesthesia inhibits the hormonal stress response more effectively than opiates.[17,18]

Acute pain has negative physiologic consequences.[19-24] These consequences include impaired ventilation and vasoconstriction of both systemic and pulmonary vascular beds leading to compromised organ function. In addition, neonates, particularly preterm neonates, exposed to noxious stimuli are at greatest risk of future neurodevelopmental impairment and altered pain sensitivity.[19-21,23,24] Long-term effects include emotional, behavioral, and learning disabilities.[19]

DETRIMENTAL EFFECTS OF OPIATE ANALGESIA

Continuous opiate infusions, although widely used, carry a risk of respiratory depression and other significant side effects that have an impact clinically. These side effects include sedation, hypotension, pruritus, nausea, vomiting, and constipation. Nausea, vomiting, and pruritus are difficult to assess in neonates and preterm infants but may be expressed as irritability, being fussy, and unsettled. Excessive sedation, in addition to the residual effects of general anesthesia, may also contribute to increased morbidity and mortality.[25,26] Paradoxically, opiates can also induce hyperalgesia leading to clinical tolerance. This tolerance is primarily the consequence of desensitization of the opiate receptors and upregulation of cAMP that requires increasing doses or additional drugs to achieve the same effect (ie, adequate analgesia).[27,28] Clinically, opiate tolerance must be differentiated from worsening pain or opiate-induced hyperalgesia.[29]

The incidence of opiate tolerance in the pediatric intensive care unit is high (35%–57%).[30–32] More disturbingly perhaps, neonates may have significant withdrawal symptoms after as little as 5 days of continuous morphine infusions.[30] Infants in early stages of development show greater vulnerability because opiate therapy may produce long-term opiate tolerance. Indirect evidence has suggested that tolerance develops earlier in preterm neonates because they, with immature hepatic enzymes, metabolize morphine to morphine-3-glucuronide (M3G). M3G has a longer half-life than morphine and accumulates to antagonize the effect of morphine.[28,30–32]

Regional anesthesia is, thus, a viable alternative and has been recommended for analgesia in neonates when possible.[1,5–9] Opinion remains divided though, not with regard to efficacy of regional anesthesia but more with the ability to safely perform regional anesthesia in newborns.[8,33–37]

BENEFICIAL EFFECTS OF REGIONAL ANESTHESIA

Neonates, particularly preterm infants, carry the greatest risk under general anesthesia given their immature organ systems (cardiovascular, central nervous, respiratory, metabolic) that are sensitive to the depressant effects of anesthetic agents. Neonatal myocardial function is particularly sensitive to both inhaled and intravenous anesthetics. When combined with general anesthesia, regional anesthesia provides profound analgesia with minimal hemodynamic effects,[38] even in the presence of comorbidities (eg, congenital heart disease, cyanotic or acyanotic, respiratory).[5,35–37] A successful regional anesthetic allows lower concentrations of inhalational agents,[1,34–37] thereby attenuating the severity of cardiovascular and respiratory depression[5] and facilitating a faster recovery. Inhalational agents have a reciprocal protective effect in that they raise the threshold of local anesthetic toxicity.[39]

Over the past decade, concerns have been raised regarding the possible detrimental effects of anesthetic agents on the developing brain. Many studies have found accelerated neuronal apoptosis with long-term cognitive and learning defects in newborn rodent and nonhuman primate models after exposure to general anesthetics.[40–57] In particular, those that interact with N-methyl-d-aspartate and γ-aminobutyric acid receptors,[40,45,50,57] such as ketamine,[44,50,54,55] propofol,[46] midazolam,[50,57] sevoflurane,[40] isoflurane,[51] morphine,[53] or nitrous oxide, have been implicated. The mechanism for anesthesia-induced apoptosis is still not entirely clear, and translating animal data to humans is very difficult. In theory, regional anesthesia alone[52] may avoid or, when used in combination with anesthesia, reduce the risk of neurotoxicity associated with general anesthetics.[37,52,57–61]

Regional anesthesia also reduces the need for muscle relaxants by providing motor blockade. Neuraxial blockade, thus, facilitates the reduction of gastroschisis,[35,62] omphalocele, and diaphragmatic hernia[35,63] by providing analgesia as well as relaxation of the abdominal musculature independent of the mode of ventilation.[5–7,33,35–37,62–65] Caudal blocks also provide muscle relaxation and have been used to reduce incarcerated inguinal hernia before definitive surgery.[66]

Neuraxial anesthesia may stimulate respiration and alter respiratory mechanics.[67,68] The effect of neuraxial blockade on ventilation depends on the level and intensity of the block, depending on the clinical situation. Neuraxial blockade may diminish abdominal and intercostal muscle activity, particularly in the compliant chest wall of neonates. On the other hand, it may improve diaphragmatic activity and excursion, thus, offsetting a loss of accessory muscle function.[36–38] The ventilatory response to carbon dioxide is also improved, resulting in more efficient ventilation and maintenance of normocarbia.[67–70] The pain relief provided by epidural analgesia improves ventilatory mechanics[37,62,68] and reduces the need for and duration of assisted or controlled ventilation after major abdominal or thoracic surgery.[6,64,65,69] As a consequence, ventilator-associated morbidity and mortality is reduced.[64,65,69]

Regional anesthesia may have salutary effects on gastrointestinal function. It enhances the early return of gastrointestinal motility,[33,59,68,71,72] particularly after gastroschisis repair.[62] In necrotizing enterocolitis, the vasodilatory effects of autonomic blockade may improve splanchnic perfusion.[34,39,73] Opiates increase intestinal smooth muscle tone that increases the risk of anastomotic leaks.[33] Lastly, oral feeding may resume earlier and speed recovery after minor surgery in the presence of a regional block.[5,10,37,39,58,59]

The immunosuppressive effect of regional anesthesia is attenuated compared with that reported with opiates.[67,71,74] Local anesthetics, but not opiates, stimulate natural killer cells that play an important role in nonspecific cellular-mediated and antitumor immunity.[71,72,74,75] Local anesthetics (bupivacaine) also confer antimicrobial activity and inhibit bacterial growth.[71]

RISKS ASSOCIATED WITH REGIONAL ANESTHESIA IN NEONATES

Opinions remain divided not on the efficacy of regional anesthesia but with the ability to safely perform regional anesthesia in neonates.[6,33,76] Some consider the risks too great for routine use by individuals who do not have the requisite expertise.[6,76] Although the risks associated with opioid and epidural analgesia in children are similar,[25,77] the risks associated with epidural analgesia and peripheral nerve blocks in neonates are less clear. The number of neonates in published surveys from the United Kingdom, Europe, Asia, and the United States are relatively small compared with children and adults.[77–89] The aggregate of published series from approximately 99 institutions yielded only one serious complication, meningitis, in the 2558 published cases.[6] The Pediatric Regional Anesthesia Network database (PRAN) has tracked outcomes of nearly 15 000 regional blocks in children from 14 large children's hospitals since 2007. Although the numbers of procedures among neonates was relatively small, there was no mortality or significant morbidity observed (**Fig. 1**).

Most of the complications, as rare as they are, occur early at the end of the needle (ie, when the anesthesiologist is still present). For example, the risk of a dural puncture is approximately 1 out of 250 and convulsions 1 out of 1250 in neonates.[6] Every effort should be made to eliminate drug errors, a feature in the UK audit.[77] Anecdotal reports of spinal cord injuries bare testimony that unfortunate disasters can occur.[61,90–92] It is generally recommended that neonatal epidurals should only be performed by those with the technical expertise despite the advent of ultrasound.[10,76]

Complications that may be observed in the NICU following placement of a regional block are even less common than those occurring at the time of placement but do occasionally occur and warrant brief discussion. Most of these complications occur in neonates that have an indwelling catheter infusing either local anesthetic alone or, in some cases, local anesthetic and a narcotic. In this setting, the complications of particular importance to the neonatologist include infection including epidural, anesthetic toxicity, bleeding/hematoma with compression or compartment syndrome, and evidence of direct nerve injury.

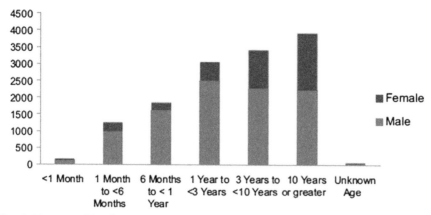

Fig. 1. Demographics for 13 725 patients in the PRAN database. (*From* Polaner DM, Taenzer AH, Walker BJ, et al. Pediatric Regional Anesthesia Network [PRAN]: a multi-institutional study of the use and incidence of complications of pediatric regional anesthesia. Anesth Analg 2012;115:1353–64; with permission.)

As previously mentioned, infection related to the placement of an indwelling catheter (typically epidural) occurs at a low rate but is potentially devastating if allowed to progress to include the neuraxia. For this reason, catheters (unless tunneled) should be removed within 72 hours of placement, whenever there is evidence of infection (fever, erythema at the insertion site) or if visibly soiled. Maintaining caudally placed epidural catheters in diapered children can be problematic and is the most common reason for premature removal of a catheter. Catheter tip colonization occurs in approximately 20% of caudal catheters, whereas it is seen in only 4% of catheters placed from the lumbar approach.[93] It is important to note that in no case in this series was colonization associated with infection.

Neonates are at a particular risk for local anesthetic toxicity because the serum free (active) fraction of local anesthetic agents is proportionately greater in neonates and young infants than older children and adults. As a consequence, the dose of anesthetic agent should be reduced to minimize the risk. Most institutions continue to use dilute bupivacaine in continuous local anesthetic infusions, although some groups use agents that are thought by some to be safer, including lidocaine, ropivacaine, or levobupivacaine, because they have less associated cardiotoxicity.

Local anesthetic overdose typically manifest in either neurotoxicity (seizures) or cardiotoxicity (malignant ventricular dysrhythmia). The former is typically short lived and without long-term sequelae. The latter, however, is a potential source of major morbidity or mortality. Because the neonatologist is likely to be called on to treat this very rare complication should it occur in the postoperative period, it is important to provide an algorithm for acute management (**Box 1**).

SPECIFIC INDICATIONS FOR REGIONAL ANESTHESIA

Spinal anesthesia was reintroduced into pediatric anesthesia in the mid-1980s in an effort to reduce the respiratory complications, especially apnea, after minor surgery in preterm and ex-preterm infants. The impact on the outcomes from anesthesia was significant.[37–39] As a result, spinal anesthesia and, more recently, caudal epidural analgesia have been advocated for high-risk neonates at risk for perioperative apnea after inguinal surgery.[5,58,77] The ex-premature infants of today differ from those of the

> **Box 1**
> **Acute management of local anesthetic toxicity**
>
> Ensure an adequate airway. Provide ventilation and supplemental oxygen as required, recognizing that acidosis may worsen toxicity.
>
> Institute cardiopulmonary resuscitation as indicated.
>
> Consider the use of intralipid 20% 1.0 to 1.5 mL/kg over 1 minute.
>
> Repeat every 3 to 5 minutes up to a total of 3 mL/kg.
>
> If successful, initiate 20% intralipid infusion at a rate of 0.25 to 0.5 mL/kg/min.
>
> Propofol should not be used as a source of lipid emulsion in this setting.

1980s. Improvements in neonatal intensive care and ventilation strategies as well as the introduction of surfactant have reduced the incidence and severity of bronchopulmonary dysplasia. A Cochrane analysis[58] investigating the perioperative risk of apnea in preterm infants anesthetized with the current inhalational agents (sevoflurane, desflurane) and remifentanil or receiving regional anesthesia for inguinal hernia surgery failed to establish the superiority of one technique over the other.[58,59]

Spinal anesthesia has been used alone or in combination with an epidural for a wide variety of surgeries, including inguinal hernia repair,[86] patent ductus arteriosus (PDA) ligation,[69] pyloromyotomy,[34] gastrostomy, gastroschisis,[62] omphalocele, bladder extrophy[88] exploratory laparotomy, lower abdominal surgery (colostomy, anoplasty, rectal biopsy, circumcision), meningomyelocele repair, and orthopedic surgery.[6–8,35,37,64,69,87]

Epidural anesthesia lumbar epidural can be used for lower abdominal, pelvic, and lower limb surgery, whereas thoracic epidural is indicated for upper abdominal or thoracic surgery.[35,37] Few dermatomes are involved in the transverse abdominal incision favored by pediatric surgeons and, thus, is easily covered by an accurately placed epidural. Epidural placement is usually performed in an anesthetized child, although it can also be performed with sedation[34] or after initial spinal blockade when indicated.[11] By far the greatest experience in epidural blockade in neonates has been gained through the use of the caudal approach to the epidural space. The caudal block remains the most frequently used regional anesthetic not only in neonates but also in children of all ages. Caudal blockade may be achieved with a single injection (**Fig. 2**) or may include placement of a catheter that may safely be left in place for up to 72 hours when infectious risk has been shown to increase. **Fig. 3** shows the frequency of catheter placement in neonates among all epidural blocks contained within the PRAN database.[80] The advantage of this approach is the ability to advance a catheter to any level (sacral, lumbar, thoracic) with a high degree of safety and certainty. Direct placement of an epidural catheter at the thoracic level poses a risk to the spinal cord and, therefore, should only be performed by experienced providers familiar with epidurals in neonates (**Fig. 4**).

Peripheral nerve blocks can be performed in neonates[94–100] to provide analgesia after surgery or for sympathetic blockade as part of the management of vascular complications associated with arterial or umbilical line placement.[94,99–102] Peripheral nerves in neonates are less myelinated; therefore, lower local anesthetic concentrations can be used successfully. For practical purposes, 0.1 to 0.2 mL/kg is sufficient to block most peripheral nerves.

Axillary or infraclavicular brachial blocks can facilitate PICC line placement[13,14] or limb salvage after arterial cannulation misadventures by vasodilating the vessel or

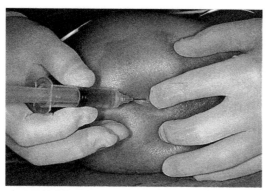

Fig. 2. Placement of a single-shot epidural regional block from the caudal approach in a neonate for a repair of hypospadias.

overcoming the vessel spasm.[94,99,101,102] Higher concentrations speed the onset and provide motor block that is useful for PICC line placement in awake neonates.[14] Femoral nerve blocks have also been used for PICC line placement in the lower limbs, for muscle biopsy,[97] skin graft, and clubfoot repair in infants.[96] This block is relatively free of complications, but the shallow joint capsule of the hip deep to the artery may be entered. Caudal block is a useful alternative for these procedures.

Paravertebral blocks are an alternative to epidural blockade for pain relief following thoracotomy both in the NICU or the operating room. Extrapleural paravertebral

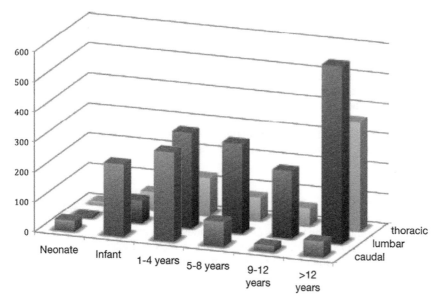

Fig. 3. A comparison of the age and site of insertion for all epidural catheter placements among patients included in the PRAN database. No mortality or persistent morbidity was observed for any child of any age (n = 6210). (*From* Polaner DM, Taenzer AH, Walker BJ, et al. Pediatric Regional Anesthesia Network [PRAN]: a multi-institutional study of the use and incidence of complications of pediatric regional anesthesia. Anesth Analg 2012;115:1353–64; with permission.)

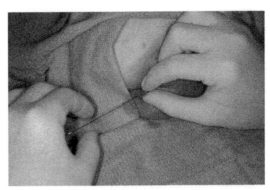

Fig. 4. Advancement of an epidural catheter from the caudal approach using an 18-gauge intravenous catheter as an introducer. The catheter tip was positioned at a low thoracic level to provide intraoperative and postoperative analgesia for a neonate undergoing resection of a thoracic mass.

catheter placement by the surgeon under direct vision immediately before chest closure has been described. Direct paravertebral placement of a catheter for continuous paravertebral blockade without ultrasound guidance is technically difficult in neonates.[103,104] Intercostal blocks can also be used for thoracotomy pain (eg, PDA ligation) or for chest tube placement.

Transabdominal plane block is becoming increasingly popular[105–108] as an alternative to epidural analgesia for intraoperative and early postoperative analgesia for selected upper (ileostomy closure)[105] or midabdominal procedures (colostomy)[106–108] involving the abdominal wall. The muscle layers are thin and compliant; the risk of penetrating the peritoneal cavity, liver, or spleen is significant if the needle is not advanced with caution.

During the past 2 decades, a substantial increase both in number and type of topical anesthetics has occurred.[109,110] Options for the prevention of neonatal pain associated with skin-breaking procedures were previously limited to injections of lidocaine. Topical anesthetics are now available as creams, gels, and a heat-activated patch system.[110] The onset time varies for each modality, and careful planning is needed to coincide with the peak effect. Indications include peripheral intravenous placement, lumbar puncture, circumcision, and heel sticks.

SUMMARY

The economic benefits of regional anesthesia include reduction in the anesthetic costs, fewer days in the NICU, earlier discharge, and more efficient use of the floor nurse's time. Although the benefits of regional anesthesia are significant, safety should remain our primary concern. However, to realize these benefits, the staff must be trained to care for neonates with epidural infusions and other regional blocks.

Although most regional anesthetic techniques are simple to perform, they should never be considered routine because of the potential risks involved.[6,111,112] Careful consideration of the indications and contraindications are warranted. Continuous infusions and nerve blocks have limited duration. It is prudent to plan subsequent analgesia as part of a multimodal approach.[1,2,111,112] In general, the more peripheral the block, the lower the risk. Epidural anesthesia should be performed by or under the guidance of an experienced practitioner.

REFERENCES

1. American Academy of Pediatrics Committee on Fetus and Newborn, American Academy of Pediatrics Section on Surgery, Canadian Paediatric Society Fetus and Newborn Committee, Batton DG, Barrington KJ, Wallman C. Prevention and management of pain in neonates: an update AAP and Canadian Pediatric Society. Pediatrics 2006;118:2231–4 Re-affirmed May 2010.
2. Berde CB, Jaksic T, Lynn AM, et al. Anesthesia and analgesia during and after surgery in neonates. Clin Ther 2005;27:900–21.
3. Bier A. Versuche uber cocainisirung des ruckenmarkes (Experiments on the cocainization of the spinal cord). Deutsche Zeitschrift fur Chirurgie 1899;51: 361–9 [in German].
4. Bainbridge WS. A report of twelve operations on infants and young children during spinal anesthesia. Arch, Pediatr 1901;18:570–4.
5. Moriarty A. In praise of the epidural space. Paediatr Anaesth 2002;12:836–7.
6. Bösenberg AT, Jöhr M, Wolf AR. Pro con debate: the use of regional vs systemic analgesia for neonatal surgery. Paediatr Anaesth 2011;21(12):1247–58.
7. Lönnqvist PA. Regional anaesthesia and analgesia in the neonate. Best Pract Res Clin Anaesthesiol 2010;24:309–21.
8. Bosenberg AT, Bland BA, Schulte-Steinberg O, et al. Thoracic epidural via the caudal route in infants. Anesthesiology 1988;69:265–9.
9. Willschke H, Bösenberg A, Marhofer P, et al. Epidural catheter placement in neonates: sonoanatomy and feasibility of ultrasonographic guidance in term and preterm neonates. Reg Anesth Pain Med 2007;32:34–40.
10. Williams RK, Adams DC, Aladjem EV, et al. The safety and efficacy of spinal anesthesia for surgery in infants: Vermont infant spinal registry. Anesth Analg 2006;102:67–71.
11. Somri M, Tome R, Yanovski B, et al. Combined spinal-epidural anesthesia in major abdominal surgery in high-risk neonates and infants. Paediatr Anaesth 2007;17:1059–65.
12. Peutrell JM, Hughes DG. Epidural anaesthesia through caudal catheters for inguinal herniotomies in awake ex-premature babies. Anaesthesia 1993;48: 128–31.
13. Messeri A, Calamandrei M. Percutaneous central venous catheterization in small infants: axillary block can facilitate the insertion rate. Paediatr Anaesth 2000;10(5):527–30.
14. Keech K, Bosenberg A. Axillary block for PICC lines in critically ill neonates. Abstract. Society Pediatric Anesthesia (SPA) Annual meeting. San Antonio, 2010.
15. Anand KJ, Sippell WG, Aynsley-Green A. Randomised trial of fentanyl anaesthesia in preterm babies undergoing surgery: effects on the stress response. Lancet 1987;1:62–6.
16. Barker DP, Rutter N. Stress severity illness and outcome in ventilated preterm infants. Arch Dis Child 1996;75:F187–90.
17. Wolf AR, Doyle E, Thomas E. Modifying the stress responses to major surgery: spinal vs extradural vs opioid analgesia. Paediatr Anaesth 1998;8:305–11.
18. Humphreys N, Bays S, Parry AJ, et al. Spinal anesthesia with an indwelling catheter reduces the stress response in pediatric open-heart surgery. Anesthesiology 2005;103:1113–20.
19. Taddio A, Katz J. The effects of early pain experience in neonates on pain responses in infancy and childhood. Paediatr Drugs 2005;7:245–57.

20. Brennan TJ. Incisional sensitivity and pain measurements: dissecting mechanisms for postoperative pain. Anesthesiology 2005;103:3–4.
21. Bouza H. The impact of pain in the immature brain. J Matern Fetal Neonatal Med 2009;22:722–32.
22. Peters CM, Eisenach JC. Contribution of the chemokine (C-C motif) ligand 2 (CCL2) to mechanical hypersensitivity after surgical incision in rats. Anesthesiology 2010;112:1250–8.
23. Walker SM, Tochiki KK, Fitzgerald M. Hindpaw incision in early life increases the hyperalgesic response to repeat surgical injury: critical period and dependence on the initial afferent activity. Pain 2009;147:99–106.
24. Fitzgerald M. The development of nociceptive circuits. Nat Rev Neurosci 2005; 6:507–20.
25. Morton NS, Errera A. APA national audit of pediatric opioid infusions. Paediatr Anaesth 2010;20:119–25.
26. Dahan A, Aarts L, Smith TW. Incidence, reversal and prevention of opioid induced respiratory depression. Anesthesiology 2010;112:226–38.
27. Anand KJ, Willson DF, Berger J, et al. Tolerance and withdrawal from prolonged opioid use in critically ill children. Pediatrics 2010;125:e1208–25.
28. Suresh S, Anand KJ. Opioid tolerance in neonates: a state-of-the-art review. Paediatr Anaesth 2001;11:511–21.
29. Colvin LA, Fallon MT. Opioid-induced hyperalgesia: a clinical challenge. Br J Anaesth 2010;104:125–7.
30. Anand KJ, Hall RW, Desai N, et al. Effects of morphine analgesia in ventilated preterm neonates: primary outcomes from the NEOPAIN randomised trial. Lancet 2004;363(9422):1673–82.
31. Bouwmeester NJ, Hop WC, van Dijk M, et al. Postoperative pain in the neonate: age-related differences in morphine requirements and metabolism. Intensive Care Med 2003;29:2009–15.
32. Menon G, Boyle EM, Bergqvist LL, et al. Morphine analgesia and gastrointestinal morbidity in preterm infants: secondary results from the NEOPAIN trial. Arch Dis Child Fetal Neonatal Ed 2008;93:F362–7.
33. Jöhr M, Berger TM. Regional anaesthetic techniques for neonatal surgery: indications and selection of techniques. Best Pract Res Clin Anaesthesiol 2004;18: 357–75.
34. Willschke H, Machata AM, Rebhandl W, et al. Management of hypertrophic pyloric stenosis with ultrasound guided single shot epidural anesthesia – a retrospective analysis of 20 cases. Paediatr Anaesth 2011;21:110–5.
35. Bösenberg AT. Epidural analgesia for major neonatal surgery. Paediatr Anaesth 1998;8:479–83.
36. Murrell D, Gibson PR, Cohen RC. Continuous epidural analgesia in newborn infants undergoing major surgery. J Pediatr Surg 1993;28:548–53.
37. Williams RK, McBride WJ, Abajian JC. Combined spinal and epidural anaesthesia for major abdominal surgery in infants. Can J Anaesth 1997;44:511–4.
38. Oberlander TF, Berde CB, Lam KH, et al. Infants tolerate spinal anesthesia with minimal overall autonomic changes: analysis of heart rate variability in former premature infants undergoing hernia repair. Anesth Analg 1995;80:20–7.
39. Hoehn T, Jetzek-Zader M, Blohm M, et al. Early peristalsis following epidural analgesia during abdominal surgery in an extremely low birth weight infant. Paediatr Anaesth 2007;17:176–9.
40. Istaphanous GK, Loepke AW. General anesthetics and the developing brain. Curr Opin Anaesthesiol 2009;22:368–73.

41. Sanders RD, Davidson A. Anesthetic induced neurotoxicity of the neonate: time for clinical guidelines? Paediatr Anaesth 2009;19:1141–6.

42. Perouansky M, Hemmings HC. Neurotoxicity of general anesthetics. Anesthesiology 2009;11:1365–71.

43. Wang C, Slikker W Jr. Strategies and experimental models for evaluating anesthetics: effects on the developing nervous system. Anesth Analg 2008;106: 1643–58.

44. Slikker W Jr, Zou X, Hotchkiss CE, et al. Ketamine-induced neuronal cell death in the perinatal rhesus monkey. Toxicol Sci 2007;98:145–58.

45. Davidson A, Soriano SG. Does anaesthesia harm the developing brain–evidence or speculation? Paediatr Anaesth 2004;14:199–200.

46. Cattano D, Young C, Straiko MM, et al. Subanesthetic doses of propofol induce neuroapoptosis in the infant mouse brain. Anesth Analg 2008;106:1712–4.

47. Rizzi S, Carter LB, Ori C, et al. Clinical anesthesia causes permanent damage to the fetal guinea pig brain. Brain Pathol 2008;18:198–210.

48. Bhutta AT, Anand KJ. Vulnerability of the developing brain. Neuronal mechanisms. Clin Perinatol 2002;29:357–72.

49. Lu LX, Yon J, Carter LB, et al. General anesthesia activates BDNF-dependent neuroapoptosis in the developing rat brain. Apoptosis 2006;11(9):1603–15.

50. Young C, Jevtovic-Todorovic V, Qin Y, et al. Potential of ketamine and midazolam, individually or in combination, to induce apoptotic neurodegeneration in the infant mouse brain. Br J Pharmacol 2005;146(2):189–97.

51. Johnson SA, Young C, Olney JW. Isoflurane-induced neuroapoptosis in the developing brain of nonhypoglycemic mice. J Neurosurg Anesthesiol 2008;20: 21–8.

52. Yahalom B, Athiraman U, Soriano SG, et al. Spinal anesthesia in infant rats: development of a model and assessment of neurologic outcomes. Anesthesiology 2011;114:1325–35.

53. Bajic D, Commons KG, Soriano SG. Morphine-enhanced apoptosis in selective brain regions of neonatal rats. Int J Dev Neurosci 2013;31(4):258–66.

54. Soriano SG. Neurotoxicity of ketamine: known unknowns. Crit Care Med 2012; 40(8):2518–9.

55. Liu JR, Liu Q, Li J, et al. Noxious stimulation attenuates ketamine-induced neuroapoptosis in the developing rat brain. Anesthesiology 2012;117(1):64–71.

56. McCann ME, Soriano SG. Perioperative central nervous system injury in neonates. Br J Anaesth 2012;109(Suppl 1):i60–7.

57. Soriano SG. Thinking about the neurotoxic effects of sedatives on the developing brain. Pediatr Crit Care Med 2010;11(2):306–7.

58. Craven PD, Badawi N, Henderson-Smart DJ, et al. Regional (spinal, epidural, caudal) versus general anaesthesia in preterm infants undergoing inguinal herniorrhaphy in early infancy. Cochrane Database Syst Rev 2003;(3):CD003669.

59. Gerber AC, Weiss M. Awake spinal or caudal anaesthesia in preterms for herniotomies: what is the evidence based benefit compared with general anaesthesia? Curr Opin Anaesthesiol 2003;16:315–20.

60. Sale SM, Read JA, Stoddart PA, et al. Prospective comparison of sevoflurane and desflurane in formerly premature infants undergoing inguinal herniotomy. Br J Anaesth 2006;96:774–8.

61. Henderson K, Sethna NF, Berde CB. Continuous caudal anesthesia for inguinal hernia repair in former preterm infants. J Clin Anesth 1993;5:129–33.

62. Raghavan M, Montgomerie J. Anesthetic management of gastroschisis–a review of our practice over the past 5 years. Paediatr Anaesth 2008;18:1055–9.

63. Hodgson RE, Bösenberg AT, Hadley LG. Congenital diaphragmatic hernia repair—impact of delayed surgery and epidural analgesia. S Afr J Surg 2000; 38:31–4.
64. Bösenberg AT, Hadley GP, Wiersma R. Oesophageal atresia: caudothoracic epidural anaesthesia reduces the need for postoperative ventilatory support. Pediatr Surg Int 1992;7:289–91.
65. Krishnan K, Marcus R. Epidural analgesia for tracheo-oesophageal fistula repair. Abstract. APAGBI Scientific meeting. Cardiff, 2006.
66. Brindley N, Taylor R, Brown S. Reduction of incarcerated inguinal hernia in infants using caudal epidural anaesthesia. Pediatr Surg Int 2005;21:715–7.
67. Hatch DJ, Hulse MG, Lindahl SG. Caudal analgesia in children: influence of ventilatory efficiency during halothane anaesthesia. Anaesthesia 1984;39: 873–8.
68. Von Ungern-Sternberg BS, Regli A, Frei FJ, et al. The effect of caudal block on functional residual capacity and ventilation homogeneity in healthy children. Anaesthesia 2006;61:758–63.
69. Shenkman Z, Hoppenstein D, Erez I, et al. Continuous lumbar/thoracic epidural analgesia in low-weight paediatric surgical patients: practical aspects and pitfalls. Pediatr Surg Int 2009;25:623–34.
70. Aspirot A, Pulingandla PS, Bouchard S, et al. A contemporary evaluation of surgical outcome in neonate and infants undergoing lung resection. J Pediatr Surg 2008;43:508–12.
71. Borgeat A, Aguirre J. Update on local anaesthetics. Curr Opin Anaesthesiol 2010;23:466–71.
72. Hollmann MW, Durieux ME. Local anesthetics and the inflammatory response. Anesthesiology 2000;93:858–75.
73. Udassin R, Eimerl D, Schiffman J, et al. Epidural anesthesia accelerates the recovery of post ischemic bowel motility in the rat. Anesthesiology 1994;80(4): 832–6.
74. Holmann MW, Durieux ME, Graf BM. Novel local anaesthetics and novel indications for local anaesthetics. Curr Opin Anaesthesiol 2001;14:741–9.
75. Forget P, de Kock M. Could anesthesia, analgesia and sympathetic modulation affect neoplastic recurrence after surgery? A systematic review centered over the modulation of natural killer cells activity. Ann Fr Anesth Reanim 2009;109: 1464–9.
76. Jöhr M. Regional anesthesia in newborn infants, infants and children–what prerequisites must be met? Anaesthesiol Reanim 2003;28:69–73.
77. Llewellyn N, Moriarty A. National paediatric epidural audit. Paediatr Anaesth 2007;17:520–32.
78. Giaufré E, Dalens B, Gombert A. Epidemiology and morbidity of regional anesthesia in children: a one-year prospective survey of the French-language society of pediatric anesthesiologists. Anesth Analg 1996;83:904–12.
79. Ecoffey C, Lacroix F, Giaufré E, et al. Epidemiology and morbidity of regional anesthesia in children: a follow-up one-year prospective survey of the French-Language Society of Paediatric Anaesthesiologists (ADARPEF). Paediatr Anaesth 2010;20:1061–9.
80. Polaner DM, Taenzer AH, Walker BJ, et al. Pediatric Regional Anesthesia Network (PRAN): a multi-institutional study of the use and incidence of complications of pediatric regional anesthesia. Anesth Analg 2012;115:1353–64.
81. Lacroix F. Epidemiology and morbidity of regional anaesthesia in children. Curr Opin Anaesthesiol 2008;21(3):345–9.

82. Rochette A, Dadure C, Raux O, et al. A review of pediatric regional anesthesia practice during a 17-year period in a single institution. Paediatr Anaesth 2007; 17:874–80.
83. Osaka Y, Yamashita M. Intervertebral epidural anesthesia in 2,050 infants and children using the drip and tube method. Reg Anesth Pain Med 2003;28:103–7.
84. Hasan MA, Howard RF, Lloyd-Thomas AR. Depth of epidural space in children. Anaesthesia 1994;49:1085–7.
85. Courrèges P, Lecoutre D, Poddevin F, et al. Epidural anesthesia in children under 3 months of age. Apropos of 49 cases. Cah Anesthesiol 1996;44:403–8.
86. Webster AC, McKishnie JD, Watson JT, et al. Lumbar epidural anaesthesia for inguinal hernia in low birth weight infants. Can J Anaesth 1993;40:670–5.
87. Valairucha S, Seefelder C, Houck CS. Thoracic epidural catheters placed by the caudal route in infants: the importance of radiographic confirmation. Paediatr Anaesth 2002;12:424–8.
88. Kost-Byerly S, Jackson EV, Yaster M, et al. Perioperative anesthetic and analgesic management of newborn bladder exstrophy repair. J Pediatr Urol 2008; 4:280–5.
89. Lundblad M, Lönnqvist P, Eksborg S, et al. Segmental distribution of high-volume caudal anesthesia in neonates, infants, and toddlers as assessed by ultrasonography. Paediatr Anaesth 2011;21(2):121–7.
90. Kasai T, Yaegashi K, Hirose M, et al. Spinal cord injury in a child caused by an accidental dural puncture with a single-shot thoracic epidural needle. Anesth Analg 2003;96:65–7.
91. Breschan C, Krumpholz R, Jost R, et al. Intraspinal haematoma following lumbar epidural anaesthesia in a neonate. Paediatr Anaesth 2001;11:105–8.
92. Flandin-Bléty C, Barrier G. Accidents following extradural analgesia in children. The results of a retrospective study. Paediatr Anaesth 1995;5:41–6.
93. McNeely JK, Farber NE, Rusy LM, et al. Epidural analgesia improves outcome following pediatric fundoplication. A retrospective analysis. Reg Anesth 1997; 22(1):16–23.
94. Breschan C, Kraschl R, Jost R, et al. Axillary brachial plexus block for treatment of severe forearm ischemia after arterial cannulation in an extremely low birth-weight infant. Paediatr Anaesth 2004;14:681–4.
95. Abouleish AE, Chung DH, Cohen M. Caudal anesthesia for vascular access procedures in two extremely small premature neonates. Pediatr Surg Int 2005; 21:749–51.
96. Bösenberg AT, Kimble FW. Infraorbital nerve block in neonates for cleft lip repair anatomical study and clinical application. Br J Anaesth 1995;74:506–8.
97. Sethuraman M, Neema PK, Rathod RC. Combined monitored anesthesia care and femoral nerve block for muscle biopsy in children with myopathies. Paediatr Anaesth 2008;18:691.
98. Oberndorfer U, Marhofer P, Bösenberg A, et al. Ultrasonographic guidance for sciatic and femoral nerve blocks in children. Br J Anaesth 2007;98:797–801.
99. Hack WW, Vos A, Okken A. Incidence of forearm and hand ischaemia related to radial artery cannulation in newborn infants. Intensive Care Med 1990;16:50–3.
100. Willschke H, Bosenberg A, Marhofer P, et al. Ultrasonographic-guided ilioinguinal-iliohypogastric nerve block in pediatric anesthesia: what is the optimal volume. Anesth Analg 2006;102:1680–4.
101. Lagade MR, Poppers PJ. Stellate ganglion block: a therapeutic modality for arterial insufficiency of the arm in premature infants. Anesthesiology 1984; 61(2):203–4.

102. Elias M. Continuous cervico-thoracic sympathetic ganglion block: therapeutic modality for arterial insufficiency of the arm of a neonate. Middle East J Anesthesiol 2001;16:359–63.

103. Karmakar MK, Booker PD, Franks R, et al. Continuous extrapleural paravertebral infusion of bupivacaine for post-thoracotomy analgesia in young infants. Br J Anaesth 1996;76:811–5.

104. Cheung SL, Booker PD, Franks R, et al. Serum concentrations of bupivacaine during prolonged continuous paravertebral infusion in young infants. Br J Anaesth 1997;79(1):9–13.

105. Jacobs A, Thies KC. Ultrasound-guided transversus abdominis plane block for reversal of ileostomy in a 2-kg premature neonate. Paediatr Anaesth 2009;19: 1237–8.

106. Visoiu M, Boretsky KR, Goyal G, et al. Postoperative analgesia via transversus abdominis plane (TAP) catheter for small weight children-our initial experience. Paediatr Anaesth 2012;22(3):281–4.

107. Bielsky A, Efrat R, Suresh S. Postoperative analgesia in neonates after major abdominal surgery: 'TAP' our way to success! Paediatr Anaesth 2009;19:541–2.

108. Fredrickson MJ, Seal P. Ultrasound-guided transversus abdominis plane block for neonatal abdominal surgery. Anaesth Intensive Care 2009;37:469–72.

109. Lehr VT, Taddio A. Topical anesthesia in neonates: clinical practices and practical considerations. Semin Perinatol 2007;31:323–9.

110. Yamada J, Stinson J, Lamba J, et al. A review of systematic reviews on pain interventions in hospitalized infants. Pain Res Manag 2008;13:413–20.

111. Polaner DM, Drescher J. Pediatric regional anesthesia: what is the current safety record. Paediatr Anaesth 2011;21:737–42.

112. Bösenberg A, Lönnqvist P. The potential future or just a way of trespassing the safety limits of pediatric regional anesthesia? Paediatr Anaesth 2011;21(2): 95–7.

Sedation and Analgesia to Facilitate Mechanical Ventilation

Michael E. Nemergut, MD, PhD[a,b,*], Myron Yaster, MD[c,d],
Christopher E. Colby, MD[e]

KEYWORDS

- NICU • Sedation • Analgesia • Anesthesia • Mechanical ventilation • Intubation

KEY POINTS

- Intubation and mechanical ventilation have associated physiologic changes consistent with pain and stress.
- The provision of sedatives and analgesics can mollify the stress response, improve intubation conditions, and is recommended for elective intubations.
- The prophylactic delivery of sedatives for mechanical ventilation has not been demonstrated to improve short-term neurologic outcomes in neonates.

INTRODUCTION

Historically, newborns, particularly premature infants, have been undertreated for pain, particularly pain related to the performance of procedures. In its extreme, in the past this led to newborns undergoing surgery without anesthesia. We now know from both clinical and preclinical research that newborns are, in fact, more

Disclosures: M.E.N, C.E.C: None; Myron Yaster currently serves on the Data and Safety Monitoring Board for Purdue and Endo Pharmaceuticals. Over the past 3 years, he has been both a consultant and/or a primary investigator on several clinical trials sponsored by Purdue Pharma, Endo Pharmaceuticals, Hospira, Cadence Pharmaceuticals, and AstraZeneca Pharmaceuticals. Additionally, he or a family member is a stockholder (5K) for Sucampo Pharmaceuticals, Johnson and Johnson, Cadence, and Pfizer. Current funding: Blaustein Pain Foundation and Richard J. Traystman Endowed Chair.

[a] Department of Anesthesiology, The Mayo Clinic, 200 First Street Southwest, Mary Brigh 7-252, Rochester, MN 55905, USA; [b] Department of Pediatrics and Adolescent Medicine, The Mayo Clinic, 200 First Street Southwest, Mary Brigh 7-252, Rochester, MN 55905, USA; [c] Department of Anesthesiology and Critical Care Medicine, The Johns Hopkins University, 1800 Orleans Street, Bloomberg Children's Center 6320, Baltimore, MD 21287, USA; [d] Department of Pediatrics, The Johns Hopkins University, 1800 Orleans Street, Bloomberg Children's Center 6320, Baltimore, MD 21287, USA; [e] Departments of Pediatrics and Adolescent Medicine, The Mayo Clinic, 200 First Street Southwest, Marian Hall MN-515, Rochester, MN 55905, USA
* Corresponding author. Department of Anesthesiology, The Mayo Clinic, 200 First Street Southwest, Mary Brigh 7-252, Rochester, MN 55905.
E-mail address: nemergut.michael@mayo.edu

sensitive to pain than older infants, children, and adults and that the failure to treat pain and distress is associated with short- and long-term adverse consequences. Thus, regardless of age, health care professionals have an ethical obligation to provide safe and effective pain relief to patients with ongoing pain or undergoing painful procedures. Indeed, in 2013, it would be unacceptable for a newborn to undergo surgery without anesthesia, although the current debate regarding the safety of anesthetic agents in the very young has prompted some to, once again, question the need for sedatives and analgesics for neonates.[1] Nevertheless, the decision to and methods for treating all pains and painful conditions in neonates are unclear.

Approximately one-fifth of all infants admitted to the neonatal intensive care unit (NICU) require intubation and mechanical ventilation.[2] These ubiquitous procedures are known to cause pain, distress, and sleep deprivation in older children and adults. Although intubation and mechanical ventilation are both painful, the pain they produce is quite different. Intubation and tracheal suction can be considered acute, procedure-related pain. Mechanical ventilation, on the other hand, can be considered a form of chronic pain. The goals for the use of analgesia and sedation are, therefore, also quite different. The former requires episodic intervention, the latter prolonged drug administration. These differences have a profound impact on therapeutic decision making.

WHY TREAT PAIN?

Over the past 20 years, there has been an explosion of research in this area. Although recommendations have been published in favor of routine and preemptive amelioration of neonatal pain,[3,4] there remains considerable variation in clinical practice, particularly with regard to the use of sedatives and analgesics for intubation and mechanical ventilation.[5–7] This variation is not surprising because there is little evidence to guide practitioners in the safe use of these drugs in neonates. Indeed, there are virtually no analgesics or sedatives labeled by the US Food and Drug Administration, or its European counterpart the European Medicines Agency, for use in newborns. Further, there are limited pharmacokinetic/pharmacodynamic data and little to no studies including long-term neurodevelopmental assessment of survivors of the pain experienced in the neonatal period. This, coupled with the difficulty in pain assessment and legitimate concerns about safety, has produced a therapeutic conundrum for practitioners. Furthermore, babies requiring intensive care are unable to express pain/discomfort like older children or even full-term healthy neonates and may even lack the strength to avoid painful interventions by withdrawal, making pain assessment in this population difficult. However, this does not mean that they do not experience pain. There is an overwhelming body of evidence to suggest that neonates do indeed feel pain.[8–10]

It has been well documented, in all patients capable of self-reporting, that intubation with mechanical ventilation is a significant source of discomfort for patients in the ICU.[11] Although guidelines for the provision of sedatives/analgesics have been available for adult patients from the American Society of Critical Care Medicine for more than 15 years,[12,13] similar practice parameters do not exist for the neonatal population, and considerable variation exists in this age group. One recent study evaluated the use of opioids in pediatric critical care settings.[14] This group reported tremendous variation in clinical practice across multiple age groups, including neonates, with up to a 100-fold difference in the doses of opioids used, including starting dose, average daily dose, and peak infusion rate.[14]

NEONATAL STRESS RESPONSE

Although it is incontrovertible that neonatal pain management is essential for perioperative acute pain, whether it is needed for tracheal intubation and mechanical ventilation is less clear. Circumcision in term, male neonates has historically been used as a model to study the response of neonates to both anesthetized and unanesthetized procedural pain. In response to this procedure, these patients have associated changes in vital signs,[15] serum cortisol,[16] transcutaneous partial pressure of oxygen,[15,17] and short-[18] and long-term[19] behavior changes consistent with both a pain response and implicit memory formation. As procedures become proportionately more invasive, serum concentrations of a variety of stress hormones have been repeatedly demonstrated to increase (**Table 1**).[20] These effects are ameliorated by analgesics and have been associated with improved clinical outcomes.[15,19,21] Importantly, it has been reported that the number of painful procedures experienced by neonates correlates with increased somatic complaints in later childhood, suggesting that neonatal pain may produce long-standing deficits despite the presence of explicit amnesia (**Box 1**).[22,23] Nevertheless, a recent study evaluating the treatment of procedural pain in the NICU suggests that treatment barriers remain; of the more than 40,000 painful procedures evaluated, approximately 80% were untreated.[24]

Similar effects have been described in neonates in response to acute medical illness. In preterm neonates with respiratory failure, it was found that the levels of stress hormones correlated with the degree of respiratory dysfunction and that failure to reduce these values was associated with increased mortality.[25] Mechanical ventilation has been associated with higher corticotropin levels as well as altered responses to the corticotropin-releasing hormone test; these responses are augmented in neonates requiring more invasive modes of assisted ventilation, such as high-frequency oscillatory ventilation and intermittent positive-pressure ventilation, relative to neonates requiring less invasive respiratory support, such as supplemental oxygen or continuous positive airway pressure.[26] Mechanical ventilatory support is associated with increased levels of catecholamines,[27,28] which can be significantly altered by the provision of opioids[28,29] and changing the ventilation mode to improve synchrony.[27] Together these data demonstrate the response of neonates to various forms of stress and suggest that intubation and mechanical ventilation is a significant contributor to this response. Reducing the premature and sick infants' response to intubation and mechanical ventilation requires commitment, planning, and coordination at many levels.

Tracheal intubation is associated with dramatic changes in blood pressure, heart rate, and catecholamine release, all of which have been associated with adverse

Table 1 Physiologic and endocrine response to pain in neonates	
Parameter	**Neonatal Response**
Blood pressure, heart rate, respiratory rate	Increased
Oxygen saturation	Decreased
Protein, carbohydrate, and fat mobilization	Increased
Epinephrine	Increased
Norepinephrine	Increased
Cortisol	Increased
Glucagon	Increased
Insulin	Increased (no change in preterm neonates)

Box 1
Reported consequences of undertreated pain in neonates

1. Hypertension, tachycardia, tachypnea, hypoxemia

2. Increased pain responses to future painful stimuli

3. Increased somatic pain complaints in childhood

---

outcomes. Treatment should increase the likelihood of intubation success and prevent ventilator asynchrony, thereby facilitating mechanical ventilation. On the other hand, these same drugs can cause hypotension, respiratory depression, and prolonged ventilator dependence. They may also enhance neuronal cell death, produce paradoxic hyperalgesia, induce withdrawal, and have unknown long-term effects.

PAIN ASSESSMENT

To effectively study, evaluate, and manage pain in neonates, it is necessary to develop and use widely accepted assessment tools. Although neonates cannot self-report, they can mount significant physiologic, behavioral, and hormonal responses to acute and painful surgical and medical procedures. Some of these behaviors include changes in vital signs (eg, heart/respiratory rates and blood pressure), agitated body movement, vocal responses (eg, crying), facial grimacing, and limb position. Validated scales incorporating these measures include the Neonatal Infant Pain Scale, the Premature Infant Pain Profile, and the Crying, Requires Oxygen for saturation, Increased vital signs, Expression, Sleepless tool.[30–32] How reliable these measures are in chronic neonatal painful conditions such as mechanical ventilation is unknown.[33] The most commonly used tool, the Neonatal Pain, Agitation, and Sedation Scale (N-PASS) assesses both pain and sedation numerically using 5 indicators: crying/irritability, behavior/state, facial expression, extremities/tone, and vital signs.[34] Within each category, examples of criteria are provided to assist in the assignment of a numerical value. The N-PASS can be viewed at the following Web site: www.n-pass. com.

NEONATAL TRACHEAL INTUBATION

Neonatal tracheal intubation occurs both under emergent and nonemergent circumstances. Recent position statements acknowledge the need to proceed with intubation of the trachea without premedication in emergent contexts or in neonates with airway anomalies.[35,36] However, many neonatal tracheal intubations occur nonemergently, allowing an opportunity to consider premedication. Laryngoscopy and tracheal intubation are known to be painful and to induce apnea, hypoxemia, and bradycardia while increasing systemic and intracranial pressure.[37,38] Along with the skills required to successfully intubate the trachea and mechanically ventilate neonatal patients, an evidence-based approach for drug selection is essential to optimize the quality of these procedures.

NONPHARMACOLOGIC TREATMENT

Numerous nonpharmacologic techniques have been studied for the alleviation of neonatal procedural pain. These techniques include, but are not limited to, sucrose,[39–41] skin-to-skin contact,[42] swaddling,[43] and massage.[44] These techniques have reported efficacy for the treatment of several painful procedures and are considered to be extremely safe.[45] However, their applicability has been limited to single, mild to moderately painful procedures, excluding tracheal intubation. Their utility for repeated or chronically stimulating conditions, such as mechanical ventilation, is not known; although techniques such as swaddling are widely used in mechanically ventilated neonates, their effect remains unclear.

OPIOIDS

There are few who would suggest that direct laryngoscopy and endotracheal tube placement does not cause pain and discomfort in all patients. Providing adequate analgesia for this invasive procedure is indicated to provide patient comfort, avoid hypertension, and optimize intubating conditions. The ideal analgesic would have rapid pharmacodynamics with minimal side effects. Opioids share many of these features and are commonly used to facilitate tracheal tube placement and maintenance.

Opioids act at μ receptors in the central nervous system, mimicking endogenous opioid peptides and endorphins to produce analgesia, most commonly morphine, fentanyl, and remifentanil. Administration of intravenous morphine results in peak analgesia in 15 minutes,[46] whereas clearance of morphine is gestational age dependent, with a longer half-life observed in premature infants.[47] Fentanyl has a rapid onset of action (<3 minutes) and, when given in small doses (1–2 μg/kg), a short duration of action ($\sim$60 minutes).[48] Clearance of fentanyl is also positively correlated with gestational age and birth weight.[49] Remifentanil has onset and offset times (half-life <5 minutes) even more rapid than fentanyl, and experience in the neonatal population is growing.[50–52]

N-METHYL-D-ASPARTIC ACID RECEPTOR ANTAGONISTS

The only N-methyl-D-aspartic acid (NMDA) receptor antagonist in common clinical practice is ketamine. In older children, it produces a dissociated anesthetic state with potent analgesia, amnesia, and bronchodilation. It produces minimal cardiorespiratory depression making it ideal in hemodynamically unstable patients.[53] Finally, it increases systemic vascular resistance more than pulmonary vascular resistance making it among the safest anesthetic/analgesics in patients with congenital heart disease. Nevertheless, it has several detrimental side effects, including: increased salivation (with the potential to induce laryngospasm), myoclonic jerking (which is often mistaken for convulsions), and elevation of intracranial pressure (which may have catastrophic consequences in patients with intracranial hypertension). The safety and efficacy of use in the neonatal population has not been well established.

γ-AMINOBUTYRIC ACID RECEPTOR AGONISTS

Benzodiazepines (eg, midazolam, diazepam, lorazepam), barbiturates (eg, phenobarbital, pentobarbital), and propofol are used extensively for sedation, anxiolysis, amnesia, and as anticonvulsants. All of these drugs facilitate the action of the inhibitory neurotransmitter γ-aminobutyric acid (GABA) causing neuronal inhibition. They have no analgesic properties.[54] Midazolam is the most widely used benzodiazepine to facilitate neonatal endotracheal intubation and assisted ventilation. The pharmacokinetics vary between individual neonates, and clearance seems to be positively correlated with gestational age.[55]

Phenobarbital is a barbiturate that targets GABA receptors in the central nervous system and is minimally sedating.[56] Barbiturates that have been studied for endotracheal intubation in neonates include thiopental and methohexital.[57,58] The pharmacokinetics of thiopental in neonates suggest a half-life of nearly 15 hours.[59] Unfortunately, this drug is no longer available in the United States.

Propofol is a unique agent with several mechanisms of action, including activation of GABA receptors, inhibition of NMDA receptors, modulation of slow calcium channels, and sodium channel blockade.[60,61] Pharmacokinetic studies of propofol in neonates suggest lower clearance in neonates compared with older pediatric populations. It seems that both gestational and postnatal age contribute to the variability of propofol clearance.[62]

The safety profile of propofol in pediatric patients is well documented both inside and outside the operating room.[63] Early reports of the use of propofol as an induction agent for endotracheal intubation in preterm infants suggested a reassuring safety profile.[64] However, more recent data suggest that propofol used for this indication in this population should be approached with caution because of its significant cardiovascular side effects.[65,66] The literature describing the potential adverse effects of sedative agents is extensive in older children and adults as well as in neonates (**Table 2**).[35,50,54,55,58,59,65–67]

NEUROTOXICITY

The possible neurotoxic potential of sedatives began through mechanistic studies of fetal alcohol syndrome. Exposure of developing rodents to ethanol, a known GABA-receptor agonist and NMDA-receptor antagonist, was found to induce widespread neuroapoptosis of the central nervous system.[68] These data have been reproduced in a variety of species with virtually every commonly used agent that uses these receptors, including benzodiazepines, propofol, barbiturates, and ketamine.[69,70]

Table 2 Side effects of analgesics and sedatives in neonates	
Medication	**Side Effects in Neonates**
Morphine	Respiratory depression
Fentanyl	Respiratory depression Hypotension Muscle rigidity Hypothermia
Remifentanil	Respiratory depression Muscle rigidity
Ketamine	Respiratory depression Salivation Myoclonic jerking Increased intracranial pressure
Midazolam	Respiratory depression Hypotension Decreased cerebral blood flow Exposure to benzyl alcohol
Methohexital	Twitching Hypotension
Thiopental	Hypotension Prolonged clearance
Propofol	Hypotension Respiratory depression

Neurotoxicity has been reported in neonatal nonhuman primates,[71–76] with long-term cognitive deficits.[77] Several retrospective studies have found an association between early anesthetic exposure and neurocognitive deficits in humans,[78–82] which have caused great concern among the scientific and regulatory communities. Although this subject remains an active area of research, prospective data in humans are lacking, a causal relationship remains unknown, and there are no data that dictate a change in clinical practice (**Box 2**).

VAGOLYTIC AGENTS

Vagolytic agents prevent vagal-induced bradycardia and decrease oral secretions. Atropine, an antimuscarinic agent, has been shown to be effective in preventing bradycardia during endotracheal intubation in neonates.[83,84] Glycopyrrolate has also been shown to be effective as a vagolytic in the neonatal population, which may have an added benefit in that it does not cross the blood-brain barrier and will, therefore, not induce pupillary and neurocognitive changes.[85]

ALPHA-2 ADRENERGIC RECEPTOR AGONISTS

Clonidine and dexmedetomidine are alpha-2 adrenergic receptor agonists with sedative, anxiolytic, and analgesic properties.[86] Clonidine has reported utility for ameliorating withdrawal symptoms in infants born to drug-addicted mothers and to newborns iatrogenically tolerant and dependent to opioids.[87] Dexmedetomidine is 800 times more selective than clonidine. Because of its unusual quality of providing sedation/analgesia, easy arousal, and no respiratory depression, dexmedetomidine is becoming an increasingly common sedative adjunct for critically ill patients, with reduced ventilation times and less delirium being reported in adult patients.[88,89] Although frequently used in pediatric patients, dexmedetomidine has been the subject of few randomized trials[90]; reports in the neonatal population is restricted to operative use,[91] imaging studies,[92] cardiac catheterization,[93] and case reports.[94] Although this agent has been reported to protect against the purported neurotoxic properties of sedatives/anesthetics,[95] a clear role for this agent has yet to be established by the available literature.

NEUROMUSCULAR BLOCKADE

Muscle relaxation is another component of both optimizing intubation conditions as well as eliminating ventilator dyssynchrony when common sedative strategies fail, particularly with techniques such as high-frequency oscillatory ventilation. The primary

---

Box 2
Evidence for neurotoxicity

1. Numerous commonly used sedatives induce histologic degeneration of developing rodent brains.

2. Histologic degeneration has also been reported in neonatal monkeys, with associated long-term neurobehavioral deficits.

3. Several retrospective human studies have reported an association between early anesthetic exposure and neurocognitive deficits.

4. Prospective human data are absent, and causation remains speculative.

effect is achieved by inducing paralysis of all striated skeletal muscle, thereby preventing laryngospasm and providing the laryngoscopist with an optimal view of the larynx for rapid tracheal tube placement. A secondary effect of neuromuscular blockade is a decrease in intracranial pressure, an effect that may be further enhanced by decreasing the time for tracheal tube placement (**Box 3**).[84,96] Neuromuscular blockers can be classified as nondepolarizing (mivacurium, vecuronium, and rocuronium) and depolarizing (succinylcholine). Succinylcholine is contraindicated in patients with hyperkalemia, suspected muscular dystrophy, or a family history of malignant hyperthermia.

Muscle relaxants demonstrate distinct pharmacokinetic profiles in neonates relative to adults. Succinylcholine is highly water soluble, and a higher dose is recommended for neonates given their larger volume of distribution. The nondepolarizing agents may have a longer duration of action resulting from reduced renal or hepatic function in neonates. The duration of muscle relaxants range from ultrashort (5 minutes) to long (60 minutes) (**Table 3**). Significant interpatient pharmacodynamic differences for muscle relaxation are observed in the neonatal population.[97]

CLINICAL TRIALS: GABA-RECEPTOR AGONISTS

Several studies have attempted to identify the optimal medications to improve physiologic stability and short-term outcomes during elective intubation of the trachea. Many demonstrated improved conditions when neuromuscular relaxation is combined with other analgesics in the setting of laryngoscopy and tracheal intubation.[83,98–100] Although succinylcholine has been shown to be effective, concern for its rare but potentially lethal side effects has resulted in increasing interest in the nondepolarizing agents. Studies have suggested that mivacurium is effective, although it is no longer commercially available. Rocuronium has recently been demonstrated as a safe and effective alternative.[99] Sugammadex, a new reversal agent, may soon be approved for use in the United States, allowing virtually immediate reversal of muscle relaxation induced by rocuronium.[101] Vagolytic agents improve physiologic stability during intubation, and both atropine and glycopyrrolate have been shown to be safe and effective in term and preterm infants.[84,99]

Midazolam is suboptimal for both premedication for tracheal tube placement and residence. A small, randomized double-blind study evaluated 8 patients with a total of 16 intubation attempts. One group was placebo only (n = 3), another atropine (0.01 mg/kg) plus placebo (n = 6), and the third group was atropine (0.01 mg/kg) plus midazolam (0.1 mg/kg) (n = 7). The study was terminated when infants

---

Box 3
Neuromuscular blockade

Advantages

1. Averts laryngospasm and chest-wall rigidity

2. Optimizes direct laryngoscopy independent of the induction agent

3. Precludes ventilator dyssynchrony

Precautions

1. Succinylcholine can induce fatal hyperkalemia, bradycardia, and malignant hyperthermia.

2. It is contraindicated if mask ventilation is presumed to be difficult.

3. It is not possible to fully assess comfort in the setting of neuromuscular blockade.

Table 3
Duration of action for muscle relaxants

Medication	Duration of Action
Succinylcholine	Ultrashort
Mivacurium	Short
Atracurium	Intermediate
Vecuronium	Intermediate
Rocuronium	Intermediate
Pancuronium	Long

randomized to the midazolam group had clinically significant increases in the number of desaturations requiring cardiopulmonary resuscitation.[102]

Although midazolam is a common agent to facilitate sedation for mechanical ventilation, relatively few studies have evaluated the effectiveness of this agent (**Box 4**). The largest study, the Neonatal Outcome and Prolonged Analgesia in Neonates (NOPAIN) trial, a multicenter, randomized, double-blind, placebo-controlled trial of 67 premature infants randomized to 3 groups (placebo, morphine alone, and midazolam alone), evaluated the effect of these agents on sedation, pain, and short-term neurologic outcomes.[65] Although the midazolam group exhibited lower pain scores in response to suctioning, the same group exhibited prolonged hospital stays and increased rates of poor neurologic outcomes (severe intraventricular hemorrhage [IVH], periventricular leukomalacia, or death) relative to both controls and the morphine-only group. These data were included in a recent Cochrane review on the use of midazolam for sedation in the NICU, which could only combine 2 additional studies for analysis (totaling 146 neonates) and found increased NICU length of stay when midazolam was used.[103–105] Although all studies included for review reported higher sedation scores, none of the scales used had been validated in preterm infants such that the effectiveness could not be evaluated. These investigators, therefore, found no evidence to promote the use of midazolam for sedation in the NICU, and concerns over the safety of this agent remain.

Other studies investigating the use GABA agents have included a nonblinded placebo-controlled study with thiopental (6 mg/kg) or placebo given 1 minute before laryngoscopy. The thiopental group had less vital-sign derangements and required less total time for intubation.[57] In another observational study of 18 neonates, methohexital (2.6 mg/kg) was given and patients were intubated when unresponsive to stimuli. All study participants were intubated within 2 minutes. There were no significant changes in blood pressure, although 8 out of 18 infants experienced a drop in oxygen saturation that lasted greater than 30 seconds.[58] Neither thiopental nor methohexital

Box 4
Midazolam for intubation and mechanical ventilation

1. Midazolam has been reported to decrease responses to noxious stimuli.

2. Midazolam has not been reported to improve intubation conditions when given as monotherapy.

3. Midazolam is associated with poor neurologic outcomes and prolonged hospital stays when used for sedation for mechanical ventilation.

are commonly used as a primary sedative for mechanical ventilation in neonates, and trials with these agents have yet to be reported.

CLINICAL TRIALS: OPIOIDS

Current evidence would suggest that morphine as a single agent for premedication is not effective in improving physiologic stability or intubating conditions. A randomized, double-blind, placebo-controlled trial of 34 preterm patients compared morphine (0.2 mg/kg) with placebo when laryngoscopy was attempted 5 minutes after morphine administration. In this study, there were no differences observed in physiologic stability, procedure duration, or intubation attempts. However, the interval between morphine administration and laryngoscopy may not have been sufficient to observe any clinical differences.[106]

Premedication with morphine (100 μg/kg), atropine (10 μg/kg), and succinylcholine (1 mg/kg) was compared with awake intubations in 20 neonates. The time to intubation was reduced in the treatment group by nearly 9 minutes, and the control group required twice as many attempts. Oral injury was observed in 5 of the control neonates and one in the treatment group. There was a greater decrease in heart rate in the control group, but no differences in oxygen saturation were observed.[107]

A double-blind randomized study with 20 preterm patients compared morphine (150 μg/kg) versus remifentanil (1 μg/kg), with both groups receiving midazolam (200 μg/kg). The probability of achieving excellent intubating conditions was increased 24-fold in the group who received remifentanil. No reintubation attempts were necessary in the remifentanil group, whereas 40% of patients in the morphine required a reintubation attempt. Neither chest wall rigidity nor physiologic instability was noted in either group.[108]

Further evidence against using morphine as a premedication was obtained in a study of preterm infants. Patients were randomized to undergo rapid sequence intubation (RSI) using glycopyrrolate, thiopental, succinylcholine, and remifentanil or to receive only atropine and morphine. The doses of medications in the RSI group included glycopyrrolate (5 μg/kg), thiopental (2 mg/kg if <1000 g or 3 mg/kg if ≥1000 g), succinylcholine (2 mg/kg), and remifentanil (1 μg/kg). The patients randomized to the morphine group received morphine (0.3 mg/kg) and atropine (0.01 mg/kg). The neonates receiving RSI had superior intubating conditions and a significantly shorter procedure duration. The morphine group had a prolonged heart rate decrease and mean arterial blood pressure increase during intubation, followed by lower mean arterial blood pressure 3 hours after intubation.[85] Subgroup analyses of 28 patients in the study also had ongoing blood pressure monitoring and 2-channel amplitude integrated electroencephalogram (aEEG). RSI was associated with aEEG depression lasting less than 3 hours, whereas patients from the morphine group had aEEG depression with a discontinuous background for 24 hours.[109]

To evaluate the efficacy and safety of remifentanil in comparison with fentanyl and succinylcholine, a randomized controlled trial of stable term and preterm infants was performed in 30 patients. Infants in the intervention arm received remifentanil (3 μg/kg) and the control group received fentanyl (2 μg/kg) and succinylcholine (2 mg/kg); both groups also received atropine (20 μg/kg). The median time to successful intubation was not different between groups, but the intubation conditions were rated as more favorable with fentanyl/succinylcholine. Although not statistically significant, chest wall rigidity was observed more commonly with remifentanil. The degree of oxygen saturation, heart rate, and blood pressure changes were not significantly different between the two groups.[110]

The preemptive use of morphine in mechanically ventilated neonates has been evaluated in several randomized clinical trials. Among the first to suggest clinical benefit, the NOPAIN trial reported decreased rates of periventricular leukomalacia, severe IVH, and death when morphine was prophylactically infused into mechanically ventilated premature neonates.[65] Other small, randomized controlled trials reported improved ventilator synchrony and serum stress markers in response to morphine.[28,29,111] In contrast, 2 large, placebo-controlled trials could not demonstrate the benefit of morphine for intubated neonates found in smaller trials. The Neurologic Outcomes and Preemptive Analgesia in Neonates trial was a large, multicenter, double-bind, placebo-controlled trial of 898 premature neonates randomized to either morphine or placebo.[112] All infants received open-label morphine as needed for analgesia. These investigators found no significant effect of morphine on the incidence of periventricular leukomalacia, severe intraventricular hemorrhage, or death, although patients receiving open-label morphine in both groups had a higher incidence of worse composite outcomes. Furthermore, increased episodes of hypotension were reported in morphine-treated neonates. A second study evaluated the effect of morphine on both pain relief and neurologic outcomes in 150 neonates receiving mechanical ventilation.[113] These investigators found that routine use of morphine neither improved pain scores nor influenced the incidence of poor, short-term neurologic outcomes. In addition, the 5-year follow-up of these patients demonstrated decreased intelligence-quotient scores for the infants randomized to the morphine group.[114]

Fentanyl has been used extensively in the neonatal population for more than 20 years and has been reported to offer many of the benefits of morphine, with more rapid pharmacokinetics and a potentially improved side-effect profile.[115] In single doses, fentanyl has been reported to decrease pain and physiologic stress markers in mechanically ventilated premature infants.[116] These effects have also been reported for fentanyl delivered by continuous infusion in 3 small, randomized controlled trials in intubated neonates,[117–119] with increased ventilator settings reported in one trial.[119] These data have been included in 2 meta-analyses on the use of opioids for NICU sedation.[120,121] Although both studies reported small decreases in pain scores when opioids were given prophylactically, they found insufficient evidence to recommend routine use of opioids for sedation in the NICU because no significant differences in mortality, neurodevelopmental outcomes, and duration of mechanical ventilation were found. In addition, increased times to establish full enteral feeding were reported when morphine was used in premature infants (**Box 5**).

Box 5
Opioids for intubation and mechanical ventilation

1. As a monotherapy, the effectiveness of select opioids for optimizing intubation conditions seems to be that remifentanil is the most effective, followed by fentanyl and then morphine.

2. In the setting of neuromuscular blockade, the aforementioned distinction is lost.

3. The slow onset/offset of morphine is not congruent to the stimulus of direct laryngoscopy, and prolonged hemodynamic changes have been reported.

4. Decreased stress, decreased pain, and improved ventilator synchrony have been reported in response to opioid infusions in mechanically ventilated neonates.

5. Preemptive opioid infusions are reported to increase the duration of mechanical ventilation, promote hypotension, and delay full enteral feeding but not prevent early adverse neurologic events.

Although remifentanil has been used for neonatal anesthesia for more than 10 years,[122] there are relatively few reports on its use for sedation for mechanical ventilation in neonates and only one randomized trial. Two observational studies, without a comparison group, have described the use of remifentanil for sedation in intubated neonates, which reported the drug to be both effective and safe.[123,124] One double-blind controlled study randomized 24 term neonates to receive midazolam with either fentanyl or remifentanil.[125] Although there were no significant differences in the incidence of adverse events, a shorter time to extubate was reported for the remifentanil group. Although the pharmacokinetics of remifentanil suggest promise as a sedative adjunct in the NICU, conclusions regarding its effectiveness are overtly tempered by the limited data on its use.

CLINICAL TRIALS: PROPOFOL

Although small, randomized studies of premedication with ketamine have been performed in the older pediatric population,[126] none have been published in the neonatal population. In contrast, propofol has been studied in neonates. Propofol (2.5 mg/kg) was compared with the combination of succinylcholine (2 mg/kg), morphine (0.1 mg/kg), and atropine (0.01 mg/kg) for premedication in preterm neonates. Hypnosis or muscle relaxation were achieved within 60 seconds in both groups, but the time to achieve successful intubation was more than twice as fast with propofol. Blood pressure and heart rates were not different, but intraprocedural oxygen saturations were significantly lower in infants in the morphine group. Trauma was less common and recovery time was shorter in the propofol group.[64]

In a double-blinded, randomized, controlled trial in preterm infants comparing the use of remifentanil (1 μg/kg) and propofol (2 mg/kg) with remifentanil and midazolam (200 μg/kg), no differences were observed regarding conditions for laryngoscopy or the number of attempts, suggesting that propofol could be a valid alternative to midazolam for endotracheal intubation in this population.[127]

One observational study evaluated intubation in term and preterm infants when propofol (2.0 mg/kg) or fentanyl (1.5 μg/kg) was used. More than 86% of patients were intubated successfully on the first attempt in both groups. However, in 7 out of 21 patients in the propofol group, hypotension and oxygen saturations as low as 60% were observed, which improved with mask ventilation and fluid resuscitation.[128]

Another observational study of propofol (1 mg/kg) for intubation in preterm neonates with a gestational age of 29 to 32 weeks and respiratory distress was stopped early because of cardiovascular instability. Although propofol generally offered good intubating conditions, even low propofol doses (1 mg/kg) caused a decline in mean arterial blood pressure from 38 mm Hg (range 29–42 mm Hg) before premedication to 24 mm Hg (22–40 mm Hg) 10 minutes after propofol administration.[67] Lastly, the onset of persistent fetal circulation after the administration of propofol for endotracheal intubation has been reported.[129]

At present, no randomized trials have been reported studying the use of propofol for ICU sedation in mechanically ventilated neonates. A recent Cochrane review has been published evaluating the use of propofol for procedural sedation in neonates; however, only one study was included consisting of only 63 neonates undergoing endotracheal intubation, and no practice recommendations were made.[130] Given concern for propofol-infusion syndrome (PRIS) in children and adults and that a case report of PRIS has been reported after a brief-period of propofol exposure in a premature neonate,[131] the safety of this agent has yet to be established in this age group.

SUMMARY

Although clear conclusions regarding the use of various medications for sedation in neonates cannot be drawn, the American Academy of Pediatrics Committee on Fetus and Newborn, Section on Anesthesiology and Pain Medicine has provided guidance. The section advises the use of premedication for nonurgent neonatal intubations. The use of sedatives without analgesics should be avoided, and muscle relaxants should only be given after administering an analgesic. No specific medication recommendations were given based on the available evidence.[36]

The Canadian Pediatric Society has developed a position statement with slightly different conclusions. They too recommend premedication for all nonemergent neonatal intubations, also advising that vagolytic agents be strongly considered. Rapid-acting analgesic agents should be given, suggesting that the best choice is fentanyl. Rapid-acting muscle relaxation should be considered with succinylcholine, which is currently considered to be the best choice.[35]

Nevertheless, it is apparent that best practices for pharmaceutical intervention for intubation and mechanical ventilation have not been established. The key questions that must be answered include the following:

1. Are there adverse long-term outcomes from failing to provide adequate analgesia to mechanically ventilated patients?
2. Are adverse long-term outcomes ameliorated by effective analgesia?
3. What are the long-term consequences of using analgesics and sedative hypnotics over prolonged periods of time?
4. Do combinations of analgesics and hypnotics increase or decrease short- and long-term outcomes?
5. Once these therapies are initiated, how and when do we stop?

Most studies include single-center experience with a limited number of patients; few long-term follow-up studies have been reported. Although there is consistent evidence that opioids can ameliorate physiologic and hormonal indices of stress, their provision has not reliably altered short-term clinical outcomes in mechanically ventilated neonates. Nevertheless, the relief of stress is a relevant outcome in and of itself; whether this benefit merits their inherent risk remains with the provider.

REFERENCES

1. Davidson AJ. Neurotoxicity and the need for anesthesia in the newborn: does the emperor have no clothes? Anesthesiology 2012;116(3):507–9.
2. Wilson A, Gardner MN, Armstrong MA, et al. Neonatal assisted ventilation: predictors, frequency, and duration in a mature managed care organization. Pediatrics 2000;105(4 Pt 1):822–30.
3. Prevention and management of pain and stress in the neonate. American Academy of Pediatrics. Committee on Fetus and Newborn. Committee on Drugs. Section on Anesthesiology. Section on Surgery. Canadian Paediatric Society. Fetus and Newborn Committee. Pediatrics 2000;105(2):454–61.
4. Batton DG, Barrington KJ, Wallman C. Prevention and management of pain in the neonate: an update. Pediatrics 2006;118(5):2231–41.
5. Eriksson M, Gradin M. Pain management in Swedish neonatal units–a national survey. Acta Paediatr 2008;97(7):870–4.
6. Kahn DJ, Richardson DK, Gray JE, et al. Variation among neonatal intensive care units in narcotic administration. Arch Pediatr Adolesc Med 1998;152(9):844–51.

7. Lago P, Guadagni A, Merazzi D, et al. Pain management in the neonatal intensive care unit: a national survey in Italy. Paediatr Anaesth 2005;15(11): 925–31.

8. Anand KJ. Pharmacological approaches to the management of pain in the neonatal intensive care unit. J Perinatol 2007;27(Suppl 1):S4–11.

9. Anand KJ. Consensus statement for the prevention and management of pain in the newborn. Arch Pediatr Adolesc Med 2001;155(2):173–80.

10. Anand KJ, Hickey PR. Pain and its effects in the human neonate and fetus. N Engl J Med 1987;317(21):1321–9.

11. Gelinas C, Fortier M, Viens C, et al. Pain assessment and management in critically ill intubated patients: a retrospective study. Am J Crit Care 2004;13(2): 126–35.

12. Jacobi J, Fraser GL, Coursin DB, et al. Clinical practice guidelines for the sustained use of sedatives and analgesics in the critically ill adult. Crit Care Med 2002;30(1):119–41.

13. Shapiro BA, Warren J, Egol AB, et al. Practice parameters for intravenous analgesia and sedation for adult patients in the intensive care unit: an executive summary. Society of Critical Care Medicine. Crit Care Med 1995;23(9): 1596–600.

14. Anand KJ, Clark AE, Willson DF, et al. Opioid analgesia in mechanically ventilated children: results from the multicenter measuring opioid tolerance induced by fentanyl study. Pediatr Crit Care Med 2013;14(1):27–36.

15. Williamson PS, Williamson ML. Physiologic stress reduction by a local anesthetic during newborn circumcision. Pediatrics 1983;71(1):36–40.

16. Talbert LM, Kraybill EN, Potter HD. Adrenal cortical response to circumcision in the neonate. Obstet Gynecol 1976;48(2):208–10.

17. Rawlings DJ, Miller PA, Engel RR. The effect of circumcision on transcutaneous PO2 in term infants. Am J Dis Child 1980;134(7):676–8.

18. Marshall R, Stratton W, Moore J, et al. Circumcision I: effects upon newborn behavior. Infant Behavior Development 1980;3:1–14. http://dx.doi.org/10.1016/S0163-6383(80)80003-8.

19. Taddio A, Katz J, Ilersich AL, et al. Effect of neonatal circumcision on pain response during subsequent routine vaccination. Lancet 1997;349(9052):599–603.

20. Anand KJ, Aynsley-Green A. Measuring the severity of surgical stress in newborn infants. J Pediatr Surg 1988;23(4):297–305.

21. Anand KJ, Hickey PR. Halothane-morphine compared with high-dose sufentanil for anesthesia and postoperative analgesia in neonatal cardiac surgery. N Engl J Med 1992;326(1):1–9.

22. Grunau RV, Whitfield MF, Petrie JH. Pain sensitivity and temperament in extremely low-birth-weight premature toddlers and preterm and full-term controls. Pain 1994;58(3):341–6.

23. Grunau RV, Whitfield MF, Petrie JH, et al. Early pain experience, child and family factors, as precursors of somatization: a prospective study of extremely premature and full-term children. Pain 1994;56(3):353–9.

24. Carbajal R, Rousset A, Danan C, et al. Epidemiology and treatment of painful procedures in neonates in intensive care units. JAMA 2008;300(1):60–70.

25. Barker DP, Rutter N. Stress, severity of illness, and outcome in ventilated preterm infants. Arch Dis Child Fetal Neonatal Ed 1996;75(3):F187–90.

26. Ng PC, Lam CW, Lee CH, et al. Reference ranges and factors affecting the human corticotropin-releasing hormone test in preterm, very low birth weight infants. J Clin Endocrinol Metab 2002;87(10):4621–8.

27. Quinn MW, de Boer RC, Ansari N, et al. Stress response and mode of ventilation in preterm infants. Arch Dis Child Fetal Neonatal Ed 1998;78(3):F195–8.

28. Quinn MW, Wild J, Dean HG, et al. Randomised double-blind controlled trial of effect of morphine on catecholamine concentrations in ventilated pre-term babies. Lancet 1993;342(8867):324–7.

29. Quinn MW, Otoo F, Rushforth JA, et al. Effect of morphine and pancuronium on the stress response in ventilated preterm infants. Early Hum Dev 1992;30(3): 241–8.

30. Lawrence J, Alcock D, McGrath P, et al. The development of a tool to assess neonatal pain. Neonatal Netw 1993;12(6):59–66.

31. Stevens B, Johnston C, Petryshen P, et al. Premature infant pain profile: development and initial validation. Clin J Pain 1996;12(1):13–22.

32. Krechel SW, Bildner J. CRIES: a new neonatal postoperative pain measurement score. Initial testing of validity and reliability. Paediatr Anaesth 1995;5(1):53–61.

33. Pillai Riddell RR, Stevens BJ, McKeever P, et al. Chronic pain in hospitalized infants: health professionals' perspectives. J Pain 2009;10(12):1217–25.

34. Hummel P, Puchalski M, Creech SD, et al. Clinical reliability and validity of the N-PASS: neonatal pain, agitation and sedation scale with prolonged pain. J Perinatol 2008;28(1):55–60.

35. Barrington K. Premedication for endotracheal intubation in the newborn infant. Paediatr Child Health 2011;16(3):159–71.

36. Kumar P, Denson SE, Mancuso TJ. Premedication for nonemergency endotracheal intubation in the neonate. Pediatrics 2010;125(3):608–15.

37. Marshall TA, Deeder R, Pai S, et al. Physiologic changes associated with endotracheal intubation in preterm infants. Crit Care Med 1984;12(6):501–3.

38. Raju TN, Vidyasagar D, Torres C, et al. Intracranial pressure during intubation and anesthesia in infants. J Pediatr 1980;96(5):860–2.

39. Hatfield LA, Chang K, Bittle M, et al. The analgesic properties of intraoral sucrose: an integrative review. Adv Neonatal Care 2011;11(2):83–92 [quiz: 93–4].

40. Stevens B, Yamada J, Ohlsson A. Sucrose for analgesia in newborn infants undergoing painful procedures. Cochrane Database Syst Rev 2010;(1): CD001069.

41. Yamada J, Stinson J, Lamba J, et al. A review of systematic reviews on pain interventions in hospitalized infants. Pain Res Manag 2008;13(5):413–20.

42. Cong X, Ludington-Hoe SM, McCain G, et al. Kangaroo care modifies preterm infant heart rate variability in response to heel stick pain: pilot study. Early Hum Dev 2009;85(9):561–7.

43. Morrow C, Hidinger A, Wilkinson-Faulk D. Reducing neonatal pain during routine heel lance procedures. MCN Am J Matern Child Nurs 2010;35(6):346–54 [quiz: 354–6].

44. Jain S, Kumar P, McMillan DD. Prior leg massage decreases pain responses to heel stick in preterm babies. J Paediatr Child Health 2006;42(9):505–8.

45. Meek J, Huertas A. Cochrane review: non-nutritive sucking, kangaroo care and swaddling/facilitated tucking are observed to reduce procedural pain in infants and young children. Evid Based Nurs 2012;15(3):84–5.

46. Goodman LS, Gilman A, Brunton LL, et al. Goodman & Gilman's the pharmacological basis of therapeutics. 11th edition. New York: McGraw-Hill; 2006.

47. Scott CS, Riggs KW, Ling EW, et al. Morphine pharmacokinetics and pain assessment in premature newborns. J Pediatr 1999;135(4):423–9.

48. Simons SH, Anand KJ. Pain control: opioid dosing, population kinetics and side-effects. Semin Fetal Neonatal Med 2006;11(4):260–7.

49. Saarenmaa E, Neuvonen PJ, Fellman V. Gestational age and birth weight effects on plasma clearance of fentanyl in newborn infants. J Pediatr 2000;136(6): 767–70.

50. Hume-Smith H, McCormack J, Montgomery C, et al. The effect of age on the dose of remifentanil for tracheal intubation in infants and children. Paediatr Anaesth 2010;20(1):19–27.

51. Penido MG, Garra R, Sammartino M, et al. Remifentanil in neonatal intensive care and anaesthesia practice. Acta Paediatr 2010;99(10):1454–63.

52. Pereira e Silva Y, Gomez RS, Barbosa RF, et al. Remifentanil for sedation and analgesia in a preterm neonate with respiratory distress syndrome. Paediatr Anaesth 2005;15(11):993–6.

53. Cravero JP, Havidich JE. Pediatric sedation–evolution and revolution. Paediatr Anaesth 2011;21(7):800–9.

54. Blumer JL. Clinical pharmacology of midazolam in infants and children. Clin Pharmacokinet 1998;35(1):37–47.

55. Lee TC, Charles BG, Harte GJ, et al. Population pharmacokinetic modeling in very premature infants receiving midazolam during mechanical ventilation: midazolam neonatal pharmacokinetics. Anesthesiology 1999;90(2): 451–7.

56. Rho JM, Donevan SD, Rogawski MA. Direct activation of GABAA receptors by barbiturates in cultured rat hippocampal neurons. J Physiol 1996;497(Pt 2): 509–22.

57. Bhutada A, Sahni R, Rastogi S, et al. Randomised controlled trial of thiopental for intubation in neonates. Arch Dis Child Fetal Neonatal Ed 2000; 82(1):F34–7.

58. Naulaers G, Deloof E, Vanhole C, et al. Use of methohexital for elective intubation in neonates. Arch Dis Child Fetal Neonatal Ed 1997;77(1):F61–4.

59. Bach V, Carl P, Ravlo O, et al. A randomized comparison between midazolam and thiopental for elective cesarean section anesthesia: III. Placental transfer and elimination in neonates. Anesth Analg 1989;68(3):238–42.

60. Haeseler G, Karst M, Foadi N, et al. High-affinity blockade of voltage-operated skeletal muscle and neuronal sodium channels by halogenated propofol analogues. Br J Pharmacol 2008;155(2):265–75.

61. Kotani Y, Shimazawa M, Yoshimura S, et al. The experimental and clinical pharmacology of propofol, an anesthetic agent with neuroprotective properties. CNS Neurosci Ther 2008;14(2):95–106.

62. Allegaert K, Peeters MY, Verbesselt R, et al. Inter-individual variability in propofol pharmacokinetics in preterm and term neonates. Br J Anaesth 2007;99(6): 864–70.

63. Cravero JP, Beach ML, Blike GT, et al. The incidence and nature of adverse events during pediatric sedation/anesthesia with propofol for procedures outside the operating room: a report from the Pediatric Sedation Research Consortium. Anesth Analg 2009;108(3):795–804.

64. Ghanta S, Abdel-Latif ME, Lui K, et al. Propofol compared with the morphine, atropine, and suxamethonium regimen as induction agents for neonatal endotracheal intubation: a randomized, controlled trial. Pediatrics 2007;119(6): e1248–55.

65. Anand KJ, Barton BA, McIntosh N, et al. Analgesia and sedation in preterm neonates who require ventilatory support: results from the NOPAIN trial. Neonatal Outcome and Prolonged Analgesia in Neonates. Arch Pediatr Adolesc Med 1999;153(4):331–8.

66. Nauta M, Onland W, De Jaegere A. Propofol as an induction agent for endotracheal intubation can cause significant arterial hypotension in preterm infants. Paediatr Anaesth 2011;21(6):711–2.
67. Welzing L, Kribs A, Eifinger F, et al. Propofol as an induction agent for endotracheal intubation can cause significant arterial hypotension in preterm neonates. Paediatr Anaesth 2010;20(7):605–11.
68. Ikonomidou C, Bittigau P, Ishimaru MJ, et al. Ethanol-induced apoptotic neurodegeneration and fetal alcohol syndrome. Science 2000;287(5455):1056–60.
69. Brambrink AM, Orfanakis A, Kirsch JR. Anesthetic neurotoxicity. Anesthesiol Clin 2012;30(2):207–28.
70. Stratmann G. Review article: neurotoxicity of anesthetic drugs in the developing brain. Anesth Analg 2011;113(5):1170–9.
71. Brambrink AM, Back SA, Riddle A, et al. Isoflurane-induced apoptosis of oligodendrocytes in the neonatal primate brain. Ann Neurol 2012;72(4):525–35.
72. Brambrink AM, Evers AS, Avidan MS, et al. Ketamine-induced neuroapoptosis in the fetal and neonatal rhesus macaque brain. Anesthesiology 2012;116(2):372–84.
73. Brambrink AM, Evers AS, Avidan MS, et al. Isoflurane-induced neuroapoptosis in the neonatal rhesus macaque brain. Anesthesiology 2010;112(4):834–41.
74. Slikker W Jr, Zou X, Hotchkiss CE, et al. Ketamine-induced neuronal cell death in the perinatal rhesus monkey. Toxicol Sci 2007;98(1):145–58.
75. Zou X, Liu F, Zhang X, et al. Inhalation anesthetic-induced neuronal damage in the developing rhesus monkey. Neurotoxicol Teratol 2011;33(5):592–7.
76. Zou X, Patterson TA, Sadovova N, et al. Potential neurotoxicity of ketamine in the developing rat brain. Toxicol Sci 2009;108(1):149–58.
77. Paule MG, Li M, Allen RR, et al. Ketamine anesthesia during the first week of life can cause long-lasting cognitive deficits in rhesus monkeys. Neurotoxicol Teratol 2011;33(2):220–30.
78. DiMaggio C, Sun LS, Kakavouli A, et al. A retrospective cohort study of the association of anesthesia and hernia repair surgery with behavioral and developmental disorders in young children. J Neurosurg Anesthesiol 2009;21(4):286–91.
79. DiMaggio C, Sun LS, Li G. Early childhood exposure to anesthesia and risk of developmental and behavioral disorders in a sibling birth cohort. Anesth Analg 2011;113(5):1143–51.
80. Flick RP, Katusic SK, Colligan RC, et al. Cognitive and behavioral outcomes after early exposure to anesthesia and surgery. Pediatrics 2011;128(5):e1053–61.
81. Sprung J, Flick RP, Katusic SK, et al. Attention-deficit/hyperactivity disorder after early exposure to procedures requiring general anesthesia. Mayo Clin Proc 2012;87(2):120–9.
82. Wilder RT, Flick RP, Sprung J, et al. Early exposure to anesthesia and learning disabilities in a population-based birth cohort. Anesthesiology 2009;110(4):796–804.
83. Barrington KJ, Finer NN, Etches PC. Succinylcholine and atropine for premedication of the newborn infant before nasotracheal intubation: a randomized, controlled trial. Crit Care Med 1989;17(12):1293–6.
84. Kelly MA, Finer NN. Nasotracheal intubation in the neonate: physiologic responses and effects of atropine and pancuronium. J Pediatr 1984;105(2):303–9.
85. Norman E, Wikstrom S, Hellstrom-Westas L, et al. Rapid sequence induction is superior to morphine for intubation of preterm infants: a randomized controlled trial. J Pediatr 2011;159(6):893–9.e1.

86. Gerlach AT, Dasta JF. Dexmedetomidine: an updated review. Ann Pharmacother 2007;41(2):245–52.

87. Agthe AG, Kim GR, Mathias KB, et al. Clonidine as an adjunct therapy to opioids for neonatal abstinence syndrome: a randomized, controlled trial. Pediatrics 2009;123(5):e849–56.

88. Jakob SM, Ruokonen E, Grounds RM, et al. Dexmedetomidine vs midazolam or propofol for sedation during prolonged mechanical ventilation: two randomized controlled trials. JAMA 2012;307(11):1151–60.

89. Riker RR, Shehabi Y, Bokesch PM, et al. Dexmedetomidine vs midazolam for sedation of critically ill patients: a randomized trial. JAMA 2009;301(5):489–99.

90. Hosokawa K, Shime N, Kato Y, et al. Dexmedetomidine sedation in children after cardiac surgery. Pediatr Crit Care Med 2010;11(1):39–43.

91. Dilek O, Yasemin G, Atci M. Preliminary experience with dexmedetomidine in neonatal anesthesia. J Anaesthesiol Clin Pharmacol 2011;27(1):17–22.

92. Mason KP, Zurakowski D, Zgleszewski SE, et al. High dose dexmedetomidine as the sole sedative for pediatric MRI. Paediatr Anaesth 2008;18(5):403–11.

93. Munro HM, Tirotta CF, Felix DE, et al. Initial experience with dexmedetomidine for diagnostic and interventional cardiac catheterization in children. Paediatr Anaesth 2007;17(2):109–12.

94. O'Mara K, Gal P, Ransommd JL, et al. Successful use of dexmedetomidine for sedation in a 24-week gestational age neonate. Ann Pharmacother 2009;43(10):1707–13.

95. Sanders RD, Xu J, Shu Y, et al. Dexmedetomidine attenuates isoflurane-induced neurocognitive impairment in neonatal rats. Anesthesiology 2009;110(5):1077–85.

96. Friesen RH, Honda AT, Thieme RE. Changes in anterior fontanel pressure in preterm neonates during tracheal intubation. Anesth Analg 1987;66(9):874–8.

97. Johnson PN, Miller J, Gormley AK. Continuous-infusion neuromuscular blocking agents in critically ill neonates and children. Pharmacotherapy 2011;31(6):609–20.

98. Dempsey EM, Al Hazzani F, Faucher D, et al. Facilitation of neonatal endotracheal intubation with mivacurium and fentanyl in the neonatal intensive care unit. Arch Dis Child Fetal Neonatal Ed 2006;91(4):F279–82.

99. Feltman DM, Weiss MG, Nicoski P, et al. Rocuronium for nonemergent intubation of term and preterm infants. J Perinatol 2011;31(1):38–43.

100. Roberts KD, Leone TA, Edwards WH, et al. Premedication for nonemergent neonatal intubations: a randomized, controlled trial comparing atropine and fentanyl to atropine, fentanyl, and mivacurium. Pediatrics 2006;118(4):1583–91.

101. Yang LP, Keam SJ. Sugammadex: a review of its use in anaesthetic practice. Drugs 2009;69(7):919–42.

102. Attardi DM, Paul DA, Tuttle DJ, et al. Premedication for intubation in neonates. Arch Dis Child Fetal Neonatal Ed 2000;83(2):F161.

103. Ng E, Taddio A, Ohlsson A. Intravenous midazolam infusion for sedation of infants in the neonatal intensive care unit. Cochrane Database Syst Rev 2012;(6):CD002052.

104. Arya V, Ramji S. Midazolam sedation in mechanically ventilated newborns: a double blind randomized placebo controlled trial. Indian Pediatr 2001;38(9):967–72.

105. Jacqz-Aigrain E, Daoud P, Burtin P, et al. Placebo-controlled trial of midazolam sedation in mechanically ventilated newborn babies. Lancet 1994;344(8923):646–50.

106. Lemyre B, Doucette J, Kalyn A, et al. Morphine for elective endotracheal intubation in neonates: a randomized trial [ISRCTN43546373]. BMC Pediatr 2004;4:20.
107. Oei J, Hari R, Butha T, et al. Facilitation of neonatal nasotracheal intubation with premedication: a randomized controlled trial. J Paediatr Child Health 2002; 38(2):146–50.
108. Pereira e Silva Y, Gomez RS, Marcatto Jde O, et al. Morphine versus remifentanil for intubating preterm neonates. Arch Dis Child Fetal Neonatal Ed 2007;92(4): F293–4.
109. Norman E, Wikstrom S, Rosen I, et al. Premedication for intubation with morphine causes prolonged depression of electrocortical background activity in preterm infants. Pediatr Res 2013;73(1):87–94.
110. Choong K, AlFaleh K, Doucette J, et al. Remifentanil for endotracheal intubation in neonates: a randomised controlled trial. Arch Dis Child Fetal Neonatal Ed 2010;95(2):F80–4.
111. Dyke MP, Kohan R, Evans S. Morphine increases synchronous ventilation in preterm infants. J Paediatr Child Health 1995;31(3):176–9.
112. Anand KJ, Hall RW, Desai N, et al. Effects of morphine analgesia in ventilated preterm neonates: primary outcomes from the NEOPAIN randomised trial. Lancet 2004;363(9422):1673–82.
113. Simons SH, van Dijk M, van Lingen RA, et al. Routine morphine infusion in preterm newborns who received ventilatory support: a randomized controlled trial. JAMA 2003;290(18):2419–27.
114. de Graaf J, van Lingen RA, Simons SH, et al. Long-term effects of routine morphine infusion in mechanically ventilated neonates on children's functioning: five-year follow-up of a randomized controlled trial. Pain 2011;152(6):1391–7.
115. Saarenmaa E, Huttunen P, Leppaluoto J, et al. Advantages of fentanyl over morphine in analgesia for ventilated newborn infants after birth: a randomized trial. J Pediatr 1999;134(2):144–50.
116. Guinsburg R, Kopelman BI, Anand KJ, et al. Physiological, hormonal, and behavioral responses to a single fentanyl dose in intubated and ventilated preterm neonates. J Pediatr 1998;132(6):954–9.
117. Lago P, Benini F, Agosto C, et al. Randomised controlled trial of low dose fentanyl infusion in preterm infants with hyaline membrane disease. Arch Dis Child Fetal Neonatal Ed 1998;79(3):F194–7.
118. Lago P, Benini F, Salvadori S, et al. Effect of administering low-dose fentanyl infusion on respiratory dynamics in the premature ventilated for respiratory distress syndrome-a randomized double-blind trial. Pediatr Res 1999;45(4): 308a.
119. Orsini AJ, Leef KH, Costarino A, et al. Routine use of fentanyl infusions for pain and stress reduction in infants with respiratory distress syndrome. J Pediatr 1996;129(1):140–5.
120. Bellu R, de Waal K, Zanini R. Opioids for neonates receiving mechanical ventilation: a systematic review and meta-analysis. Arch Dis Child Fetal Neonatal Ed 2010;95(4):F241–51.
121. Bellu R, de Waal KA, Zanini R. Opioids for neonates receiving mechanical ventilation. Cochrane Database Syst Rev 2008;(1):CD004212.
122. Marsh DF, Hodkinson B. Remifentanil in paediatric anaesthetic practice. Anaesthesia 2009;64(3):301–8.
123. Giannantonio C, Sammartino M, Valente E, et al. Remifentanil analgosedation in preterm newborns during mechanical ventilation. Acta Paediatr 2009;98(7): 1111–5.

124. Stoppa F, Perrotta D, Tomasello C, et al. Low dose remifentanyl infusion for analgesia and sedation in ventilated newborns. Minerva Anestesiol 2004;70(11): 753–61.

125. Welzing L, Oberthuer A, Junghaenel S, et al. Remifentanil/midazolam versus fentanyl/midazolam for analgesia and sedation of mechanically ventilated neonates and young infants: a randomized controlled trial. Intensive Care Med 2012;38(6):1017–24.

126. Tarkkila P, Viitanen H, Mennander S, et al. Comparison of remifentanil versus ketamine for paediatric day case adenoidectomy. Acta Anaesthesiol Belg 2003; 54(3):217–22.

127. Penido MG, de Oliveira Silva DF, Tavares EC, et al. Propofol versus midazolam for intubating preterm neonates: a randomized controlled trial. J Perinatol 2011; 31(5):356–60.

128. Papoff P, Mancuso M, Caresta E, et al. Effectiveness and safety of propofol in newborn infants. Pediatrics 2008;121(2):448 [author reply: 448–9].

129. Veyckemans F. Propofol for intubation of the newborn? Paediatr Anaesth 2001; 11(5):630–1.

130. Shah PS, Shah VS. Propofol for procedural sedation/anaesthesia in neonates. Cochrane Database Syst Rev 2011;(3):CD007248.

131. Sammartino M, Garra R, Sbaraglia F, et al. Propofol overdose in a preterm baby: may propofol infusion syndrome arise in two hours? Paediatr Anaesth 2010; 20(10):973–4.

Neurodevelopmental Implications of the Use of Sedation and Analgesia in Neonates

Andrew Davidson, MBBS, MD, FANNZCA[a],*, Randall P. Flick, MD, MPH[b]

KEYWORDS

- Neonates • Sedation • Analgesia • Neurotoxicity • Neurodevelopment

KEY POINTS

- In animal models, commonly used general anesthetics and sedatives can cause accelerated neuronal apoptosis and other morphologic changes in the developing brain.
- The clinical relevance of the laboratory findings is unknown, and many factors limit the translation of these findings.
- Increasing evidence shows that neonates who have surgery and anesthesia are at greater risk for adverse neurobehavioral outcome.
- Many possible explanations exist for the association between surgery in the neonatal period and the increased risk of poor neurobehavioral outcome, with the putative neurotoxicity of anesthetics being only one possible explanation.
- Withholding adequate anesthesia and analgesia is associated with adverse outcome, and thus no firm recommendations to alter current practice based on the preclinical or clinical findings can be recommended.

INTRODUCTION

Neonates are exposed to anesthetics, sedatives, and analgesics for surgery and to facilitate the performance of a variety of investigative procedures. Neonates in the intensive care unit may also be exposed to sedatives to assist mechanical ventilation. The fetus may also be exposed to anesthetics or analgesics if the mother has surgery or during pregnancy or labor.

Increasing concern exists about the potential effect of sedative, analgesic, and, in particular, anesthetic agents on the developing brain. A wealth of preclinical data shows that some of these agents can trigger accelerated apoptosis and other

[a] Department of Anaesthesia and Pain Management, Royal Children's Hospital, Flemington Road, Parkville, Melbourne, Victoria 3052, Australia; [b] Mayo Clinic Children's Center, Mayo Clinic, 200 First Street SW, Rochester, MN 55905, USA
* Corresponding author.
E-mail address: andrew.davidson@rch.org.au

Clin Perinatol 40 (2013) 559–573
http://dx.doi.org/10.1016/j.clp.2013.05.009   **perinatology.theclinics.com**

changes in the developing brain of animals. In some cases, exposure to these agents may result in long-term neurobehavioral change. However, many challenges exist to translating these data to humans. Some clinical human studies have found an association between exposure to these agents and an increased risk of adverse neurobehavioral outcome; however, many confounding factors exist, and it is by no means certain that the link is causative. To further complicate the issue, reason also exists to believe that increasing stress and pain from withholding these agents may increase the risk of altered neurobehavioral outcomes. This article outlines the relevant animal data, possible mechanisms, human studies, and challenges translating these findings to clinical practice.

DEVELOPMENT

The brain undergoes considerable development in the fetus and infant. One aspect of that development is a growth and then decline in the number of neurons and the number of synapses. Neurons are removed through apoptosis, a form of organized cell death. Apoptosis is a basic physiologic process whereby unwanted cells can be removed, such as the tail of a tadpole. This pruning of neurons and synapses is activity-dependent. Thus, it is plausible that drugs that alter neuronal activity will have some impact on neuronal cell number and morphology. In addition to this indirect effect, γ-aminobutyric acid (GABA), N-methyl-d-aspartate (NMDA), and opioid receptors also have a direct role in neuronal migration, differentiation, and maturation. During development these receptors differ in subtype and/or function, providing a clue regarding why effects may be seen in particular developmental periods.

EARLY ANIMAL DATA

Initial concerns about occupational exposure to anesthetics in pregnant health care workers led to limited research in the 1970s. These studies showed that delayed synaptogenesis and subsequent behavioral abnormalities could be observed in rats born after exposure to repeated subanesthetic doses of halothane during pregnancy.[1,2]

RECENT RODENT DATA

The first substantial data linking anesthetic agents to apoptosis arose after investigation of the mechanisms of neuronal injury caused by exposure to alcohol and antiepileptic drugs. Blockade of NMDA receptors with the antagonist MK801 (an agent similar to ketamine) resulted in widespread neuronal apoptosis in the brains of 7-day-old rats.[3] Subsequently, the same group showed that a combination of midazolam, nitrous oxide, and isoflurane administered to 7-day-old rats for 6 hours caused widespread apoptotic neurodegeneration, changes in hippocampal synaptic function, and persistent memory and learning impairments.[4]

Many more studies have since showed increased levels of neuronal apoptosis in newborn rodents after exposure to general anesthetics, such as ketamine, propofol, sevoflurane, isoflurane, and desflurane. Apoptosis is also seen after exposure to nitrous oxide and benzodiazepines.[4–11] The effect of anesthetics on apoptosis depends on age at exposure, dose and duration of exposure, and number of exposures (single vs multiple). It is greatest during early postnatal development in animals; in rats it is greatest at 7 days of age. Prolonged and repeated exposure increases the effect. Some evidence also shows that exposure to a combination of different types of anesthetic may be greater than single-agent exposure.

Some rodent studies have shown long-term cognitive, behavioral, and learning effects in animals exposed to anesthetics in the neonatal period. The pattern of neurobehavioral effect, however, is inconsistent and has not been shown in all experiments. This variability in neurobehavioral outcome is consistent with variability in the brain region affected by different agents (see later discussion).[4,11–13]

For many reasons, translation of these animal data to humans is challenging. Two factors that influence translation are the experimental condition and the potential for greater neuroplasticity in humans. For example, newborn rats exposed to 4 hours of sevoflurane had significant memory impairment if housed in normal cages; but if the rats were housed in an enriched environment after exposure, no evidence was seen of a difference in memory between rats exposed to anesthetic and those not exposed. Examination of only those rats that were not exposed showed that memory performance was also better in the enriched group compared with those kept in normal cages.[14] This experiment is important because it demonstrates that neurobehavioral development is dependent on many factors. The possibility exists that the effect of anesthesia is insignificant compared with more powerful social and environmental determinants of development.

NONHUMAN PRIMATE DATA

Interspecies differences are a significant barrier in translation to humans. Thus the most relevant animal data are those described in nonhuman primates. Increased apoptosis has been observed in newborn monkeys exposed to 24 hours of ketamine during late gestation and those exposed to 24 hours of ketamine at 5 days of age. However, no increase in apoptosis was seen in those exposed at 35 days of age.[15] This group also found no increase in 5-day-old monkeys exposed to only 3 hours of ketamine. In contrast, another group did find an increase in apoptosis after exposure to 5 hours of ketamine.[16] Although monkeys are more similar to humans than rodents, pharmacologic differences remain that make translation difficult. Monkeys require a far greater dose of ketamine to induce anesthesia; however, if the apoptosis is caused by the functional effect of anesthesia, then this dose difference may not be important. As with rodents, long-term neurobehavioral changes have also been demonstrated in monkeys. Five-day-old monkeys exposed to 24 hours of ketamine had learning difficulties when tested at 2 to 3 years of age.[17]

A 5-hour exposure of isoflurane has also been shown to cause increased apoptosis in the newborn monkey.[18] In newborn monkeys the apoptosis was greater with isoflurane, whereas in the fetus ketamine caused greater apoptosis, highlighting species-specific differences in anesthetic effects. These studies also showed that ketamine and isoflurane cause apoptosis in different regions of the brain depending on the age of exposure. This variation according to age and agent may help explain the variation between studies in degree of long-term neurobehavioral outcome. The variation in affected region also makes the clinical outcome difficult to predict in human studies.

OTHER EFFECTS ON THE DEVELOPING BRAIN

General anesthetics have a variety of other effects on the developing brain apart from inducing apoptosis.

- Dendritic arborization and spine formation: propofol, ketamine, isoflurane, sevoflurane, and desflurane produce changes in neuronal dendritic spine morphology.[19–22] Changes are seen in dendritic arborization and spine density. The effect varies with age. In 5- and 10-day-old animals, anesthetics cause a decrease in the number of dendritic spines, whereas in 15-, 20-, and 30-day-old animals an increase in the number of dendritic spines occurs. These effects are seen in older animals and without accelerated apoptosis. This finding implies that anesthetics may have subtle effects over a broader age range than that the range at which accelerated apoptosis typically occurs.

- Changes in the neuronal cytoskeleton: the mechanism underlying these changes involves the p75[NTR] receptor and subsequent RhoA activation.[23] These changes may be linked to the changes seen in dendritic morphology.
- Altered neurogenesis and abnormal reentry into the cell cycle[24,25]
- Impaired mitochondrial function.[26]

Accelerated apoptosis and these other effects may all be linked with common underlying mechanisms.

POSSIBLE MECHANISMS FOR ANESTHESIA-INDUCED NEURONAL CHANGES

Several possible mechanisms explain how general anesthetics may induce apoptosis and other changes in the developing brain. One explanation is that the changes are linked to anesthesia-induced neuronal inactivity. During development, excess neurons are removed via apoptosis, and neuronal survival is dependent on activity. Similarly, dendritic and synaptic development is linked to activity. Active axons release tissue plasminogen activator (tPA) and pro–brain-derived neurotrophic factor (proBDNF).[27] The tPA cleaves plasmin to plasminogen. The plasminogen converts proBDNF to BDNF. BDNF acts at the TrkB receptor on the dendrite to promote cell survival. If the axon is not active, proBDNF but not tPA is released. Without tPA present, plasmin is not converted to plasminogen, and thus proBDNF is not converted to BDNF. The proBDNF then acts on the p75[NTR] receptor on the dendrite, resulting in cell death via apoptosis (**Fig. 1**).

It would seem plausible that general anesthetics may lead to neuronal inactivity via their activity at GABA. In adults, GABA is generally an inhibitory neurotransmitter; however, several reasons exist as to why GABA activity alone may not underlie the accelerated apoptosis.

- During early development, GABA receptors are excitatory rather than inhibitory.
- Giving a GABA antagonist with a general anesthetic does not reverse the accelerated apoptosis.[28]
- Apoptosis is seen with agents, such as ketamine, that have no GABA activity.

Thus it is unlikely that accelerated apoptosis is a direct GABA effect. Similarly, it is unlikely that the anesthetic state per se is the sole cause, because both xenon and dexmedetomidine, can lead to anesthetic-like states with no apoptosis.[28,29]

Another suggested mechanism is that anesthetic-induced NMDA blockade produces an acute upregulation of the NMDA receptor, and that when the anesthetic exposure ceases, subsequent excitotoxic neurotoxicity occurs.[30] However, NMDA receptor activity is unlikely the sole mechanism, because

- Apoptosis occurs with agents that have no action on NMDA receptors
- Apoptosis does not occur with NMDA antagonists agents such as xenon
- Cell death can occur during the period of NMDA blockade
- Both racemic and s-ketamine have similar degrees of toxicity.[31]

Without a clear understanding of the mechanisms, it is very difficult to know how to translate the animal data to clinical situations.

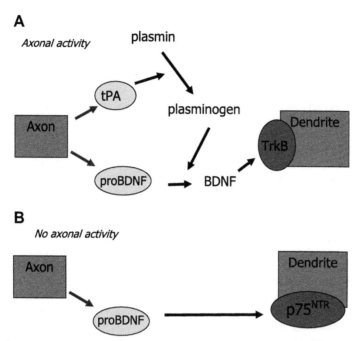

Fig. 1. (*A*) With axonal action potentials, the axon releases tPA and proBDNF; tPA cleaves plasmin to plasminogen, which converts proBDNF to BDNF; and BDNF acts on dendritic TrkB to promote cell survival. (*B*) With no axonal action potentials, proBDNF continues to be released, whereas no release of tPA occurs. proBDNF then acts directly on dendritic p75^{NTR}, resulting in cell death.

TRANSLATING THE ANIMAL DATA TO HUMAN CLINICAL SCENARIOS

Many factors make the translation of animal data difficult.

- Age of exposure: considerable controversy exists about how ages in animals equate to ages or developmental periods in humans. Because the human brain develops differently, it is simply impossible to say a particular age in a rat represents a particular age in a human. A 5- to 7-day-old rat may correspond to a late-trimester human fetus or a neonate, but this is by no means certain. Furthermore, although apoptosis may be confined to approximately 5 to 7 days after birth in a rodent, the changes in dendritic morphology are found within a far wider period.
- Dose: the dose of intravenous agents required to produce anesthesia varies hugely across species. Some animals require almost 50 times more ketamine on a milligram per kilogram basis to produce anesthesia. Without a clear understanding of the mechanisms, whether this dose difference is relevant is impossible to determine. In contrast, the dose of inhalational agents such as isoflurane changes very little across species.
- Duration of exposure: the brain develops over a few weeks in a rat, whereas in humans it develops over years. A 5-hour exposure in a rat covers a significant proportion of the animal's period of development. Thus a 5-hour exposure in a rat may not have the same effect as a 5-hour exposure in a human.
- Plasticity: given that the brain develops over a longer period in humans, there may be more time for recovery, and a period of accelerated apoptosis may be

easily "repaired." However, one can also argue that the human brain is far more complex than a rodent's and a period of injury may have critical effects on downstream development. In general, the long-term effects of injury to the developing brain are known to depend on the nature, location, and timing of the injury; whether the accelerated apoptosis seen with general anesthetics falls into one of these critical patterns of injury is not known.

- Modifying effects of environment: the animal experiments are conducted in very controlled environments. The neurobehavioral effects of anesthetic exposure are not seen in rodents that were raised in enriched environments. Humans are exposed to many factors that may influence development (hence the normal variation in human neurobehavioral outcomes). If a simple environmental intervention overwhelms any effect in rodents, then it is plausible that the wealth of exposures in humans may also overwhelm any effect of anesthesia exposure.
- Translating the neurobehavioral effects: neurobehavioral tests in rodents and even in monkeys tend to be fairly crude. It is plausible that anesthesia exposure may have subtle effects in humans that cannot be detected in animal models.
- Experimental conditions: it is well-known that sedation and anesthesia may result in hypoxia, hypotension, or hyper/hypocarbia; all of which may have deleterious effects on the brain. Human neonates undergoing anesthesia or sedation are carefully monitored to avoid these. Newborn rodents are difficult to monitor. Some experiments have results of blood gas analysis that suggest the animals do not have significant respiratory dysfunction; however, in most experiments a significant proportion of the animals die during anesthesia, implying that some degree of physiologic derangement must occur. In contrast, respiratory and hemodynamic parameters are carefully monitored and controlled in the nonhuman primate experiments.
- Surgical stimulation: most of the animal experiments are conducted without surgery. Surgical stimuli may be important, because the stimulus may influence the balance of neuronal activity, and the inflammatory and humoral effect of surgery may also influence outcome. One limited study reported no effect of surgical stimulation (tail clamping) on degree of apoptosis,[14] whereas another found that surgical stimulus did reduce the degree of apoptosis.[32] Similarly, untreated pain can cause morphologic changes, and small analgesic doses of ketamine may reduce those morphologic changes without inducing apoptosis.[33] The influence of surgery may depend on the degree of surgery and dose of anesthetic.

OTHER AGENTS

Most research has focused on general anesthetics, particularly ketamine. Fewer data exist regarding other sedative and analgesic agents. Benzodiazepines, chloral hydrate, and barbiturates all act via NMDA or GABA receptors, and therefore it would not be surprising if they had effects on neuronal development similar to general anesthetics; however, the effects cannot always be predicted given the poor understanding of the mechanisms. Not all agents acting on GABA or NMDA receptors have been found to cause increased apoptosis.

Benzodiazepines

Midazolam is often used for sedation in neonates. Single doses of 9 mg/kg of midazolam or 5 mg/kg of diazepam does not increase apoptosis in neonatal rats[4,34]; however, 10 mg/kg of diazepam does result in increased apoptosis.[34,35] In another study 5 mg/kg of diazepam caused increased neuronal apoptosis in mice but did not result in subsequent learning deficits.[36] Similarly neonatal exposure to midazolam did not result in learning deficits.[37] Apoptosis is greater when ketamine and diazepam are given together.[36]

Chloral Hydrate

One preliminary study found that 100 mg/kg of chloral hydrate causes accelerated neuronal apoptosis in neonatal mice.[38]

Barbiturates

Exposure to pentobarbital or phenobarbital causes neuronal injury in neonatal rodents and results in learning deficits.[39,40]

Dexmedetomidine

Dexmedetomidine acts on NMDA or GABA receptors. It does not accelerate neuronal apoptosis, and reduces isoflurane-induced apoptosis and learning deficits.[28,41] Similarly it does not impair hippocampal synaptic plasticity.[42]

Opioid Analgesics

Opioid receptors are crucial to normal brain development, and therefore it would be expected that opioids would have some impact neuronal morphology or apoptosis. Several studies have examined the effect of chronic administration of opioids during pregnancy. In rodents, chronic prenatal exposure to heroin increases neuronal apoptosis and results in learning deficits.[43] Perinatal methadone and morphine exposure also results in a variety of short-term and long-term neurobehavioral effects.[44,45] Chronic morphine exposure in newborn rats impairs normal development,[46,47] including an altered response to pain in later life.[48]

Opioids have been shown to have many different effects at a cellular level. Perinatal morphine causes altered dendritic architecture and neuronal density[49] and reduces μ-receptor density.[50] Perinatal administration of either methadone or buprenorphine reduces the content of the neurotrophic factor nerve growth factor.[51] Fewer data are available on apoptosis. One group suggested that chronic opioid exposure will increase susceptibility to neuronal apoptosis.[52] Another study comparing 30 μg/kg fentanyl followed by 15 μg/kg/hr for 4 hours versus 1 mg/kg of midazolam followed by 4 hours of 0.55% isoflurane and 75% nitrous oxide in neonatal pigs showed significantly less neuronal apoptosis in the fentanyl group.[53]

Other Analgesics

No data exist on the neurodevelopmental effects of simple analgesics, such as paracetamol and nonsteroidal anti-inflammatory drugs. However, given that they do not act on receptors involved in neuronal development, they are unlikely to have significant neurodevelopmental effects. Furthermore, no data are available on the long-term effects of tramadol. Tramadol acts on a variety of receptors that may influence neuronal development, including opioid receptors. Thus, further investigation into the effect of tramadol is warranted.

HUMAN DATA: THE ASSOCIATION BETWEEN SURGERY/ANESTHESIA AND INCREASED RISK OF POOR NEUROBEHAVIORAL OUTCOME

Several cohort studies show an association between surgery in infancy and an increased risk of adverse neurobehavioral outcomes; however, because of the many confounding factors, the precise role of anesthesia, analgesia, and sedation is very difficult to determine. Children with esophageal atresia have more learning, emotional, and behavioral problems than those in the general population.[54] Extremely low-birth-weight babies who have acute intra-abdominal abnormalities requiring a laparotomy have also been found to have an increased risk of neurobehavioral outcome.[55] Similarly, another study found an association between the need for any type of surgery requiring general anesthesia and an increased risk of poor sensori-neural outcome in extremely preterm or low-birth-weight infants.[56] Several other studies have found an association between major surgery and an increased risk of poor neurobehavioral outcome.[57–59] Even infants who have a relatively minor procedure, such as pyloric stenosis repair, have an increased risk of poor outcome.[60]

In determining whether anesthesia causes an increased risk of poor neurobehavioral outcome, the possible confounding factors include

- Presence of coexisting conditions: infants requiring surgery are more likely to have malformations and chromosomal disorders that may be associated with an increased risk of poor neurobehavioral outcome.
- Prematurity: prematurity is associated with a variety of conditions that require surgery, and may increase the risk of poor neurobehavioral outcome.
- Surgery may be required in septic infants or infants with other acute conditions. These conditions may also increase risk of poor outcome.
- Surgery itself may result in inflammatory or stress responses that increase the risk of poor outcome.
- Surgery and anesthesia may be associated with hemodynamic, respiratory, and metabolic instability that may contribute to the poor outcome.

Other unknown confounding factors may also be present.

Several studies have attempted to examine the association between surgery and anesthesia in the clinical setting, each of which rely on retrospective examinations of existing databases created for purposes other than the study of this question. Most of the published studies originate from research groups at Columbia University and the Mayo Clinic. Additional studies have been conducted using large national databases that exist primarily in Europe.

The first of these studies published by Wilder and colleagues from the Mayo Clinic examined an existing cohort of children born between 1976 and 1982 whose complete medical and school records were retrospectively reviewed for evidence of any type of learning disability (LD).[61] These studies were conducted to determine the incidence of LD in a birth cohort. The cohort was subsequently re-examined to determine whether those who were exposed to anesthesia before 4 years of age were more likely to have any type of LD than those not so exposed. The authors found that those with a single exposure were not at increased risk, although those with 2 or more exposures were at significantly increased risk, and that risk increased with duration of exposure.

To reduce the potential for confounding from comorbid conditions, the authors re-examined the cohort using a case cohort design in which exposed cases were matched to unexposed controls regarding known risk factors for LD (eg, maternal education, prematurity, birthweight, gender).[62] In addition, the analysis was adjusted for 2 separate measures of comorbidity, providing reassurance that the findings were not related to an excess of disease in the exposed group. The findings of this study were very similar to those of the previous study; the children exposed 2 or more times before their third birthday were at nearly twice the risk for LD as those not exposed. A subsequent study using this cohort, examined for the risk of attention deficit hyperactivity disorder, found similar results while controlling for comorbidity using a propensity analysis.[63]

Di Maggio and colleagues[64,65] examined a birth cohort from 1999 through 2002 enrolled in the New York Medicaid program. They found an association between anesthesia for inguinal hernia repair and risk of subsequent diagnosis of a behavioral and developmental disorder. In the cohort, they compared 383 children who had a hernia repair before 3 years of age with a sample of 5050 age-matched children without a history of hernia repair.[64] After correcting for age, sex, and complicating birth-related conditions, children who had hernia repair were more than twice as likely to be diagnosed with developmental or behavioral disorder (hazard ratio [HR], 2.3; 95% confidence interval [CI], 1.3–4.1).

To further reduce the influence of confounding factors, they also performed a study with twin siblings in the same database.[65] Among 10,450 twin siblings, 138 twin pairs had one twin who underwent a hernia repair and one who had not. Among these 138, development or behavioral disorders were diagnosed in 11 siblings who did not undergo a hernia repair and 9 that did, resulting in an odds ratio for adverse outcome of 0.9 (95% CI, 0.6–1.4). Unfortunately, these numbers are too small to draw any conclusions. In evaluating the entire twin sibling population, they found results similar to those of their previous study: an increased risk for developmental and behavioral disorders in children who had surgery (HR, 1.6; 95% CI, 1.4–1.8). The risk increased if the child had more than one surgical episode, increasing from 1.1 (95% CI, 0.8–1.4) for a single surgical episode to 2.9 (95% CI, 2.5–3.1) for 2 and 4.0 (95% CI, 3.5–4.5) for 3 or more operations.

In Denmark, another study also examined the risk of poor outcome and hernia repair. Academic performance was evaluated in 2689 children who underwent a hernia repair in infancy, and compared with that of a randomly selected age-matched group of 14,575 children.[66] Those who underwent a hernia repair scored worse than those in the control group. However, after correcting for sex, birthweight, and parental and maternal age and education, no difference was seen in academic performance between those who had surgery and those who did not. In a smaller but similar study using school records in Iowa, researchers examined children who had undergone surgery in infancy and who had no other risk factors for neurobehavioral delay.[67] The mean of their school test scores was similar to the population average; however, a higher percentage of children who underwent surgery scored below the fifth percentile.

A monozygotic twin study was performed in The Netherlands. The twins who underwent surgery before 3 years of age scored lower on educational achievement and had more cognitive problems than those who did not undergo surgery.[68] However, no difference was seen between twin pairs in which one twin had surgery and the other did not. This finding suggests that a genetically based need for surgery is linked to poor outcome rather than the surgery itself.

Several other studies examining older children have also found a link between multiple surgical episodes and an increased risk of poor neurobehavioral outcome.[61–63,69]

LIMITATIONS OF THESE COHORT STUDIES

Interpretation of these cohort studies has several limitations:

- Confounding: the biggest issue is that many other factors increase the need for exposure to anesthetic or sedative agents that are themselves associated with increased risk of poor neurobehavioral outcome. Adjustment for these factors can only partly remove this effect, and adjusting for the many likely unknown confounding factors is impossible.
- Dose and duration: the dose or duration of anesthesia or sedation at which risk may increase is unknown. Studies showing no association with short exposures

cannot rule out risk with long exposures, and studies showing increased risk with long exposure cannot inform short exposure.

- Neurobehavioral domain: which aspect of development is most likely to be affected by exposure to sedatives and anesthetics is unknown. Studies using very course outcomes, such as IQ or school performance, may miss subtle effects in subdomains. However, studies that perform a broad range of tests may detect some associations purely by chance.
- Age: the age range that is at greatest risk is unknown. Studies that find no association in populations of older children cannot rule out an effect in neonates or preterm infants.
- Neuroprotective effect: anesthetics, sedatives, and analgesics reduce pain and stress, which thus reduces the risk of poor outcome. This balance between neuroprotection and direct toxic effect may depend on the magnitude of the surgical stress and the dose of drug, making any clinical study difficult to interpret.

HUMAN DATA: NEONATAL MORPHINE EXPOSURE AND OUTCOME

Animal data suggest that morphine can improve outcome through reducing stress. Stressed animals without morphine and animals that are not stressed but are given morphine are at increased risk of poor outcome; however, those stressed and treated with morphine have a lower risk.[47]

Human trials are few and difficult to interpret. In the NEOPIAN randomized trial, babies were randomized to placebo infusion or morphine infusion, and both groups could have a rescue open-label morphine bolus. Morphine infusion did not reduce the frequency of poor outcomes, but intermittent boluses of open-label morphine were associated with an increased rate of poor outcome.[70] The poor outcome may have been caused by an increased risk of hypotension in the morphine groups.[71] This result illustrates the difficulty in unpicking all of the various factors that may interact to affect outcome.

Some animal data suggest a link between opioid use and neuronal changes, and in humans the newborns of opioid-abusing mothers have an increased risk of poor neurobehavioral outcome. However, at this stage no direct evidence links opioid use for analgesia and increased risk of adverse outcome in humans.

LABOR ANALGESIA AND ANESTHESIA

Very few data show any association between maternal exposure to anesthetics and analgesics and neurobehavioral outcome of the child. One study compared the risk of LD among children born via cesarean section with general anesthesia, cesarean section with regional anesthesia, and vaginal delivery. Of 5320 children in the cohort, 497 were delivered via cesarean section: 193 with general anesthesia and 304 with regional anesthesia. The incidence of learning was adjusted for sex, birthweight, gestational age, exposure to anesthesia before 4 years of age, and maternal education. LD risk was similar in children delivered via vagina or cesarean section with general anesthesia, but was reduced in children born via cesarean section with regional anesthesia. This study is difficult to interpret but supports the assertion that a brief perinatal exposure to general anesthetic does not increase risk of poor neurodevelopmental outcome. It is possible that a confounding factor decreases risk in those born via cesarean section with regional anesthesia.[72] It is also possible that neuraxial anesthesia reduced the stress responses to delivery, which reduced the risk of poor neurodevelopmental outcome. Thus the same group examined the association between use of neuraxial labor analgesia and development of childhood LDs in the same cohort. They found that LDs were not associated with the use of labor neuraxial analgesia.[73]

CLINICAL IMPLICATIONS

Animal data indicate that some sedatives, analgesics, and anesthetics may produce long-term effects in neonatal brain. However, these data are difficult to translate meaningfully to clinical situations. Some human data also show an association between exposure to surgery and anesthesia and poor outcomes. However, these findings are inconsistent and substantial reasons exist to doubt that the observed associations are causal.

In addition to the potential toxicity of anesthetics, sedatives, and analgesics, their benefits are also important to consider. Equally compelling evidence shows that excessive stress and untreated pain can also result in adverse developmental changes. Any change in practice must consider the potential for the unintended consequence of that change. Delaying necessary procedures or avoiding the judicious use of sedation for neonates in the intensive care unit may have consequences that are far more injurious than the theoretical risk associated with early exposure to anesthetics and sedatives. Many reasons exist for sick neonates to experience adverse neurodevelopmental outcomes; some of the risks are known and can be measured, some are known but cannot be measured, and many are unknown. The current retrospective epidemiologic studies, although carefully constructed and performed, are insufficient to assign causation to the emerging association between anesthetic/sedative exposure and adverse neurodevelopmental outcomes. Nonetheless, the observed associations are troubling and may represent an enormous public health challenge if confirmed. However, until definitive data are available, the focus should remain on providing optimal hemodynamic and respiratory stability, judicious use of sedatives/analgesics, and thoughtful decision making when considering the need for procedures requiring general anesthesia or sedation. None of these considerations are new or represent a change in established practice. Rather, this controversy serves to remind physicians that these decisions should always be made carefully, with a clear understating of the potential risks and benefits.

As ongoing and planned prospective studies are completed, physicians dedicated to the care of this most vulnerable population will be in a better position to guide future care. Unfortunately, currently no firm recommendations state that analgesics, sedatives, or anesthetics should be limited in the perinatal period, and considerably more research is needed before any recommendations can be made.

REFERENCES

1. Quimby KL, Katz J, Bowman RE. Behavioral consequences in rats from chronic exposure to 10 PPM halothane during early development. Anesth Analg 1975; 54(5):628–33.
2. Uemura E, Levin ED, Bowman RE. Effects of halothane on synaptogenesis and learning behavior in rats. Exp Neurol 1985;89(3):520–9.
3. Ikonomidou C, Bosch F, Miksa M, et al. Blockade of NMDA receptors and apoptotic neurodegeneration in the developing brain. Science 1999; 283(5398):70–4.
4. Jevtovic-Todorovic V, Hartman RE, Izumi Y, et al. Early exposure to common anesthetic agents causes widespread neurodegeneration in the developing rat brain and persistent learning deficits. J Neurosci 2003;23(3):876–82.

5. Yon JH, Daniel-Johnson J, Carter LB, et al. Anesthesia induces neuronal cell death in the developing rat brain via the intrinsic and extrinsic apoptotic pathways. Neuroscience 2005;135(3):815–27.

6. Hayashi H, Dikkes P, Soriano SG. Repeated administration of ketamine may lead to neuronal degeneration in the developing rat brain. Paediatr Anaesth 2002; 12(9):770–4.

7. Kodama M, Satoh Y, Otsubo Y, et al. Neonatal desflurane exposure induces more robust neuroapoptosis than do isoflurane and sevoflurane and impairs working memory. Anesthesiology 2011;115(5):1–13.

8. Istaphanous GK, Howard J, Nan X, et al. Comparison of the neuroapoptotic properties of equipotent anesthetic concentrations of desflurane, isoflurane, or sevoflurane in neonatal mice. Anesthesiology 2011;114(3):578–87.

9. Liang G, Ward C, Peng J, et al. Isoflurane causes greater neurodegeneration than an equivalent exposure of sevoflurane in the developing brain of neonatal mice. Anesthesiology 2010;112(6):1325–34.

10. Lu Y, Wu X, Dong Y, et al. Anesthetic sevoflurane causes neurotoxicity differently in neonatal naive and Alzheimer disease transgenic mice. Anesthesiology 2010; 112(6):1404.

11. Fredriksson A, Ponten E, Gordh T, et al. Neonatal exposure to a combination of N-methyl-D-aspartate and gamma-aminobutyric acid type A receptor anesthetic agents potentiates apoptotic neurodegeneration and persistent behavioral deficits. Anesthesiology 2007;107(3):427–36.

12. Stratmann G. Neurotoxicity of anesthetic drugs in the developing brain. Anesth Analg 2011;113(5):1170–9.

13. Stratmann G, Sall JW, May LD, et al. Isoflurane differentially affects neurogenesis and long-term neurocognitive function in 60-day-old and 7-day-old rats. Anesthesiology 2009;110(4):834–48.

14. Shih J, May LDV, Gonzalez HE, et al. Delayed environmental enrichment reverses sevoflurane-induced memory impairment in rats. Anesthesiology 2012; 116(3):586.

15. Slikker W Jr, Zou X, Hotchkiss CE, et al. Ketamine-induced neuronal cell death in the perinatal rhesus monkey. Toxicol Sci 2007;98(1):145–58.

16. Brambrink AM, Evers AS, Avidan MS, et al. Ketamine-induced neuroapoptosis in the fetal and neonatal rhesus macaque brain. Anesthesiology 2012;116(2): 372.

17. Paule MG, Li M, Allen RR, et al. Ketamine anesthesia during the first week of life can cause long-lasting cognitive deficits in rhesus monkeys. Neurotoxicol Teratol 2011;33(2):220–30.

18. Brambrink AM, Evers AS, Avidan MS, et al. Isoflurane-induced neuroapoptosis in the neonatal rhesus macaque brain. Anesthesiology 2010;112:834–41.

19. Briner A, De Roo M, Dayer A, et al. Volatile anesthetics rapidly increase dendritic spine density in the rat medial prefrontal cortex during synaptogenesis. Anesthesiology 2010;112(3):546–56.

20. De Roo M, Klauser P, Briner A, et al. Anesthetics rapidly promote synaptogenesis during a critical period of brain development. PLoS One 2009;4(9):e7043.

21. Vutskits L, Gascon E, Tassonyi E, et al. Effect of ketamine on dendritic arbor development and survival of immature GABAergic neurons in vitro. Toxicol Sci 2006;91(2):540–9.

22. Vutskits L, Gascon E, Tassonyi E, et al. Clinically relevant concentrations of propofol but not midazolam alter in vitro dendritic development of isolated gamma-aminobutyric acid-positive interneurons. Anesthesiology 2005;102(5):970–6.

23. Lemkuil BP, Head BP, Pearn ML, et al. Isoflurane neurotoxicity is mediated by p75ntr-rhoa activation and actin depolymerization. Anesthesiology 2011; 114(1):49–57.
24. Sall JW, Stratmann G, Leong J, et al. Isoflurane inhibits growth but does not cause cell death in hippocampal neural precursor cells grown in culture. Anesthesiology 2009;110(4):826–33.
25. Soriano SG, Liu Q, Li J, et al. Ketamine activates cell cycle signaling and apoptosis in the neonatal rat brain. Anesthesiology 2010;112(5):1155–63.
26. Sanchez V, Feinstein SD, Lunardi N, et al. General anesthesia causes long-term impairment of mitochondrial morphogenesis and synaptic transmission in developing rat brain. Anesthesiology 2011;115(5):992–1002.
27. Head BP, Patel HH, Niesman IR, et al. Inhibition of p75 neurotrophin receptor attenuates isoflurane-mediated neuronal apoptosis in the neonatal central nervous system. Anesthesiology 2009;110(4):813–25.
28. Sanders RD, Xu J, Shu Y, et al. Dexmedetomidine attenuates isoflurane-induced neurocognitive impairment in neonatal rats. Anesthesiology 2009;110(5):1077–85.
29. Ma D, Williamson P, Januszewski A, et al. Xenon mitigates isoflurane-induced neuronal apoptosis in the developing rodent brain. Anesthesiology 2007; 106(4):746–53.
30. Wang C, Sadovova N, Hotchkiss C, et al. Blockade of N-methyl-D-aspartate receptors by ketamine produces loss of postnatal day 3 monkey frontal cortical neurons in culture. Toxicol Sci 2006;91(1):192.
31. Braun S, Gaza N, Werdehausen R, et al. Ketamine induces apoptosis via the mitochondrial pathway in human lymphocytes and neuronal cells. Br J Anaesth 2010;105(3):347–54.
32. Liu J-R, Liu Q, Li J, et al. Noxious stimulation attenuates ketamine-induced neuroapoptosis in the developing rat brain. Anesthesiology 2012;117(1):64–71.
33. Anand KJ, Garg S, Rovnaghi CR, et al. Ketamine reduces the cell death following inflammatory pain in newborn rat brain. Pediatr Res 2007;62(3):283–90.
34. Bittigau P, Sifringer M, Genz K, et al. Antiepileptic drugs and apoptotic neurodegeneration in the developing brain. Proc Natl Acad Sci U S A 2002;99(23): 15089–94.
35. Ikonomidou C, Bittigau P, Ishimaru MJ, et al. Ethanol-induced apoptotic neurodegeneration and fetal alcohol syndrome. Science 2000;287(5455):1056.
36. Fredriksson A, Archer T, Alm H, et al. Neurofunctional deficits and potentiated apoptosis by neonatal NMDA antagonist administration. Behav Brain Res 2004;153(2):367–76.
37. Xu H, Liu ZQ, Liu Y, et al. Administration of midazolam in infancy does not affect learning and memory of adult mice. Clin Exp Pharmacol Physiol 2009;36(12): 1144–8.
38. Cattano D, Straiko MM, Olney JW. Chloral hydrate induces and lithium prevents neuroapoptosis in the infant mouse brain. Anesthesiology 2008;109:A315.
39. Tachibana K, Hashimoto T, Kato R, et al. Long-lasting effects of neonatal pentobarbital administration on spatial learning and hippocampal synaptic plasticity. Brain Res 2009;1388:69–76.
40. Kim JS, Kondratyev A, Tomita Y, et al. Neurodevelopmental impact of antiepileptic drugs and seizures in the immature brain. Epilepsia 2007;48(Suppl 5):19–26.
41. Sanders RD, Sun P, Patel S, et al. Dexmedetomidine provides cortical neuroprotection: impact on anaesthetic-induced neuroapoptosis in the rat developing brain. Acta Anaesthesiol Scand 2009;54(6):710–6.

42. Tachibana K, Hashimoto T, Kato R, et al. Neonatal administration with dexmedetomidine does not impair the rat hippocampal synaptic plasticity later in adulthood. Paediatr Anaesth 2012;22(7):713–9.

43. Wang Y, Han TZ. Prenatal exposure to heroin in mice elicits memory deficits that can be attributed to neuronal apoptosis. Neuroscience 2009;160(2):330–8.

44. Slamberova R, Schindler CJ, Pometlova M, et al. Prenatal morphine exposure differentially alters learning and memory in male and female rats. Physiol Behav 2001;73(1–2):93–103.

45. Lin CS, Tao PL, Jong YJ, et al. Prenatal morphine alters the synaptic complex of postsynaptic density 95 with N-methyl-D-aspartate receptor subunit in hippocampal CA1 subregion of rat offspring leading to long-term cognitive deficits. Neuroscience 2009;158(4):1326–37.

46. McPherson RJ, Gleason C, Mascher-Denen M, et al. A new model of neonatal stress which produces lasting neurobehavioral effects in adult rats. Neonatology 2007;92(1):33–41.

47. Boasen JF, McPherson RJ, Hays SL, et al. Neonatal stress or morphine treatment alters adult mouse conditioned place preference. Neonatology 2009; 95(3):230–9.

48. Rozisky JR, Medeiros LF, Adachi LS, et al. Morphine exposure in early life increases nociceptive behavior in a rat formalin tonic pain model in adult life. Brain Res 2011;1367:122–9.

49. Hammer RP Jr, Ricalde AA, Seatriz JV. Effects of opiates on brain development. Neurotoxicology 1989;10(3):475–83.

50. Tempel A. Visualization of mu opiate receptor downregulation following morphine treatment in neonatal rat brain. Brain Res Dev Brain Res 1991; 64(1–2):19–26.

51. Wu VW, Mo Q, Yabe T, et al. Perinatal opioids reduce striatal nerve growth factor content in rat striatum. Eur J Pharmacol 2001;414(2–3):211–4.

52. Dawson G, Dawson SA, Goswami R. Chronic exposure to kappa-opioids enhances the susceptibility of immortalized neurons (F-11kappa 7) to apoptosis-inducing drugs by a mechanism that may involve ceramide. J Neurochem 1997;68(6):2363–70.

53. Rizzi S, Ori C, Jevtovic-Todorovic V. Timing versus duration: determinants of anesthesia-induced developmental apoptosis in the young mammalian brain. Ann N Y Acad Sci 2010;1199:43–51.

54. Bouman NH, Koot HM, Hazebroek FW. Long-term physical, psychological, and social functioning of children with esophageal atresia. J Pediatr Surg 1999; 34(3):399–404.

55. Chacko J, Ford WD, Haslam R. Growth and neurodevelopmental outcome in extremely-low-birth-weight infants after laparotomy. Pediatr Surg Int 1999; 15(7):496–9.

56. Doyle LW, Callanan C, Carse E, et al. Surgery and the tiny baby: sensorineural outcome at 5 years of age. J Paediatr Child Health 1996;32(2):167–72.

57. Laing S, Walker K, Ungerer J, et al. Early development of children with major birth defects requiring newborn surgery. J Paediatr Child Health 2011;47(3): 140–7.

58. Gischler SJ, Mazer P, Duivenvoorden HJ, et al. Interdisciplinary structural follow-up of surgical newborns: a prospective evaluation. J Pediatr Surg 2009;44(7): 1382–9.

59. Ludman L, Spitz L, Lansdown R. Intellectual development at 3 years of age of children who underwent major neonatal surgery. J Pediatr Surg 1993;28(2):130–4.

60. Walker K, Halliday R, Holland AJ, et al. Early developmental outcome of infants with infantile hypertrophic pyloric stenosis. J Pediatr Surg 2010;45(12):2369–72.

61. Wilder RT, Flick RP, Sprung J, et al. Early exposure to anesthesia and learning disabilities in a population-based birth cohort. Anesthesiology 2009;110(4): 796–804.

62. Flick RP, Katusic SK, Colligan RC, et al. Cognitive and behavioral outcomes after early exposure to anesthesia and surgery. Pediatrics 2011;128(5):e1053–61.

63. Sprung J, Flick RP, Katusic SK, et al. Attention-deficit/hyperactivity disorder after early exposure to procedures requiring general anesthesia. Mayo Clin Proc 2012;87(2):120–9.

64. Di Maggio C, Sun L, Kakavuoli A, et al. A retrospective cohort study of the association of anesthesia and hernia repair surgery with behavioral and developmental disorders in young children. J Neurosurg Anesthesiol 2009;21:286–91.

65. Di Maggio C, Sun L, Li G. Early childhood exposure to anesthesia and risk of developmental and behavioral disorders in a sibling birth cohort. Anesth Analg 2011;113(5):1143–51.

66. Hansen TG, Pedersen JK, Henneberg SW, et al. Academic performance in adolescence after inguinal hernia repair in infancy: a nationwide cohort study. Anesthesiology 2011;114(5):1076–85.

67. Block RI, Thomas JJ, Bayman EO, et al. Are anesthesia and surgery during infancy associated with altered academic performance during childhood? Anesthesiology 2012;117(3):494–503.

68. Bartels M, Althoff RR, Boomsma DI. Anesthesia and cognitive performance in children: no evidence for a causal relationship. Twin Res Hum Genet 2009; 12(3):246–53.

69. Ing C, DiMaggio C, Whitehouse A, et al. Long-term differences in language and cognitive function after childhood exposure to anesthesia. Pediatrics 2012; 130(3):e476–85.

70. Anand KJ, Hall RW, Desai N, et al. Effects of morphine analgesia in ventilated preterm neonates: primary outcomes from the NEOPAIN randomised trial. Lancet 2004;363(9422):1673–82.

71. Hall RW, Kronsberg SS, Barton BA, et al. Morphine, hypotension, and adverse outcomes among preterm neonates: who's to blame? Secondary results from the NEOPAIN trial. Pediatrics 2005;115(5):1351–9.

72. Sprung J, Flick RP, Wilder RT, et al. Anesthesia for cesarean delivery and learning disabilities in a population-based birth cohort. Anesthesiology 2009; 111(2):302–10.

73. Flick RP, Lee K, Hofer RE, et al. Neuraxial labor analgesia for vaginal delivery and its effects on childhood learning disabilities. Anesth Analg 2011;112(6): 1424–31.

Genetic Contributions to Labor Pain and Progress

Ruth Landau, MD

KEYWORDS

- Genetics • Polymorphism • *OPRM1* • *ADRB2* • Labor pain

KEY POINTS

- Phenotyping labor pain and childbirth experience is extraordinarily complex. Therefore, genotyping to find meaningful associations with labor pain perception and neuraxial analgesic response remains challenging.
- The μ-opioid receptor gene (*OPRM1*) influences pain perception and response to opioids; however, this effect may be different according to the pain modality, the opioid chosen, and the mode of administration.
- The catechol-O-methyltransferase gene (*COMT*) influences pain perception and may impact the response to labor analgesia.
- Studies on the β2-adrenergic receptor gene (*ADRB2*) demonstrate a slow haplotype (Arg16/Gln27 double homozygosity) that seems to confer protection from preterm labor and delivery but results in prolonged labor.
- The oxytocin receptor gene (*OXTR*) is an obvious candidate in the context of labor and delivery; future studies are likely to find associations with implications for the management of labor pain and obstetric outcomes.

INTRODUCTION

Since the completion of the Human Genome Project more than a decade ago, anesthesiologists and pain specialists have been somewhat disillusioned after the promise that pharmacogenomics would transform their practice and result in personalized medicine.[1–4] Indeed, recommendations based on pharmacogenetic testing to help clinicians tailor regimens for safe and effective anesthesia and analgesia are still awaited. Working toward this translation, the pharmacogenetics research network recently

The author declares receiving funding for research projects that are not related with the topic of this review from the Millennium Research Institute (Millennium Laboratories).
Ruth Landau is the recipient of the Swiss National Foundation Research grant (SNF #3200B0-114129) that funded, in part, the *OPRM1* genetic research conducted in Switzerland.
Department of Anesthesiology and Pain Medicine, University of Washington Medical Center, 1959 NE Pacific Street, Suite BB 1415B, Seattle, WA 98195-6540, USA
E-mail address: rulandau@u.washington.edu

Clin Perinatol 40 (2013) 575–587
http://dx.doi.org/10.1016/j.clp.2013.05.014
0095-5108/13/$ – see front matter © 2013 Elsevier Inc. All rights reserved.

established a pharmacogenomics knowledge base (PharmGKB)[5] with the goal "to collect, encode, and disseminate knowledge about the impact of human genetic variations on drug response, curate primary genotype and phenotype data, annotate gene variants and gene-drug-disease relationships via literature review, and summarize important pharmacogenetic genes and drug pathways." Recently formed, the Clinical Pharmacogenetics Implementation Consortium[6] has established clinical recommendations for dosing based on genetic testing for 8 different drugs, out of which only codeine prescription according to the CYP2D6 genotype[7] may be relevant to the practice of anesthesiologists, pain doctors, pediatricians, obstetricians, or perinatologists. In addition, the current body of knowledge on the contribution of genetics on labor pain and analgesia or the progress of labor remains scarce.

This review aims to describe association studies that have examined the influence of variants within 4 genes on labor pain and the response to opioids in laboring women as well as the progress of labor; the genes include the μ-opioid receptor gene (*OPRM1*), the catechol-*O*- methyltransferase gene (*COMT*), the β_2 adrenergic receptor gene (*ADRB2*), and the oxytocin receptor gene (*OXTR*) (**Table 1**). In addition, some of the challenges inherent to the design and conduct of genetic associations studies, such as defining a crisp phenotype and selecting the appropriate candidate genes, is described.

LABOR PAIN AND PROGRESS

Clearly, the pain of childbirth is the most severe pain most women will endure in their lifetimes.[8] The International Association for the Study of Pain emphasized in their 2007–2008 report during the "Global Year against pain in women – real women, real pain"[9] that (1) the importance of treating pain within the pregnant population and the substantial public health impact if pain is neglected, (2) the alarmingly high rate of acute or chronic pain after delivery, and (3) labor pain as a clinical model for studying acute pain. Nonetheless, despite undeniable advances in our understanding of the physiology of labor pain that have resulted in the ability to provide safe and effective labor analgesia to most women in the developed world, evaluating and measuring labor pain and the response to analgesia remains a remarkable challenge.[10] During 9 months of pregnancy, women's expectations regarding the birthing process are extraordinarily diverse and influenced by many factors. In no other field of medicine is the experience of a painful process described in such divergent ways: natural, beautiful, and worthwhile to the point of being exhilarating on the one hand and overwhelmingly painful, horrible, distressing, and traumatic on the other. For the subset of women who know from the start they want to deliver with minimal discomfort by means of an epidural, providing an ideal labor analgesic is currently quite simple to achieve effectively. Nonetheless, for women who are either undecided or think they prefer a natural and unmedicated childbirth, the sense of disappointment and guilt often supersedes the benefits of pain relief if they ultimately fail and request a labor epidural analgesia, no matter how successful the analgesia.[11]

Therefore, it is no surprise when one realizes that a standard tool, such as a numeric pain score, used in all clinical pain studies does not capture very well the essence of labor pain. Other challenges that are specific to obstetric pain relate to the dynamic nature of labor and labor progress and the consequent changes in nociception that occur over time; pain of first-stage labor is conducted by thin afferent, *visceral* sympathetic fibers, entering the spinal cord at thoracic and lumbar roots (T10-L1), whereas second-stage labor pain is conducted via thicker *somatic* nerve fibers entering the spinal cord at sacral roots S2 to S4. The dynamic component of labor pain has

Table 1
Most studied genetic variants in the context of labor pain, labor analgesia response, and labor progress

Genetic Variants	Clinical Context	Intervention	Outcome	Reference
OPRM1 p.118A/G	Labor analgesia (CSE)	Spinal fentanyl (2.5–30.0 mcg)	Analgesia requested at higher cervical rate & lower ED_{50} (1.5–2.0 fold) in women with G118	Landau et al,[31] 2008
OPRM1 p.118A/G	Labor analgesia (CSE)	Spinal fentanyl (25 mcg)	No effect of G118 on duration of spinal analgesia	Wong et al,[32] 2010
OPRM1 p.118A/G	Labor analgesia (IV)	IV fentanyl (1.5 mg/kg)	Underpowered	Landau et al,[34] 2013
OPRM1 p.118A/G	Labor analgesia (epidural)	Epidural sufentanil (16–27 mcg)	Lower ED_{50} in women with G118	Camorcia et al,[33] 2012
OPRM1 p.118A/G	Labor pain & progress	NONMEM analysis	Underpowered (also for experimental pain)	Reitman et al,[58] 2011
OPRM1 p.118A/G	Labor pain	Analgesia (all types)	No difference in labor pain behaviors: Similar cervical dilatation on arrival in labor room Similar epidural rate (in the order of 30%)	Pettersson et al,[29] 2012
COMT p.472 G/A	Labor analgesia (IV)	IV fentanyl (1.5 mg/kg)	Less effective in Met/Met women (A472 homozygotes)	Landau et al,[34] 2013
COMT rs 4633	Labor progress	NONMEM analysis	Increased duration of latent phase of first stage labor	Terkawi et al,[68] 2012
ADRB2 Arg16	Preterm labor	Delivery <37 wk	Arg16 homozygotes protected from delivery <37 wk	Landau et al,[63] 2002
ADRB2 Glu27	Preterm labor	Delivery <37 wk	Glu27 allele increases risk for delivery <37 wk	Ozkur et al,[64] 2002
ADRB2 Arg16	Preterm labor	Tocolysis (IV hexoprenaline)	Better response to β-agonist in Arg16 homozygotes	Landau et al,[66] 2005
ADRB2 Arg16-Gln27	Labor progress	NONMEM analysis	Slowest haplotype for progression of first stage of labor	Miller et al,[67] 2011
ADRB2 Gln27	Labor progress	NONMEM analysis	Slower transition into active phase of first stage of labor	Reitman et al,[58] 2011
OXTR rs 53576	Labor progress	NONMEM analysis	Increased duration of latent phase of first stage of labor	Terkawi et al,[68] 2012

Abbreviations: CSE, combined spinal epidural; ED_{50}, median effective dose; IV, intravenous; NONMEM, nonlinear mixed effects modeling.

been integrated in a recent mathematical modeling technique that attempts to integrate multiple parameters to predict the intensity of pain over the course of labor.[12] Nonetheless, one of the major hurdles in labor pain studies relies on the subjective, individual ability of women to quantify their pain during labor. We have made numerous assumptions: asking women to score their pain on a 0 to 10 scale would result in a meaningful and relevant response; if women experienced severe pain, they would request an epidural; if women requested an epidural earlier in the process of labor, they were surely hurting more than women requesting an epidural at a later stage in labor; if women required more analgesic medication, they may have a poorer response to analgesia; and finally, if women had not requested any medication, they either had better coping skills or hurt less. We have also assumed that we could accurately measure pain scores, average these scores for each woman enrolled in a study, and compare these averaged scores between women and infer into which category (more pain, less pain) women belong. Last, analyzing and interpreting findings from such studies is a grueling and often-perplexing task for the obstetric anesthesiologist invested in evaluating labor pain and analgesia. Ultimately, obstetric factors greatly influence the amount of medication and analgesia women will want to take and agree to receive, based on the belief that the ability to effectively push and deliver the baby may come at the expense of some discomfort and pain. Therefore, any study that has considered overall analgesic consumption during labor and delivery, whether by means of systemic opioids or neuraxial analgesia, as a surrogate to measure pain during childbirth is likely to be meaningless and misconstruing the complexity of the labor pain experience. Labor pain and analgesic requirements in the peripartum period may well be the most intricate pain phenotype to evaluate and surely requires multidimensional tools not yet widely used to evaluate obstetric or acute postoperative pain as clinical models of acute pain.

OPRM1 Polymorphism, Pain Perception, and Analgesia

Among the myriad of candidate genes that have been considered important in opioid response, *OPRM1* is probably the most studied. A common polymorphism of *OPRM1* is a single nucleotide substitution at position 118, with an adenine substitution by a guanine (A118G) reported to occur with an allelic frequency of 10% to 30% among Caucasians,[13] a higher prevalence among Asians,[14] and a lower one in African Americans.[15] Despite numerous studies in the last 2 decades to identify the mechanism by which the altered receptor influences opioid analgesia, several hypothesis remain unconfirmed. In vitro studies have suggested that A118G polymorphism (p.118A/G) affects receptor binding characteristics[16,17] or messenger RNA expression levels[18]; however, under some experimental conditions, no effect on function[19] or expression levels[20] was confirmed. In a recent humanized mouse model exploring signal transduction pathways that mediate opioid pharmacology, sensory neurons expressing the 118GG gene displayed reduced morphine (but not fentanyl) potency and efficacy compared with the 118AA version, suggesting an effect at the level of the sensory neurons.[21]

OPRM1 and Experimental Pain Perception

Human volunteers (men and women) carrying a G118 allele have been shown to have a *lower* sensitivity to pressure pain (ie, higher tolerance threshold to pressure pain) compared with A118 homozygotes.[22] However, the association between genotype and pain perception is not that simple; a significant interaction between sex and genotype for heat pain ratings at 49°C was identified, indicating that the variant G118 allele was associated with *lower* pain ratings among men but *higher* pain ratings among women. A study in a Han Chinese cohort of healthy female volunteers demonstrated that pressure pain threshold is influenced by another polymorphism of *OPRM1* but not p.118A/G.[23] Other studies assessing the influence of genetic variants on experimental pain demonstrated no effect of the *OPRM1* A118G genotype on pain processing[24] or lower pain tolerance thresholds to single electrical nerve stimulation in individuals carrying the G118 allele.[25] It has been determined that the effect size of various determinants for experimental pain perception is greatest for heat sensitization by capsaicin, followed by gender (higher pain sensitivity in women) and a more modest effect size for genetic determinants.[26] Therefore, cautious interpretation of experimental pain tests should take into account the noxious stimulus, the gender, as well as possible linkage disequilibrium with other polymorphisms that may represent the true functional genetic variant. In a recent study evaluating the response to different experimental modalities in healthy individuals, there was no significant effect of the *OPRM1* genotype on pain sensitivity in the entire sample; but when examining each ethnic group separately (Caucasians, Hispanics, and African Americans), a lower pain sensitivity was found among Caucasians carrying the G118 allele, whereas there was a trend in the opposite direction among Hispanics, no measurable effect among African Americans (the G allele is underrepresented in this ethnicity), and there were no Asian women in that study.[27] Also, because the G118 allele is extremely common among Asians, studies comparing pain sensitivity between Caucasians and Asians will be of interest. It remains to be determined whether haplotype structure, gene-gene interactions, or DNA methylation[28] rather then the A118G genotype itself are key to explain these interethnic differences in pain sensitivity; nonetheless, this ethnicity-dependent genetic association may contribute to some of the discrepancies reported in clinical studies as underlined in the paragraphs that follow.

OPRM1 and Labor Pain

In a large cohort of Swedish women, labor pain–related behaviors, characterized by the cervical rate on arrival in the labor room and the use of any type of analgesia (nitrous oxide, epidural, systemic opioids, acupuncture) were not found to be associated with a particular genotype of *OPRM1*.[29] In other terms, women did not seem to have different thresholds for labor pain or epidural request based on the p.118A/G genotype; but the response to labor analgesia once provided was not evaluated. Of note, the overall epidural rate was relatively low (30%), and the epidurals were placed at a relatively advanced stage in labor (at approximately 6 cm of cervical dilatation); therefore, the lack of difference in epidural use is more likely to reflect a local clinical practice than a lack of genetic contribution. The same investigators also reported that a previously described pain-protective haplotype (3 single nucleotide polymorphisms [SNPs]) of the guanosine triphosphate cyclohydrolase gene (*GCH1*) did not seem to drastically alter labor pain–related behaviors.[30]

OPRM1 and Spinal Fentanyl for Labor Analgesia

The first clinical study evaluating any genetic influence on labor pain and analgesic response is most likely the one conducted in a Swiss cohort of nulliparous women requesting neuraxial analgesia early in labor evaluating p.118A/G. Using the up-down sequential allocation model to identify differences in analgesic requirement according to p.118A/G, women carrying the G118 allele required substantially *lower* doses of spinal fentanyl, with a 1.5-fold difference compared with wild-types.[31] This finding was replicated with a different pharmacologic study design using random-dose allocation, with a 2-fold difference between genetic groups.[31] Of note, cervical dilatation at the time of the analgesia request was significantly *less* in women who were A118 homozygous than that in women carrying 1 or 2 variant alleles (118AG or 118GG). The finding of lower analgesic requirements at a more advanced stage in labor at the time of the analgesic request suggests that women carrying the G118 allele have a *higher* pain tolerance, which allows them to wait longer before requesting analgesia. This finding is of interest because women received the combined spinal-epidural analgesic when they requested pain relief, in other words, at the time they experienced painful contractions. Because it has previously been demonstrated that epidural analgesic requirements increase with the progress of labor and cervical dilatation, the expectation would be that women carrying the G118 allele should have greater analgesic requirements because of the greater cervical dilatation at which they requested analgesia; the finding that these women required *less* fentanyl may actually underestimate the true effect of the genotype. Because the provision of optimal labor analgesia remains an ongoing challenge for obstetric anesthesiologists, with minimal motor impairment and opioid-related side effects, such as pruritus and fetal bradycardia (which seem to be dose dependent), this significant difference in median effective dose (ED_{50}) according to genotype may be relevant from a clinical standpoint. Therefore, one may presume that genotyping may help improve the delivery of neuraxial labor analgesia because a 1.5- to 2.0-fold difference in spinal fentanyl dose is not trivial. Another clinical study in a North American cohort determined that the duration of spinal fentanyl analgesia is not influenced by p.118A/G.[32] Taken together, these studies suggest that this common polymorphism of *OPRM1* influences spinal fentanyl potency without affecting the duration of analgesic action.

OPRM1 and Epidural Sufentanil

Using the same methodology, another recent study in Caucasian women demonstrated a similar pharmacogenetic association of p.118A/G with opioid potency during labor analgesia, although with a more modest clinical effect. In nulliparous women receiving early epidural analgesia, a lower dose requirement (ED_{50}) for epidural sufentanil was found among those carrying the G allele.[33]

OPRM1 and Intravenous Fentanyl

The benefits of intravenous fentanyl for labor analgesia have not been well studied, but fentanyl is offered to women trying to delay or avoid altogether receiving neuraxial analgesia. The rationale for studying the influence of p.118A/G in this clinical context would be to examine the hypothesis that the analgesic response to intravenous versus spinal fentanyl, under similar clinical conditions (ie, labor pain) may be influenced differently by this genetic variant. A recent study attempted to explore this question and determine whether the response to intravenous fentanyl and subsequently spinal fentanyl if women went on to request a combined spinal-epidural analgesic would be different in women carrying the G118 allele of *OPRM1*.[34] In this North American cohort, most women were Caucasian, and intravenous analgesic success was found to be relatively low (only 20% of women reported a pain score of less than 10 out of 100 at 15 minutes after dosing). Genotypes of p.118A/G in combination with p.472G/A (158Val/Met) of the *COMT* gene seemed to have an impact on the analgesic outcome; intravenous fentanyl was least effective in women with the A/A-Met/Met combination of *OPRM1* and *COMT*, which was carried by 18% of women in this cohort. The study was not sufficiently powered to explore the hypothesis that spinal and systemic opioid dynamics are different and determine whether enhanced analgesia in response to spinal fentanyl in the presence of the variant *OPRM1* G118 allele may not exist in response to intravenous fentanyl.

As already mentioned earlier, these findings in laboring women are in disagreement with most if not all other studies examining p.118A/G and opioid analgesia,[35] whether one evaluates postoperative intravenous fentanyl consumption,[36–38] spinal morphine for postcesarean pain,[32,39] intravenous morphine for postoperative pain,[40,41] or oral morphine for chronic cancer pain.[42–44] Potential explanations other than ethnicity for such discrepant results are that labor pain is different from that experienced in other clinical settings (experimental, postoperative, or chronic pain) or that the response to systemic rather than spinal fentanyl is affected differently by *OPRM1* genotype. One could speculate that human spinal cord receptor function and signal transduction is selectively more altered by the G118 variant than supraspinal receptors. Another potential explanation and factor to bare in mind is the different nature of the nociceptive stimulus in labor versus other painful syndromes. Indeed, similar disparate results in human genetic studies of pain sensitivity have been shown to occur with other polymorphisms commonly assessed in pain studies.[45]

COMT GENE, EXPERIMENTAL PAIN, OPIOID LABOR ANALGESIA, AND LABOR PROGRESS

Among the usual candidate genes proposed, the p.472G/A (158Val/Met) of *COMT* that regulates the metabolism of dopamine and noradrenaline is identified as inferring an increased risk for the development of chronic pain disorders,[46,47] acute postoperative pain,[48,49] chronic postsurgical pain,[50] and opioid-induced hyperalgesia.[51] High COMT activity, as found with the Val158 allele, is associated with improved dopaminergic transmission and confers an advantage in the processing of aversive stimuli or stressful conditions (warrior strategy), whereas Met158 alleles are associated with an advantage in memory and attention tasks (worrier strategy).[52]

COMT and Experimental Pain Perception

Individuals homozygous for the Met158 allele display increased pain sensitivity and lower μ-opioid system activation during sustained pain.[45,53,54] Opioid-induced hyperalgesia has been suggested to occur in Met158 individuals, when pain sensitivity was evaluated following remifentanil.[51] The effect of the *COMT* genotype on pain processing seems to become apparent only when pain modulation is challenged, such as occurs after repeated pain stimulation, as confirmed in a functional magnetic resonance imaging study investigating brain responses to thermal pain stimuli.[55] In a cohort of women with fibromyalgia, Met158 homozygotes displayed lower pressure pain thresholds and higher cold pain sensitivity.[56]

COMT and IV Fentanyl for Labor Analgesia

The average decrease in pain scores 15 minutes after a unique dose of intravenous fentanyl was lowest among Met/Met158 women compared with women carrying Val/Met or Val/Val of p.472G/A of *COMT*; that genotype with the poorer analgesic response was carried by 31% of women enrolled in this North American cohort (data mentioned earlier).[34] Although there is no doubt that intravenous fentanyl for labor analgesic is not a common practice, such findings my have useful clinical implications, such as not offering intravenous fentanyl in labor to women who will most likely not benefit from it.

COMT and Labor Progress

Demographic, obstetric, and genetic factors have been shown to be associated with the time required to progress to full cervical dilation. Using the previously validated nonlinear mixed effects modeling (NONMEM) to predict the pain and labor progress of the first stage of labor in nulliparous women,[57] 8 SNPs on 3 different genes (ADRB2, COMT, and OXTR) were examined in a cohort of 233 Saudi Arabian nulliparas. One of the 3 COMT SNPs evaluated, rs 4633 (different from p.472G/A at rs 4680), and one of OXTR SNPs, rs 53576, were associated with increased duration of the latent phase of first stage of labor, resulting in longer labors (in the order of 5 hours for COMT and 2 hours for OXTR, respectively). These findings contrast with results from other studies that found no effect of OXTR SNPs on the duration of first stage labor[58] or risk of dystocia.[59] In addition, ADRB2 genotype/haplotype was not associated with labor progress once demographic factors were accounted for (see later discussion). Lastly, data combining all the genetic variants (joined allelic combination) for each woman in the cohort were not reported, so one cannot infer the overall importance of a genetic contribution to the progress of labor.

ADRB2 HAPLOTYPE, PRETERM LABOR, AND LABOR PROGRESS

The ADRB2 gene and in particular 2 polymorphisms, p.16Arg/Gly and p.27Gln/Glu, found in strong linkage disequilibrium have been extensively evaluated in numerous studies with relevant clinical effects in the context of asthma[60] and cardiac perioperative outcomes.[61]

The influence of these genetic variants on preterm delivery, preterm labor, as well as the progress of labor is also of interest. The preterm birth phenotype has been defined as having 5 components (maternal conditions that are present before presentation for delivery, fetal conditions that are present before presentation for delivery, placental pathologic conditions, signs of the initiation of parturition, and the pathway to delivery)[62]; therefore, the exact contribution and the weight carried by each genetic variants remains to be determined. Homozygosity for Arg16 confers protection from preterm delivery, whereas the Glu27 variant seems to increase the risk for preterm delivery.[63–65] Furthermore, a pharmacogenetic effect with a better response to $\beta_2$agonist therapy (hexoprenaline) for tocolysis in women who are Arg16 homozygous with idiopathic preterm labor between 24 and 34 weeks' gestation has been demonstrated in a cohort of Swiss women.[66] This improved response to tocolysis had a significant impact on neonatal outcomes, with higher birth weights and less neonatal intensive care unit admissions for respiratory or other complications caused by prematurity in babies born to mothers with that genotype.

In a large trial evaluating the impact of ADRB2 genotype/haplotype on preterm labor, a subanalysis confirmed the hypothesis that Arg16 homozygosity of ADRB2 is associated with a slower rate of labor progress in successful term and late-preterm labor when compared with women with all other genotypes.[67] In this North American cohort, women with Arg16Arg-Gln27Gln (double homozygous) progressed at the slowest rate of active labor (slow haplotype), and women with Gly16Gly-Glu27Glu (double homozygous) progressed with the fastest cervical rate (fast haplotype).

Another smaller study from the same North American group to evaluate the effect of ADRB2 and OPRM1 on the progress of labor and labor pain using again NONMEM demonstrated that women homozygous for the variant Gln27 allele had a slower transition into the active phase of labor, resulting in prolonged labor compared with women with the other genotypes.[58] Genotype was strongly correlated with ethnicity (no Asian women included in the study was Glu27 homozygous), and labor was indeed found to be slower among Asians. The study was underpowered to detect an effect of OPRM1 on labor pain but identified that cold sensitivity was the pain modality that may predict the intensity of labor pain.

Homozygosity for Arg16 was also shown in the Saudi Arabian cohort to be associated with a later transition into active labor, but this effect was no longer significant when adjusted for demographic factors.[68]

Taken together, all studies evaluating obstetric outcomes based on the *ADRB2* genotype reported that women carrying Arg16 and/or Gln27 are conferred protection from preterm delivery and have a more quiescent uterus, resulting at the time of labor and delivery in a slower progression and prolonged labor duration. Overall, the factors influencing the progress of labor are multiple, including ethnicity and maternal weight, and genetic variability, out of which *ADRB2* is only one of many candidate genes, is unlikely to contribute in a major manner. A variety of genomic studies have examined the influence of genetic variants, and validation of biomarkers to identify women at risk for preterm labor and delivery is ongoing.[69,70] On the other extreme of the clinical spectrum, a genome-wide scan study in Sweden has identified at least 6 loci that seem to contribute to the risk of women requiring a cesarean delivery for dystocia,[59] and further prospective studies will need to validate these findings.

SUMMARY

In pain and analgesia studies, whether in the perioperative period or chronic-pain setting, defining relevant clinical outcomes (ie, identifying meaningful differences) in the context of pain and analgesic response remains the problem to solve.[71] Unfortunately, this has proven to be even more complex in the context of obstetric pain.[10] Phenotyping is critically important in all association studies, and designing clinical studies to assess the genetic contribution to pain is challenging. In addition, interpreting results, particularly when multiple genes are evaluated, requires large sample sizes and appropriate statistical analysis to avoid misconstrued findings.[72,73] Last but not least, the genetic contribution to labor pain or even that of pharmacogenetics to explain differences in analgesic response is probably not that simple and straightforward[74]; we are at the beginning of our explorations. These pharmacogenetic studies have taught us that it is futile to design clinical studies that attempt to identify one dose for one drug that will fit all because genetic variants do influence drug response in ways that have clinical implications. Unfortunately, firm recommendations to tailor opioid regimens based on our patients' individual genetic profiles are not yet available and are unlikely to become available in the near future other than for the prescription of codeine.[75]

The concept of mathematical modeling of labor progress is certainly promising and may allow investigators to identify some of the genetic contributions that are important for the progression of labor and the risk for dystocia and, therefore, predict labor outcome. Adding pain perception into that model is exciting, particularly if a pain modality easily tested with a quantitative sensory test to predict pain intensity during labor is soon identified. However, large prospective studies will be needed to thoroughly investigate this fascinating topic. Meanwhile, genome-wide association studies or exome sequencing to examine closely known and yet undiscovered genetic variants resulting in women being outliers for the various phenotypes during labor will be of interest.

REFERENCES

1. Mogil JS. Are we getting anywhere in human pain genetics? Pain 2009;146: 231–2.
2. Candiotti K. Anesthesia and pharmacogenomics: not ready for prime time. Anesth Analg 2009;109:1377–8.

3. Donahue BS, Balser JR. Perioperative genomics. Venturing into uncharted seas. Anesthesiology 2003;99:7–8.
4. Schwinn DA, Booth JV. Genetics infuses new life into human physiology: implications of the human genome project for anesthesiology and perioperative medicine. Anesthesiology 2002;96:261–3.
5. Available at: http://www.pharmgkb.org. Accessed March 27, 2013.
6. Relling MV, Klein TE. CPIC: clinical pharmacogenetics implementation consortium of the pharmacogenomics research network. Clin Pharmacol Ther 2011;89:464–7.
7. Crews KR, Gaedigk A, Dunnenberger HM, et al. Clinical Pharmacogenetics Implementation Consortium (CPIC) guidelines for codeine therapy in the context of cytochrome P450 2D6 (CYP2D6) genotype. Clin Pharmacol Ther 2012;91: 321–6.
8. Melzack R. The myth of painless childbirth (the John J. Bonica lecture). Pain 1984;19:321–37.
9. Available at: http://www.iasp-pain.org. Accessed March 27, 2013.
10. Carvalho B, Cohen SE. Measuring the labor pain experience: delivery still far off. Int J Obstet Anesth 2013;22:6–9.
11. Kannan S, Jamison RN, Datta S. Maternal satisfaction and pain control in women electing natural childbirth. Reg Anesth Pain Med 2001;26:468–72.
12. Conell-Price J, Evans JB, Hong D, et al. The development and validation of a dynamic model to account for the progress of labor in the assessment of pain. Anesth Analg 2008;106:1509–15.
13. Landau R, Cahana A, Smiley RM, et al. Genetic variability of mu-opioid receptor in an obstetric population. Anesthesiology 2004;100:1030–3.
14. Tan EC, Tan CH, Karupathivan U, et al. Mu opioid receptor gene polymorphisms and heroin dependence in Asian populations. Neuroreport 2003;14:569–72.
15. Crowley JJ, Oslin DW, Patkar AA, et al. A genetic association study of the mu opioid receptor and severe opioid dependence. Psychiatr Genet 2003;13: 169–73.
16. Kroslak T, Laforge KS, Gianotti RJ, et al. The single nucleotide polymorphism A118G alters functional properties of the human mu opioid receptor. J Neurochem 2007;103:77–87.
17. Bond C, LaForge KS, Tian M, et al. Single-nucleotide polymorphism in the human mu opioid receptor gene alters beta-endorphin binding and activity: possible implications for opiate addiction. Proc Natl Acad Sci U S A 1998;95: 9608–13.
18. Zhang Y, Wang D, Johnson AD, et al. Allelic expression imbalance of human mu opioid receptor (OPRM1) caused by variant A118G. J Biol Chem 2005;280: 32618–24.
19. Beyer A, Koch T, Schroder H, et al. Effect of the A118G polymorphism on binding affinity, potency and agonist-mediated endocytosis, desensitization, and re-sensitization of the human mu-opioid receptor. J Neurochem 2004;89:553–60.
20. Oertel BG, Kettner M, Scholich K, et al. A common human micro-opioid receptor genetic variant diminishes the receptor signaling efficacy in brain regions processing the sensory information of pain. J Biol Chem 2009;284:6530–5.
21. Mahmoud S, Thorsell A, Sommer WH, et al. Pharmacological consequence of the A118G mu opioid receptor polymorphism on morphine- and fentanyl-mediated modulation of Ca(2) channels in humanized mouse sensory neurons. Anesthesiology 2011;115:1054–62.

22. Fillingim RB, Kaplan L, Staud R, et al. The A118G single nucleotide polymor-phism of the mu-opioid receptor gene (OPRM1) is associated with pressure pain sensitivity in humans. J Pain 2005;6:159–67.
23. Huang CJ, Liu HF, Su NY, et al. Association between human opioid receptor genes polymorphisms and pressure pain sensitivity in females. Anaesthesia 2008;63:1288–95.
24. Vossen H, Kenis G, Rutten B, et al. The genetic influence on the cortical pro-cessing of experimental pain and the moderating effect of pain status. PLoS One 2010;5:e13641.
25. Zwisler ST, Enggaard TP, Noehr-Jensen L, et al. The antinociceptive effect and adverse drug reactions of oxycodone in human experimental pain in relation to genetic variations in the OPRM1 and ABCB1 genes. Fundam Clin Pharmacol 2010;24:517–24.
26. Doehring A, Kusener N, Fluhr K, et al. Effect sizes in experimental pain pro-duced by gender, genetic variants and sensitization procedures. PLoS One 2011;6:e17724.
27. Hastie BA, Riley JL 3rd, Kaplan L, et al. Ethnicity interacts with the OPRM1 gene in experimental pain sensitivity. Pain 2012;153:1610–9.
28. Nielsen DA, Hamon S, Yuferov V, et al. Ethnic diversity of DNA methylation in the OPRM1 promoter region in lymphocytes of heroin addicts. Hum Genet 2010; 127:639–49.
29. Pettersson FD, Gronbladh A, Nyberg F, et al. The A118G single-nucleotide poly-morphism of human mu-opioid receptor gene and use of labor analgesia. Re-prod Sci 2012;19:962–7.
30. Dabo F, Gronbladh A, Nyberg F, et al. Different SNP combinations in the GCH1 gene and use of labor analgesia. Mol Pain 2010;6:41.
31. Landau R, Kern C, Columb MO, et al. Genetic variability of the mu-opioid recep-tor influences intrathecal fentanyl analgesia requirements in laboring women. Pain 2008;139:5–14.
32. Wong CA, McCarthy RJ, Blouin J, et al. Observational study of the effect of mu- opioid receptor genetic polymorphism on intrathecal opioid labor anal-gesia and post- cesarean delivery analgesia. Int J Obstet Anesth 2010;19: 246–53.
33. Camorcia M, Capogna G, Stirparo S, et al. Effect of mu-opioid receptor A118G polymorphism on the ED50 of epidural sufentanil for labor analgesia. Int J Ob-stet Anesth 2012;21(1):40–4.
34. Landau R, Liu SK, Blouin JL, et al. The effect of OPRM1 and COMT genotypes on the analgesic response to intravenous fentanyl labor analgesia. Anesth Analg 2013;116:386–91.
35. Walter C, Lotsch J. Meta-analysis of the relevance of the OPRM1 118A>G genetic variant for pain treatment. Pain 2009;146:270–5.
36. Fukuda K, Hayashida M, Ide S, et al. Association between OPRM1 gene poly-morphisms and fentanyl sensitivity in patients undergoing painful cosmetic sur-gery. Pain 2009;147:194–201.
37. Wu WD, Wang Y, Fang YM, et al. Polymorphism of the micro-opioid receptor gene (OPRM1 118A>G) affects fentanyl-induced analgesia during anesthesia and recovery. Mol Diagn Ther 2009;13:331–7.
38. Zhang W, Chang YZ, Kan QC, et al. Association of human mu-opioid receptor gene polymorphism A118G with fentanyl analgesia consumption in Chinese gynaecological patients. Anaesthesia 2009;65:130–5.

39. Sia AT, Lim Y, Lim EC, et al. A118G single nucleotide polymorphism of human mu-morphine consumption after intrathecal morphine for postcesarean analgesia. Anesthesiology 2008;109:520–6.

40. Chou WY, Wang CH, Liu PH, et al. Human opioid receptor A118G polymorphism affects intravenous patient-controlled analgesia morphine consumption after total abdominal hysterectomy. Anesthesiology 2006;105:334–7.

41. Coulbault L, Beaussier M, Verstuyft C, et al. Environmental and genetic factors associated with morphine response in the postoperative period. Clin Pharmacol Ther 2006;79:316–24.

42. Klepstad P, Fladvad T, Skorpen F, et al. Influence from genetic variability on opioid use for cancer pain: a European genetic association study of 2294 cancer pain patients. Pain 2011;152:1139–45.

43. Klepstad P, Rakvag TT, Kaasa S, et al. The 118 A > G polymorphism in the human mu- opioid receptor gene may increase morphine requirements in patients with pain caused by malignant disease. Acta Anaesthesiol Scand 2004; 48:1232–9.

44. Reyes-Gibby CC, Shete S, Rakvag T, et al. Exploring joint effects of genes and the clinical efficacy of morphine for cancer pain: OPRM1 and COMT gene. Pain 2007;130:25–30.

45. Diatchenko L, Nackley AG, Slade GD, et al. Catechol-O-methyltransferase gene polymorphisms are associated with multiple pain-evoking stimuli. Pain 2006; 125:216–24.

46. Belfer I, Segall S. COMT genetic variants and pain. Drugs Today (Barc) 2011;47: 457–67.

47. Tammimaki A, Mannisto PT. Catechol-O-methyltransferase gene polymorphism and chronic human pain: a systematic review and meta-analysis. Pharmacogenet Genomics 2012;22:673–91.

48. Kolesnikov Y, Gabovits B, Levin A, et al. Combined catechol-O- methyltransferase and mu-opioid receptor gene polymorphisms affect morphine postoperative analgesia and central side effects. Anesth Analg 2011;112:448–53.

49. Lee PJ, Delaney P, Keogh J, et al. Catecholamine-o-methyltransferase polymorphisms are associated with postoperative pain intensity. Clin J Pain 2011;27: 93–101.

50. Hickey OT, Nugent NF, Burke SM, et al. Persistent pain after mastectomy with reconstruction. J Clin Anesth 2011;23:482–8.

51. Jensen KB, Lonsdorf TB, Schalling M, et al. Increased sensitivity to thermal pain following a single opiate dose is influenced by the COMT val(158)met polymorphism. PLoS One 2009;4:e6016.

52. Stein DJ, Newman TK, Savitz J, et al. Warriors versus worriers: the role of COMT gene variants. CNS Spectr 2006;11:745–8.

53. Zubieta JK, Heitzeg MM, Smith YR, et al. COMT val158met genotype affects mu-opioid neurotransmitter responses to a pain stressor. Science 2003;299: 1240–3.

54. Andersen S, Skorpen F. Variation in the COMT gene: implications for pain perception and pain treatment. Pharmacogenomics 2009;10:669–84.

55. Loggia ML, Jensen K, Gollub RL, et al. The catechol-O-methyltransferase (COMT) val158met polymorphism affects brain responses to repeated painful stimuli. PLoS One 2011;6:e27764.

56. Martinez-Jauand M, Sitges C, Rodriguez V, et al. Pain sensitivity in fibromyalgia is associated with catechol-O-methyltransferase (COMT) gene. Eur J Pain 2013; 17:16–27.

57. Debiec J, Conell-Price J, Evansmith J, et al. Mathematical modeling of the pain and progress of the first stage of nulliparous labor. Anesthesiology 2009;111: 1093–110.

58. Reitman E, Conell-Price J, Evansmith J, et al. β2-adrenergic receptor genotype and other variables that contribute to labor pain and progress. Anesthesiology 2011;114:927–39.

59. Algovik M, Kivinen K, Peterson H, et al. Genetic evidence of multiple loci in dystocia–difficult labour. BMC Med Genet 2010;11:105.

60. Carroll CL, Sala KA, Zucker AR, et al. β2-adrenergic receptor haplotype linked to intubation and mechanical ventilation in children with asthma. J Asthma 2012; 49:563–8.

61. Nagele P, Liggett SB. Genetic variation, beta-blockers, and perioperative myocardial infarction. Anesthesiology 2011;115:1316–27.

62. Villar J, Papageorghiou AT, Knight HE, et al. The preterm birth syndrome: a prototype phenotypic classification. Am J Obstet Gynecol 2012;206:119–23.

63. Landau R, Xie HG, Dishy V, et al. β2-Adrenergic receptor genotype and preterm delivery. Am J Obstet Gynecol 2002;187:1294–8.

64. Ozkur M, Dogulu F, Ozkur A, et al. Association of the Gln27Glu polymorphism of the β2-adrenergic receptor with preterm labor. Int J Gynaecol Obstet 2002;77: 209–15.

65. Doh K, Sziller I, Vardhana S, et al. β2-adrenergic receptor gene polymorphisms and pregnancy outcome. J Perinat Med 2004;32:413–7.

66. Landau R, Morales MA, Antonarakis SE, et al. Arg16 homozygosity of the β2-adrenergic receptor improves the outcome after β2-agonist tocolysis for preterm labor. Clin Pharmacol Ther 2005;78:656–63.

67. Miller RS, Smiley RM, Daniel D, et al. β2-adrenoceptor genotype and progress in term and late preterm active labor. Am J Obstet Gynecol 2011;205:137.e1–7.

68. Terkawi AS, Jackson WM, Thiet MP, et al. Oxytocin and catechol-O-methyltransferase receptor genotype predict the length of the first stage of labor. Am J Obstet Gynecol 2012;207:184.e1–8.

69. Esplin MS, Merrell K, Goldenberg R, et al. Proteomic identification of serum peptides predicting subsequent spontaneous preterm birth. Am J Obstet Gynecol 2011;204:391.e1–8.

70. Gracie S, Pennell C, Ekman-Ordeberg G, et al. An integrated systems biology approach to the study of preterm birth using "-omic" technology–a guideline for research. BMC Pregnancy Childbirth 2011;11:71.

71. Landau R, Schwinn D. Genotyping without phenotyping: does it really matter? Anesth Analg 2013;116:8–10.

72. Landau R, Ortner C, Carvalho B. Challenges in interpreting joined allelic combinations of OPRM1 and COMT genes. Anesth Analg 2011;113:432.

73. Lotsch J. Basic genetic statistics are necessary in studies of functional associations in anesthesiology. Anesthesiology 2007;107:168–9.

74. Wong CA. The promise of pharmacogenetics in labor analgesia… tantalizing, but not there yet. Int J Obstet Anesth 2012;21:105–8.

75. Vuilleumier PH, Stamer UM, Landau R. Pharmacogenomic considerations in opioid analgesia. Pharmgenomics Pers Med 2012;5:73–87.

Index

Note: Page numbers of article titles are in **boldface** type.

Clin Perinatol 40 (2013) 589–599
http://dx.doi.org/10.1016/S0095-5108(13)00095-X
0095-5108/13/$ – see front matter © 2013 Elsevier Inc. All rights reserved.
perinatology.theclinics.com

Moving?

Make sure your subscription moves with you!

To notify us of your new address, find your **Clinics Account Number** (located on your mailing label above your name), and contact customer service at:

Email: journalscustomerservice-usa@elsevier.com

800-654-2452 (subscribers in the U.S. & Canada)
314-447-8871 (subscribers outside of the U.S. & Canada)

Fax number: 314-447-8029

Elsevier Health Sciences Division
Subscription Customer Service
3251 Riverport Lane
Maryland Heights, MO 63043

*To ensure uninterrupted delivery of your subscription, please notify us at least 4 weeks in advance of move.

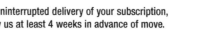

Printed and bound by CPI Group (UK) Ltd, Croydon, CR0 4YY

03/10/2024

01040489-0009